Professional and Student Portfolios for Physical Education

SECOND EDITION

Vincent J. Melograno, EdD

Cleveland State University

Includes CD-ROM portfolio builders

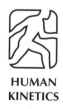

HUMAN KINETICS

Library of Congress Cataloging-in-Publication Data

Melograno, Vincent.
 Professional and student portfolios for physical education / Vincent J. Melograno. -- 2nd ed.
 p. cm.
 Includes CD-ROM portfolio builders.
 Includes bibliographical references.
 ISBN-13: 978-0-7360-5924-4 (soft cover)
 ISBN-10: 0-7360-5924-5 (soft cover)
 1. Physical fitness--Testing. 2. Portfolios in education. I. Title.
 GV436.5.M45 2006
 796.07'7--dc22
                                                                                                          2006002437

ISBN-10: 0-7360-5924-5
ISBN-13: 978-0-7360-5924-4

The Web addresses cited in this text were current as of February 16, 2006, unless otherwise noted.

Acquisitions Editor: Scott Wikgren; **Developmental Editor:** Amy Stahl; **Assistant Editor:** Bethany J. Bentley; **Technology Assistance:** Bonnie S. Mohnsen, PhD, CEO, Bonnie's Fitware Inc.; **CD-ROM Assistance:** Mary Motley, MA, Cleveland State University; **Copyeditor:** Patsy Fortney; **Proofreader:** Kathy Bennett; **Permission Manager:** Dalene Reeder; **Graphic Designer (interior and cover):** Nancy Rasmus; **Graphic Artists:** Angela K. Snyder and Yvonne Griffith; **Photo Manager:** Sarah Ritz; **Photographer (cover):** Les Woodrum; **Photographer (interior):** Sarah Ritz, unless otherwise noted. Photo on p. 40 by Dan Wendt. Photos on pp. 121 and 140 © Human Kinetics. Photos on pp. 1, 137, 144, 235, 252 courtesy of Instructional Media Services, Cleveland State University, Cleveland, OH, and Shaker Heights City School District, Shaker Heights, OH. Photos on pp. 23, 29, 49, 62, 79, 92, 157, 177, 240 courtesy of Instructional Media Services, Cleveland State University, Cleveland, OH, and Department of Health, Physical Education, Recreation, and Dance, Cleveland State University, Cleveland, OH. Photos on pp. 68, 81, 153, 246 courtesy of Department of Health, Physical Education, Recreation, and Dance, Cleveland State University, Cleveland, OH; **Art Manager:** Kelly Hendren; **Illustrators:** Kelly Hendren and Nancy Rasmus; **Printer:** Versa Press

Printed in the United States of America

10 9 8 7 6 5 4 3 2 1

Human Kinetics
Web site: www.HumanKinetics.com

United States: Human Kinetics
P.O. Box 5076
Champaign, IL 61825-5076
800-747-4457
e-mail: humank@hkusa.com

Canada: Human Kinetics
475 Devonshire Road Unit 100
Windsor, ON N8Y 2L5
800-465-7301 (in Canada only)
e-mail: orders@hkcanada.com

Europe: Human Kinetics
107 Bradford Road
Stanningley
Leeds LS28 6AT, United Kingdom
+44 (0) 113 255 5665
e-mail: hk@hkeurope.com

Australia: Human Kinetics
57A Price Avenue
Lower Mitcham, South Australia 5062
08 8277 1555
e-mail: liaw@hkaustralia.com

New Zealand: Human Kinetics
Division of Sports Distributors NZ Ltd.
P.O. Box 300 226 Albany
North Shore City
Auckland
0064 9 448 1207
e-mail: info@humankinetics.co.nz

CONTENTS

PREFACE

Schools today are being asked to address an ever-increasing array of educational and social issues. These increasing demands are competing for already limited instructional resources and valuable instructional time. In addition, schools are increasingly pressured to be more accountable and to be more productive by having higher percentages of their students meet established national, state, and local outcomes and achievement standards. For example, No Child Left Behind legislation was built on accountability and assessment principles including setting standards, measuring student progress against the standards, providing intervention for struggling students, and holding schools responsible for results.

Teaching practices and student learning of the past are not adequate to meet the demands of the 21st century. The roots for the redesign of teaching and learning for this century have been planted and established through a challenging national standards movement. Emerging from this effort are explicit standards for both teachers and students. The questions that arise are, What knowledge and skills are essential for effective teaching? and, What should students know and be able to do as a result of their education? As higher and more demanding expectations are placed on students, the need for professionals capable of teaching to achieve these standards becomes greater. In other words, student standards must be matched by teacher standards.

The standards-based reform of teaching and learning is evident in physical education at three levels. First, the second edition of the *National Standards for Beginning Physical Education Teachers* (National Association for Sport and Physical Education, 2003) presents 10 standards as the focus for competent instruction within physical education. The definition and description of each standard are supported by "acceptable" and "target" teaching outcomes as well as the dispositions, knowledge, and performances a beginning teacher must demonstrate. Second, explicit standards for K-12 students in physical education were developed through a series of projects leading to the second edition of *Moving Into the Future: National Standards for Physical Education* (National Association for Sport and Physical Education, 2004). Following a purposeful process of consensus building, the document reflects current thinking on what students should know and be able to do as a result of a quality physical education program. And third, advanced standards for experienced teachers were identified to recognize teachers who effectively enhance student learning and demonstrate the high level of knowledge, skills, dispositions, and commitments reflected in five core propositions (National Board for Professional Teaching Standards, 1999). Supporting standards of accomplished practice for physical education and corresponding knowledge, skills, dispositions, and beliefs are also available (National Board for Professional Teaching Standards, 2001). These three sets of standards are described in chapter 1 and applied in chapters 2, 3, and 4, respectively.

Concomitant to the standards-based reform in education is the dissatisfaction with traditional forms of assessment. The trend is toward authentic forms of assessment that rely on more naturalistic, performance-based approaches instead of highly inferential estimates provided by the group-administered, objectively scored, and normatively interpreted standardized tests. Authentic assessment applies to both students and teachers and is structured to provide evidence of real-life samples of learning and classroom performance, respectively. To meet this demand, teachers must develop assessment literacy—the ability to determine what to assess (learning targets) and how to assess (methods), and then to match the proper method of assessment with the intended target. Assessment *for* learning—student-involved, formative assessment—is also advanced because it produces significant learning gains. In physical education, multiple-choice, machine-scored tests or standardized sport skill or fitness tests do not seem to be good indicators of what students really learned. Likewise, multiple-choice tests of basic skills and general knowledge seem woefully inadequate to measure teaching skill. Thus, assessment systems are needed to document the degree to which established student and teacher standards are met, specific to physical education.

The pendulum of alternative educational assessment has swung toward a portfolio format. Although relatively new to education, portfolios have been used for a long time by commercial artists, journalists, architects, photographers, models, and other professionals to showcase talent, skills, style, and range of work visually. The term *portfolio assessment* is frequently used. For the purpose of this book, it should be clear that *portfolios are not an assessment method, but a device for collecting and communicating about student learning and teaching competence.* Although a portfolio can be assessed as a whole, its true purpose is to enrich the ability to learn, the desire to learn, and the learning itself. Thus, portfolios can play a significant role in keeping track of and celebrating standards-based learning and creating assessment *for* learning and authentic assessment. In general terms, a portfolio is a purposeful, integrated collection of artifacts showing effort, progress, or achievement in one or more aspects. The type of portfolio that a teacher or student will use depends on the needs the portfolio serves. Because portfolios feature work samples over time, they are well suited to demonstrate student growth and learning. Teachers can also use them, for example, to document the implementation and success of a new instructional strategy.

Given the national focus on learning and teaching standards, it follows that any accompanying portfolio system should correspond to established standards. Therefore, this second edition of *Professional and Student Portfolios for Physical Education* provides both teacher and student portfolio systems based on teacher standards and K-12 content standards, respectively. It presents guidelines, practical procedures, and tips on how to organize portfolio systems. These systems can be used for every phase of a physical educator's career as follows:

- Professional portfolio systems are presented for teacher candidates to help them become "beginning" physical education teachers. The book is recommended to higher education personnel in the business of teacher training. A portfolio system is suggested for a physical education teacher education (PETE) program.

- Because comprehensive student portfolio systems are outlined across the K-12 physical education spectrum, practicing physical education teachers will find the book useful.

- Experienced and accomplished physical education teachers will also discover the value of portfolios to help them grow professionally and maintain teaching effectiveness.

This second edition has been updated in several ways and many new features have been added.

1. *New standards.* Since the publication of the first edition, all three sets of professional teacher standards and content standards for physical education have been changed. The standards for physical education teacher candidates have been updated and expanded, content standards and grade-level student expectations for K-12 physical education have been revised, and advanced standards for practicing physical education teachers have been developed. These changes, which have had a significant impact on the basis for organizing professional and student portfolios, are identified and applied in each chapter.

2. *Expected outcomes.* Establishing targets is an important principle of learning. Thus, each chapter includes a set of expected outcomes that identifies the knowledge and skills readers will acquire by completing the chapter.

3. *Step-by-step processes.* Designing an integrated portfolio system is a complex process. For this reason, step-by-step procedures are recommended in chapters 2, 3, and 4. The steps are clearly identified throughout each chapter.

4. *Integration of assessment, learning, and teaching.* Changes in approaches to assessment, student learning styles, and the teacher roles clearly suggest that assessment, learning, and teaching must be integrated. Teachers need to develop assessment literacy and create a balance between assessment *of* learning and assessment *for* learning. Assessment *of* learning provides achievement status at a point in time, usually at the end of the learning process for grading or public record keeping. Assessment *for* learning focuses on student-involved assessment that promotes achievement during the learning process. Student portfolios may hold the key to successful integration by cultivating desirable student habits—reflecting on learning, developing self-direction and feedback, setting goals, creating new challenges, and communicating achievement results. These concepts are introduced in chapter 1 and developed further in chapter 3.

5. *Rubric development.* In standards-based education, an authentic or performance-based assessment tool is needed to define and communicate what constitutes excellence or quality. A rubric is a scoring guide designed to assess the quality of a student's performance. Rubrics are used to inform students about intended learning targets or standards and levels of quality. For this reason, scoring rubrics have emerged as a popular assessment tool in conjunction with student portfolios. The use of rubrics is fully addressed in chapter 3, which includes a discussion of the design of rubrics, criteria for determining the quality of rubrics, and an explanation of converting rubric scores to grades. Rubrics for teachers are also presented and illustrated in chapters 2 and 4.

6. *Use of technology.* The application of technology for portfolio assembly, management, and storage is a significant new feature of this second edition. Using digital protocols instead of paper-based formats has many advantages. General guidelines for creating electronic-based and Web-based portfolios, including hardware, storage, and software recommendations, are presented in chapter 1. The specific use of technology in developing student and teacher portfolios is also addressed in chapters 2, 3, and 4.

7. *CD-ROM portfolio builders.* Templates for creating electronic-based portfolios for teacher candidates, K-12 students, and practicing teachers are available on the accompanying CD-ROM. These portfolio builders provide a step-by-step process for developing professional and student portfolios. The suggested components for each portfolio can be changed and customized to fit individual needs and school settings. The templates are developed in Microsoft PowerPoint®. When completed, the portfolio can be copied to a CD for distribution and review. It can also be uploaded to the Internet for access as a Web-based portfolio.

The principles and concepts underlying the portfolio systems are treated in four chapters.

Chapter 1: Gateway to Professional and Student Portfolios

In this chapter the demand for greater educational effectiveness and accountability is analyzed with respect to teaching and learning. Various educational trends are explored as contexts for the contemporary emphasis on standards-based education and authentic forms of assessment. Student-involved, formative assessment is advanced for improving student achievement by focusing on assessment *for* learning. A rationale is offered for portfolios as the means for validating the standards-based reform of teaching and learning in physical education. Portfolios are justified as the recommended device for collecting evidence and communicating about student learning and teaching competence. The role of technology in the development and implementation of portfolio systems for teacher candidates, K-12 students, and practicing teachers is presented.

Chapter 2: Professional Portfolios for Teacher Candidates

This chapter proposes a portfolio scheme for integrating and interrelating the knowledge and skills learned in a physical education teacher education (PETE) program. General guidelines are provided for organizing the teacher candidate professional portfolio around a set of standards for the beginning physical education teacher. Strategies for implementing portfolios are identified along with processes for involvement. Guidelines for the assembly, management, and storage of portfolios are presented including the use of technology. Required and optional artifacts are suggested for each type of portfolio (introductory, presentation, and employment). Finally, formative and summative assessment procedures are described and illustrated. A sample portfolio system is included for a PETE program.

Chapter 3: Student Portfolios for K-12 Learners

The process for integrating assessment, learning, and teaching outlined in this chapter includes student-involved, classroom-level assessment. A multifaceted approach is recommended for designing student portfolio systems appropriate for K-12 school physical education programs. The process of developing portfolios includes determining the purposes and types of portfolios to use; deciding how they will be organized; dealing with production and logistics concerns; establishing a process for item selection; determining student reflection and self-assessment strategies; creating a framework for conducting conferences; and choosing assessment procedures. Exemplary materials are provided for established content standards in physical education. Sample portfolio systems are included for the elementary, middle, and high school levels.

Chapter 4: Professional Portfolios for Practicing Teachers

This chapter offers practicing physical education teachers procedures for organizing professional portfolios. Various purposes are suggested to document professional competence. Organization and management strategies are offered for professional growth and showcase portfolios including the use of technology. Guidelines are also provided for collecting and selecting artifacts and for assessing one's own portfolio. A sample portfolio system for accomplished teachers is included.

The portfolio is now widely accepted as a device for collecting, verifying, communicating, and celebrating authentic student learning and teaching competency. Professional and student portfolios offer the means for integrating assessment, learning, and teaching in a high-stakes, standards-based world. Because of technology advances, portfolio systems can be comprehensive in design, yet practical in assembly, management, access, and dissemination. This book provides all of the tools necessary for creating portfolios, including portfolio samples and CD-ROM portfolio builders. Portfolios are truly beneficial for every phase of one's career.

ACKNOWLEDGMENTS

This second edition of *Professional and Student Portfolios for Physical Education* represents the varied contributions of many others over the past eight years since the first edition. Teacher candidates and practicing teachers provided constructive feedback regarding the practical development and use of professional portfolios, school-aged children provided real-life insight into the value and benefits of personal learning portfolios, and other colleagues were always willing to offer their opinions and judgments about professional and student portfolios for physical education.

In particular, I am deeply grateful to two outstanding professionals for their expertise and contributions to the book. Bonnie Mohnsen, CEO of Bonnie's Fitware Inc., served as the technology adviser. Her reputation in the area of technology is renowned. She contributed nearly all of the material dealing with technology, and for that, I thank her. I am sincerely honored that she was willing to assist me in this endeavor. It has been a pleasure to know Bonnie for many years as a colleague, never realizing that she would support me in this writing. Mary Motley, HPERD Department, Cleveland State University, served as both a technology and portfolio adviser. She has been instrumental in the continual evolution and refinement of the professional portfolio system at Cleveland State. At the same time, she developed advanced technology skills leading to the creation of e-portfolios. She provided invaluable assistance in the structure of the CD-ROM portfolio builders that accompany this book. More cherished, however, has been Mary's friendship, respect, and support for many years, and for that, I will always be thankful.

Appreciation and thanks are extended to Scott Wikgren, a division director at Human Kinetics, for his support and commitment to this second edition. Having worked with Scott on other projects, I value his timely assistance, professional style and integrity, and personable manner. Finally, I would like to thank Amy Stahl, a developmental editor at Human Kinetics. Her organizational skills, attention to detail, and overall efficiency were evident during all phases of manuscript review, editing, and production. Her suggestions for improving the book were much appreciated. Amy demonstrated outstanding leadership in getting the book published, and for that, I am most thankful.

HOW TO USE THE CD-ROM

The three portfolio builders on the CD-ROM included with *Professional and Student Portfolios for Physical Education* offer templates to create electronic-based physical education portfolios for teacher candidates, K-12 students, and practicing teachers. The templates for these professional and student portfolios are developed in Microsoft PowerPoint®. Each portfolio builder is organized around a set of appropriate standards. The physical education teacher education (PETE) professional portfolio for teacher candidates uses the standards from *National Standards for Beginning Physical Education Teachers* (National Association for Sport and Physical Education, 2003); the K-12 physical education student portfolio uses the standards from *Moving Into the Future: National Standards for Physical Education* (National Association for Sport and Physical Education, 2004); and the professional portfolio for practicing physical education teachers uses the standards from *NBPTS Physical Education Standards* (National Board for Professional Teaching Standards, 2001).

The templates can be used for the various types of portfolios suggested in the book for teacher candidates (i.e., introductory, presentation, employment), K-12 students (i.e., personal, record-keeping, thematic, integrated, showcase or celebration of achievement, employment, scholarship), and practicing teachers (i.e., professional growth, showcase). However, the templates are particularly useful for employment, achievement, and professional growth portfolios, respectively.

Getting Started

1. Insert the *Professional and Student Portfolios for Physical Education, Second Edition, CD-ROM* into your computer's CD-ROM drive.
2. Click on the Contents link at the bottom of the CD-ROM launch page.
3. On the Contents page, click on the link for the Teacher Candidate Professional Portfolio, K-12 Student Portfolio, or Practicing Teacher Professional Portfolio. This link will take you to the instructions for creating this portfolio.
4. Read the entire Instructions document carefully before starting to create your portfolio.

It is suggested that you move the entire portfolio folder you select to your hard drive. You could also move it to your desktop to make it even easier to find. Each folder contains the files that are needed to build the portfolio. The files were developed in Microsoft Word®, except for the PowerPoint file that contains the template for actually constructing the portfolio. When you have completed the portfolio, you can copy it to a CD for distribution and review. You can also upload it to the Internet for access as a Web-based portfolio. You should have an understanding of each portfolio builder before developing your portfolios.

Instructions

Read the instructions file thoroughly before exploring the portfolio template and starting to create your portfolio. Open the file named Instructions for Teacher Candidate Portfolio, Instructions for Student Portfolio, or Instructions for Practicing Teacher Portfolio. The information will guide you in a step-by-step approach to developing the portfolio. Follow the instructions specific to each portfolio to navigate through the slides contained in each file. Printing out these instructions may be helpful. The following section describes how to begin the actual process of creating your portfolio.

PowerPoint Template With Links to Files

After reading the instructions thoroughly, you should be ready to create your portfolio. Open the appropriate portfolio folder and begin by opening the PowerPoint file named Welcome to Teacher Candidate Professional Portfolio, Welcome to K-12 Student Portfolio, or Welcome to Practicing Teacher Professional Portfolio. The components for these portfolio templates are different. This is the file you will use to develop the electronic-based portfolio. Before going any further, run the Slide Show to get a sense of the portfolio you will be building. Hyperlinks to files are already built into the individual slides.

Files

Various files correspond to the components of each portfolio. These files can be found in the portfolio folders. Hyperlinks have been created in the PowerPoint slides for easy access to and easy navigability through the files. You will need to replace these files with your own documents, graphs, spreadsheets, pictures, video clips, and presentations. You may also need to scan paper-based materials to produce digital files in word-processed or PDF formats. The following components are used to organize each portfolio:

Teacher candidate professional portfolio	K-12 student portfolio	Practicing teacher professional portfolio
• Table of contents • Introduction • Resume • Coursework • Teacher candidate standards • Lesson plan sample • Student work samples • Gallery (pictures, video clips) • Letters of recommendation • Teaching evaluations	• Table of contents • Introduction • Standards • Learning targets • Goal setting • Reflections • Journal (self-assessment) • Gallery (pictures, video clips) • Conferences • Assessment	• Table of contents • Introduction • Resume • Professional development • Standards for accomplished teachers • Lesson plan sample • Student work samples • Gallery (pictures, video clips) • Letters of recommendation • Teaching evaluations

If you already have electronic versions of your portfolio materials, creating a portfolio using the CD-ROM should be relatively quick and easy if you follow the instructions. Although the general templates for teacher candidates, students, and practicing teachers include sets of suggested components, you are free to modify and customize these PowerPoint portfolio templates to fit your unique needs and settings. The instructions provide information on how to edit, add, or remove slides and links.

To get started, click the Contents link at the bottom of the CD-ROM launch page. From the Contents page, click the link at the bottom of the page that corresponds to the resource instructions you wish to see, Teacher Candidate Professional Portfolio, K-12 Student Portfolio, or Practicing Teacher Professional Portfolio.

Gateway to Professional and Student Portfolios

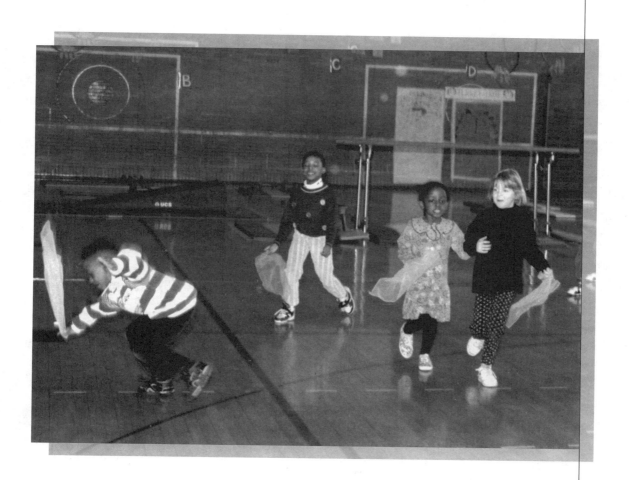

The imperative of educational reform—holding schools accountable for results—is alive and well. The challenging standards movement established the roots for the ongoing redesign of learning and teaching in this century. As expectations become more rigorous about what students should know and be able to do as a result of their education, so do the knowledge, skills, and dispositions essential for effective teaching. Standards for students must be matched by standards for teachers. Teachers must develop assessment literacy, including authentic measures of achievement and student-involved assessment *for* learning—assessment that promotes student achievement during the learning process. Students who engage in goal setting, self-assessment, record keeping, and communication are more motivated to learn. So, how do we document that both students and teachers are meeting standards?

EXPECTED OUTCOMES

This chapter establishes the foundation for the use of professional and student portfolios in physical education. After reading this chapter, you will be able to do the following:

1. Identify the dynamics of change in and the contexts for educational reform.
2. Trace the redesign of learning and teaching and the wave of educational trends and issues.
3. Describe the meaning of standards-based education and the learning and teaching standards that support such an environment.
4. Recognize the need for assessment literacy and the distinction between assessment *of* learning and assessment *for* learning.
5. Determine the importance of authentic assessment for measuring student achievement and documenting effective teaching.
6. Justify the use of portfolios to verify and communicate about student achievement and teaching competence, specific to physical education.
7. Decide how to use technology to develop electronic-based and Web-based portfolios for teacher candidates, K-12 students, and practicing teachers.

The ongoing demand for greater educational effectiveness has resulted in widespread educational reform. The wave of reform initiatives is still going strong today. This chapter traces the contexts for educational change, including the redesign of learning and teaching, and presents an analysis of some important education trends and issues. Three of these trends are particularly significant and warrant further discussion. First, the national standards movement is explored from the general perspective of standards-based education, and more specifically in terms of learning and teaching standards. Content standards for K-12 physical education students, standards for teacher candidates, and standards for practicing teachers are presented. Second, the development of assessment literacy is recommended, including assessment *for* learning and more authentic forms of assessment. Suggestions are offered for measuring student achievement and documenting effective teaching. Both of these trends are discussed relative to their impact on learning and teaching. In combination, standards-based assessment of both students and teachers offers a new vision for the future of physical education. Therefore, a rationale is offered for using portfolios to validate established student and teacher standards in physical education. Third, emerging technologies will continue to have a significant impact on education. The use of technology in developing portfolios has many advantages. Technology requirements and protocols are provided for general application to portfolio systems for teacher candidates in physical education teacher education (PETE) programs, for K-12 students in physical education, and for practicing physical education teachers.

Contexts for Educational Change

The school curriculum reflects the role of education in society and the blending of public policy and professional judgment. Although we should make every attempt to be current, sustaining the momentum of change that is found in society and schools is difficult. For that reason, we must recognize the dynamics of change and our natural reaction to change. This section begins with an analysis of the ambivalence between change as growth and renewal (the public ideal) and change as a conservative impulse (our private reality) (Kelly & Melograno, 2004).

What kind of world might we face in 5 or 10 years given expected changes in technology, biology, social values, demography, and education? Popular in today's education, for example, is the notion of preparing students to participate in the global economy of the "Information Age." Educators face a daunting task; they are engaged in a great venture of exploration, risk, discovery, and change without a comprehensive map for guidance. According to Senge and others (1999), profound change sometimes refers to external changes in technology, customers (students), or the social and political environment. But change also refers to internal attempts to adapt to changes in the environment. The timeless concern is whether internal changes in practices, views, and strategies are keeping pace with external changes.

Change is riddled with paradox—we both embrace and resist it. We know change is inevitable and needed perhaps, but our natural reaction to it is often defensive. For this reason, change is more difficult to implement than we think for several reasons. Change provokes *loss*, challenges *competence*, creates *confusion*, and causes *conflict* (Evans, 2001).

- Significant change almost always results in some kind of loss. Suppose that, after years of teaching a required personal fitness course for high school seniors, you are suddenly forced to eliminate it in favor of an elective program consisting of alternative activities (e.g., cycling, in-line skating, rock climbing). It would be hard to deny your feeling of loss.

- Change immediately threatens your sense of competence. New practices, procedures, and routines can make you feel inadequate and insecure. It is understandable that a different approach might make you feel that the personal fitness course you have been teaching is outmoded and that you have been ineffective.

- Whatever improvements change may promise, it almost always increases confusion. The previous roles, rules, and policies of the required fitness course are replaced with the confusion, loss of control, and politics associated with completely different kinds of elective activities. With this uncertainty, it is often unclear who is responsible for what. You may become confused or distressed.

- Innovation is supposed to be better for everyone, but the reality is quite different, often leading to conflict and friction. Changing from a required, fitness-based course to an elective, alternative activities program invariably produces winners and losers, at least initially. Conflict is both natural and inevitable when resources are limited and competing priorities are at stake.

Change exposes us to risks and failures. How do we respond to potential failure? We need to know ourselves and look at how others are dealing with change (coping or avoiding). Although there may be no external rewards for change, there is a professional imperative to change, the internal need to be a change agent. So what are the ingredients of the change process? And, what are the tasks of implementing the transition to improvement?

To be change agents, we must first make the case for innovation by emphasizing the seriousness of the problem and the rightness of the solution. We must challenge other teachers' acceptance of and comfort with the status quo by provoking the four dilemmas of change identified earlier. Those who are resisting change need help, however difficult and unpleasant it may be to provide it, to move from loss to commitment, from old competence to new competence, from confusion to coherence, and from conflict to consensus. Our goals as change agents are to do the following:

1. Make change meaningful (through the use of continuity, time, and personal contact).
2. Develop new behaviors, skills, beliefs, and ways of thinking (by providing training that is coherent, continuous, and personal).
3. Realign structures, functions, and roles (by clarifying responsibility, authority, and decision making).
4. Generate broad support for change (with critical mass, pressure, and the positive use of power).

The public outcry for change in education is constant. The school curriculum and teaching approaches are often criticized for their lack of relevance. However, the challenging national standards movement and the focus on high-stakes assessment have established the roots for a redesign of learning and teaching in this century. This redesign effort is explored in this section along with some education trends and issues that could potentially influence the nature of physical education curriculum and instruction.

Redesign of Learning and Teaching

In the 1980s a federal report titled *A Nation at Risk: The Imperative of Educational Reform* (National Commission on Excellence in Education, 1983) raised public concern about the condition of education in the United States. Overall, the quality of education was rated as poor. Supposedly, students were not learning, and teachers were not teaching effectively. As a result, the 1980s saw massive school improvement efforts through legislation at all levels, school effectiveness projects, and instructional intervention approaches. Many so-called reforms that became popular included magnet schools, proficiency testing, school choice, alternative schools, vouchers, charter schools, and year-round schools.

Just three years after *A Nation at Risk*, another pivotal report was issued titled *A Nation Prepared: Teachers for the 21st Century* (Carnegie Task Force on Teaching as a Profession, 1986). One of its recommendations led to the creation of the National Board for Professional Teaching Standards (NBPTS) in 1987. The mission of the NBPTS was to establish high and rigorous standards for what accomplished teachers should know and be able to do; develop and operate a national, voluntary system to assess and certify teachers who meet these standards; and advance related education reforms for the purpose of improving student learning in U.S. schools (National Board for Professional Teaching Standards, 1999).

An overwhelming set of expectations, it seemed, had been placed on schools in general, and on students and teachers in particular. It prompted a historic education summit in 1989 involving the president and the nation's governors. Educational goals were adopted and a National Education Goals Panel was established to measure their progress. *America 2000: An Education Strategy* (U.S. Department of Education, 1991) provided the elements needed to ensure that students would be prepared to function in a diverse society and to compete in a global economy. The goals stated that by the year 2000,

1. children would enter school ready to learn;
2. the high school graduation rate would be 90 percent;
3. students would leave 4th, 8th, and 12th grades having demonstrated competency in challenging subject matter;
4. teachers would receive the professional development needed to help students reach the other goals;
5. U.S. students would be first in the world in math and science;
6. every adult would be literate;
7. schools would be free of drugs and violence; and
8. schools would promote partnerships to increase parent involvement.

The other critical element of the education equation—the teacher—was not forgotten. The Interstate New Teacher Assessment and Support Consortium (INTASC) developed model standards for teachers (Darling-Hammond, 1992). Because of the general applicability of the standards for teachers of all disciplines and all levels, many professional societies, state departments of education, and university schools of education have used the standards in their attempts to define teaching excellence.

Ultimately, the shift toward student and teacher competencies led to the passage of the Goals 2000: Educate America Act (PL 103-227) in March 1994. With educational standards written into federal law, a national standards movement emerged. Through the National Education Standards Improvement Council (NESIC), students were expected to achieve the standards, given adequate support and sustained effort. Voluntary content standards were developed on a kindergarten through 12th grade (K-12) continuum across various school subjects, including physical education. In addition, a National Commission on Teaching & America's Future was appointed in 1994. After two years of intense study, it concluded "that the reform of elementary and secondary education depends first and foremost on restructuring its foundation—the teaching profession" (National Commission on Teaching & America's Future, 1996, p. 5). The commission recommended that rigorous standards be developed and enforced for teacher preparation, initial licensing, and continuing development.

Despite the unprecedented challenges of an economic recovery and the war on terrorism following the events of September 11, 2001, President George W. Bush secured passage of the landmark No Child Left Behind (NCLB) Act of 2001 (PL 107-110). The NCLB Act was the most sweeping reform of the Elementary and Secondary Education Act (ESEA) since it was enacted in 1965. This reauthorization of ESEA was built on the accountability and assessment requirements established in 1994 and the overall direction of states' education policy initiatives over the past decade: setting standards, measuring students' progress against standards, providing help for struggling students, and holding schools accountable for results. It redefined the federal role in K-12 education to help close the achievement gap between disadvantaged and minority students and their peers. The NCLB Act (accessible through its official Web site, www.NoChildLeftBehind. gov) requires statewide accountability systems covering all public schools and students. These systems must be based on challenging state standards in reading and mathematics, annual testing for all students in grades 3 through 8, and annual statewide progress objectives ensuring that all groups of students reach proficiency within 12 years. Assessment results and state progress objectives must be broken down by economic status, race, ethnicity, disability, and English proficiency to ensure that no group is left behind. School districts and schools that fail to make adequate yearly progress (AYP) toward statewide proficiency goals will, over time, be subject to improvement, corrective action, and restructuring measures aimed at getting them back on course to meet state standards.

Clearly, student learning and teaching practices of the past are not adequate to meet the demands of the 21st century. Along with the extensive school restructuring efforts, teachers are also expected to respond to forces that operate in the larger culture (e.g., substance abuse, changes in family patterns, sexually transmitted diseases, ethnic and linguistic diversity, economic inequities, and child abuse). The result has been some education trends and issues that affect the daily lives of students and teachers, including physical education.

Education Trends and Issues

Education responds constantly to societal forces that operate in the larger culture. Many people expect schools to solve our "social ills." We are confronted with substance abuse, changes in family patterns, violence, terrorist-related threats, poor fitness among youth, childhood obesity, sexually transmitted diseases, greater inequities between the "haves" and the "have-nots," a TV and video game generation, high crime rates, poor school performance, child abuse, teenage suicide, disruptive behavior, changing ethnic and linguistic diversity, and high dropout rates, to mention a few. The increased demand for accountability that has resulted from these challenges has changed education through curriculum reform, school restructuring, and teacher empowerment for school-based management decisions. For example, along with programming for students with disabilities, special attention is being given to new categories, such as students from diverse ethnic groups, at-risk students, and gifted students (Kelly & Melograno, 2004).

Although many trends in education are promising, they are accompanied by many associated issues and concerns. Future and practicing professional educators need to acknowledge, respond to, and embrace these trends and issues. The seven trends and issues that follow are addressed throughout this book in a variety of ways. For example, an emphasis on responsibility and decision making is often advocated for at-risk students. Because decision making can be enhanced through self-directed learning supported by technology, the use of an electronic-based or Web-based portfolio may be an effective learning tool for at-risk students. As you review brief descriptions of these trends and issues in this section, try to imagine how each might influence your role as a teacher, the physical education program, and student learning. Your own beliefs and values should be challenged.

Culturally Responsive Teaching

Skills are needed to accommodate the variation found in cross-cultural school settings; that is, teachers should consider cultural differences. For example, language differences are evident in school systems. Ethnic minorities account for more than 20 percent of the school-age population. Teachers do not need to be members of students' cultural group, but they must be sensitive to the cultural characteristics of students and accommodate these characteristics in the classroom. In addition to being knowledgeable about various cultures, teachers need to be aware of their own biases. They must also realize that bias and prejudice are learned responses. Teachers should respect cultural differences, believe that all students are capable of learning, and see themselves as capable of making a difference in their students' learning. These competencies could serve as performance criteria to ensure that teachers can instruct effectively in a multicultural society.

Physical education, because of its social orientation, can play a leading role in eliminating discriminatory practices and promoting multicultural understanding. Physical education and sport have a rich heritage that has evolved from cultures throughout the world. The different racial and ethnic contributions or the unique contributions of women could be highlighted. A focus on culturally responsive teaching will help physical educators respond to the issues of diversity raised by the wave of social and cultural change in the United States.

Student Diversity

The school setting has changed dramatically over the past several decades. For example, the combined minority student population in schools is approaching 50 percent and many adolescents maintain a physically inactive lifestyle, due in large part to an information-based, technological society. Change among students and schools means that teachers must be able to adjust their planning and teaching to accommodate the wide range of differences in terms of race, primary language, cultural values, religion, lifestyle, gender, sexual orientation, social class, physical and cognitive ability, and learning style. Providing *total* equity in physical education is not easy. Attempts to forge a society based on equality and mutual respect via the education system are obvious. Desegregation, legal mandates, and programming such as multicultural, bilingual, and character education make it clear that schools are playing a serious role in this *affirmative* action. Designing an individualized curriculum for a diverse class is a difficult but essential task.

Creating an affirmative curriculum may be even more challenging to the physical education teacher than it is to the regular classroom teacher. Although many teachers perceive students to be alike, this illusion of homogeneity should be replaced by the reality of heterogeneity. Developing a knowledge and awareness of student diversity is one thing. Doing something about it is another. The physical education curriculum provides opportunities for all students to experience a wide range of activities that suit individual needs. To start, it is important to know the categories that define the common characteristics of people or groups. These general terms, which seem to be socially acceptable, include gender, race, culture, social class, physical ability, cognitive ability, gifted and talented, at-risk, and learning style. There is a tendency to deal with issues of diversity by looking at single categories. However, the problems facing students, and teachers, are really complex combinations of two or more of these elements.

Inclusive Education

The concepts presented here are usually associated with special education categories. However, they are applicable to learners for whom a "regular" education is not considered appropriate, regardless of the reasons. The *full inclusion* model places and instructs all students in regular settings regardless of the type or severity of disability. Multidisciplinary teams of professionals representing different specialties (e.g., reading, math), including motor development, bring their collective skills and knowledge together to provide personal programs for each student.

The legislation that guides policies and practices for educating students with disabilities is the Individuals With Disabilities Education Act (IDEA), first passed in 1970 and reauthorized ever since. IDEA mandates that placement of students with disabilities be based on the concept of the least restrictive environment (LRE). This means that, to the maximum extent appropriate, students with disabilities are educated with students without disabilities. Inclusion has implications for subject areas such as physical education (motor development) because of the need to create an individualized curriculum. Unfortunately, many schools interpret least restrictive environment as a continuum of placements rather than as a mandate to provide appropriate support in the regular setting. Inclusion focuses on everyone's abilities and possibilities, not on deficiencies and limitations.

Developmentally Appropriate Practices

The quality of educational programs is determined by many factors (e.g., cost-effectiveness, range of activities, satisfaction, achievement). But, a primary determinant should be the degree to which principles of child and adolescent development are applied. In other words, is the program *developmentally appropriate?* By definition, developmental appropriateness is two-dimensional. Age appropriateness depends on universal, predictable sequences of growth and change that occur in all dimensions—physical, intellectual, emotional, and social. These typical developments provide a framework for program planning. Individual appropriateness refers to each person's pattern and timing of growth, as well as individual personalities, learning styles, and family backgrounds.

In physical education, developmentally appropriate practices recognize each learner's unique abilities to move, and they accommodate individual characteristics such as previous movement experiences, fitness and skill levels, and body size. A distinction is made between practices that are in the best interests of children (appropriate) and those that are counterproductive or even harmful (inappropriate). For example, appropriate practice means that the physical education curriculum has an obvious scope and sequence based on goals and objectives appropriate for all children. It includes a balance of skills, concepts, games, educational gymnastics, rhythms, and dance experiences designed to enhance cognitive, motor, affective, and physical fitness development. Inappropriate practice may be reflected in a physical education curriculum that lacks developed goals and objectives and is based primarily on the teacher's interests, preferences, and background rather than the student's.

Emphasis on Standards

Excellence in education is in the spotlight; it is a national priority. Everyone seems to know how to improve schools. For nearly three decades, the widespread reform of U.S. education has focused on what children need to know and be able to do to meet the demands of the 21st century and to prepare for their futures. The goal is to ensure that students will be ready to take their place in society, survive in a global economy, and lead healthy and productive lives. The national standards movement identified the knowledge and skills that students were expected to achieve in given subject areas.

Clearly developed, publicly stated content and performance standards provide the focus for curriculum organization. The critical first step is to define desirable learning outcomes. Next, appropriate curriculum materials (learning units) are adopted. The third step is to "link," or align, exit outcomes with objectives and then with assessment instruments. Establishing this kind of congruency is a complex task. The last step is to devise a way of managing the curriculum. During this phase, learning units are monitored and formal procedures are developed for revising the curriculum based on student achievement and teacher experience. For physical education, the content standards and corresponding student expectations and performance outcomes for grade level ranges (K-2, 3-5, 6-8, 9-12) that define the *physically educated person* are detailed later in this chapter (pages 13-14). In addition, standards for teacher candidates (pages 16-17) and practicing teachers (page 18) are presented later in this chapter.

Quality Assessment

The emphasis on world-class standards for student achievement has brought attention to account-ability-oriented, high-stakes testing. Many believe that standardized testing is the key to achieving educational excellence. However, students will not attain higher levels of achievement and schools will not become effective simply because of high standards and rigorous tests. In other words, assessment *of* learning measures status at a point in time, but it is not designed to meet the information needs of students, teachers, and parents. Day-to-day assessment *for* learning can meet these needs. Therefore, a balanced combination of high-quality standardized assessment *of* learning and high-quality assessment *for* learning will maximize student achievement and provide the information required by those seeking excellence. These distinctions are developed later in this chapter (page 19).

Quality assessment is essential to dependable information about student achievement. Teachers must understand and apply known standards of quality assessment; they must become assessment literate. Sound and productive assessment is accurate and is used to benefit students, not merely to grade and sort them. Assessment literacy is defined as the ability to match the proper method of assessment (e.g., selected response, constructed response, performance assessment) with the intended learning target (e.g., knowledge, reasoning, skill mastery, positive values) and to relate assessment techniques (e.g., rating scales, checklists, logs, peer task cards, self-reports, rubrics) with teaching models (e.g., direct, reciprocal, cooperative learning, guided discovery, tactical games). These alignments—learning targets with assessment methods and teaching models with assessment techniques—are evident within the context of student-involved, class-room-level assessment. Ultimately, teachers need to integrate learning targets, teaching patterns and models, and assessment methods and techniques. No doubt, the synthesis of these three elements is a complex and challenging task. Assessment literacy is described in greater detail later in this chapter (page 19).

Advances in Technology

Our lives are being transformed by technology. The World Wide Web has created new ways to gain information and communicate. In business, education, and everyday life, people are using personal computers, notebook computers, handheld computers, digital videodiscs (DVDs), pedometers, digital cameras, camcorders, and other technologies. Many participate regularly in electronic message systems such as interactive newsgroups, bulletin boards, chat rooms, and listservs (subscription mailing lists that allow subscribers to send and receive e-mail messages). Software programs for word processing, databases, spreadsheets, and teacher utilities (e.g., grading programs, sign makers, awards, desktop publishing) offer practical applications for curriculum development and computer-assisted instruction (CAI). Handheld computers (data-entry devices) are also becoming popular in physical education because of the need to collect data in the field (e.g., attendance, performance scores, anecdotal notes). Data in these devices can be transferred easily to a desktop computer and stored in some type of database or spreadsheet file.

Even our means of physical activity is being transformed by technology. High-tech exercise equipment is widely available, and virtual reality technology creates virtual activity experiences such as mountain climbing, scuba diving, or skiing without having to leave home. Following are some other examples of using technology to enhance and improve the physical education curriculum (Siedentop, 2004):

- Heart monitors track exercise patterns; collected data are downloaded to computers for graphic display and use by students and teachers.
- Teachers and students use the Internet to participate in newsgroups that address needs and interests related to physical activity.
- Teachers can access Web sites for information on various topics, such as lesson planning, assessment, and program promotion (e.g., www.pelinks4u.org/).
- Online technology newsletters keep students and teachers up-to-date with technology developments (e.g., www.pesoftware.com/technews/news.html).
- Courses and degree programs are offered online that require an Internet connection, e-mail account, and Web browser.
- Complete, portable fitness evaluation systems are available to students and teachers (e.g., www.polarusa.com/education/products/trifit/models/trifit620_hardware.asp).
- Pedometers are used to count steps as part of fitness monitoring and evaluation.

Imagine the physical education setting of the future. Middle school students have met a series of performance criteria for tumbling skills (e.g., forward and backward rolls, headstands, cartwheels, handstands). Now they are expected to learn the roundoff, review skills, and create a routine. The following learning centers (stations) are set up around the gymnasium for tumbling and cardiorespiratory endurance activities (Siedentop, 2004):

- A DVD player with a DVD showing sample floor exercise routines.
- Skill levels are verified through peer review of video clips.
- Students are given a choice of aerobic activity (e.g., virtual reality rowing, jump rope, interactive dance routines following a robot that provides feedback); they wear devices to record physiological data (e.g., heart rate, energy expenditure, breathing rate).
- A video recording station provides immediate feedback of attempts to perform the roundoff on a large flat-screen monitor.
- Handheld computers are used to create routines that are demonstrated by a 3D hologram.
- Routines are edited and fine-tuned for immediate playback and review.
- A virtual human provides the biomechanical principles of the roundoff.

The data collected at each learning center are entered into networked computers that are wirelessly connected to a server where student work is stored in individual folders. The teacher or student can check the folder using a personal handheld or worn (e.g., wristwatch, glasses, belt, ring) computer (Mohnsen, 2004).

Standards Movement

The roots of the educational change discussed in the preceding section were established through the challenging national standards movement. Standards provide a broad framework for the knowledge, skills, and dispositions that students and future and practicing teachers should exhibit. They describe, with varying degrees of clarity and specificity, what students and teachers are expected to know and be able to do. Standards are oriented not to the lowest common denominator, but rather to quality, excellence, and proficiency. Although the standards movement has its critics, there is widespread agreement that standards have benefits by providing clear outcomes, common direction, equity in learning goals, a consistent basis for communicating achievement, and an explicit and external basis for judging learning and teaching.

Standards create broad targets for learning, but do not prescribe process and function. There is a tendency to confuse outputs (ends) with inputs (means). Satisfactory completion of learning experiences and opportunities (means) assumes that learners have acquired the intended knowledge and skills (ends). Therefore, programs for students and teachers must consider both inputs and outputs relative to the ultimate accomplishment of the standards. Standards documents such as the ones published by national organizations and subject matter groups, and the federally funded documents in other subject areas, are now complete. The majority of these documents describe standards at levels of specificity that provide sufficient clarity for instruction. They serve as instruments of accountability even though the process used to validate standards is unclear and many standards are merely untested goals.

In an attempt to identify what students and teachers should know and be able to do, standards documents describe the requisite knowledge and skills, performance activities, curriculum goals, instructional strategies, and assessment options. For example, schools have adopted the standards, and parents want to know how their children are performing compared to the standards. In some cases, there are competing sets of standards, and they are too complex to be of any practical value. The public outcry for and political attention given to school improvement and high performance standards leaves many wondering whether we are setting ourselves up for failure. However, there is a clear expectation that standards serve as the organizing framework for curriculum design and assessment. This section presents the characteristics, benefits, and planning sequence underlying standards-based education followed by an introduction to learning and teaching standards for physical education.

Standards-Based Education

Standards play a central role in the construction of educational programs whether for K-12 curricula, teacher education preparation programs, or teacher professional development programs. Generally, there are two kinds of standards. Content standards describe *what* outcomes, expectations, or learning results are sought. Performance standards describe *how good is good enough* in terms of achievement levels, benchmarks, or indicators. These two kinds of standards form the basis of assessment including assessment activities (e.g., performance tasks, constructed response) and assessment scoring tools (e.g., rating scales, checklists, rubrics). Standards should be seen as the primary focus for classroom-level assessment rather than for large-scale assessment.

Past decades of educational reform have revealed the power of curriculum, assessment, and instruction alignment to improve levels of student achievement. Curriculum is chosen so that students can meet standards, assessment activities and tools are chosen that will identify students' progress toward meeting standards, and instructional techniques are chosen to provide opportunities for students to meet standards. Learning, rather than teaching, is primary to standards-based education (SBE). When learning is the focus, covering material is no longer the goal. Teachers are challenged to develop standards-based learning environments in which students are active participants. Standards-based education means the following (SBE Design Team, 1997):

- Standards guide all classroom decisions.
- The focus is always on student learning.
- Expectations for learning are high for all students, even those who have traditionally performed at low levels.
- The final determination of the effectiveness of instructional practices is whether they result in higher levels of achievement for students.
- Assessment results are used to inform the teacher about the effectiveness of curricular and instructional decisions.

The benefits of standards-based education include clear public expectations for programs and schools, a focus on the curriculum, rigorous academic content, high expectations demanding hard work and effort, and all students reaching high levels of achievement. In traditional schools, the planning sequence is to design the curriculum, develop instructional strategies, implement instruction, design the assessment, and assess students. To be effective, SBE requires a different approach as shown in figure 1.1. The planning sequence represents a *design down,* or backward design, approach. We start with the end in mind—the desired standards—and then derive the curriculum that will achieve them. Assessments are developed and performance levels are established before the curriculum is designed and instructional strategies are planned and implemented. Next, students are assessed and the results of assessment are used to evaluate and refine the SBE process. The absolute measure of effectiveness is whether students successfully demonstrate standards proficiency (SBE Design Team, 1997).

As a result of standards-based education, assessment practices have changed dramatically, but grading practices have evolved more slowly. Traditional grading practices also need to change to align with standards and support current assessment practices. The primary purpose of assessment under SBE is to inform learning, not to sort, select, or justify a grade. Assessment literacy, including assessment for learning and authentic assessment, are discussed later in this chapter (page 19). Many issues and concerns are associated with grading, such as the basis for grades, achievement versus behavior, sources of information, number crunching, record keeping, and the degree of student involvement. The following guidelines are suggested for grading in standards-based systems (O'Connor, 2002):

1. Relate grading procedures to learning goals (i.e., standards), not to methods of assessment (e.g., skill test, project, written exam).

2. Use criterion-referenced performance standards as reference points to determine grades. Students who reach the performance standard get the grade; there is no bell curve.

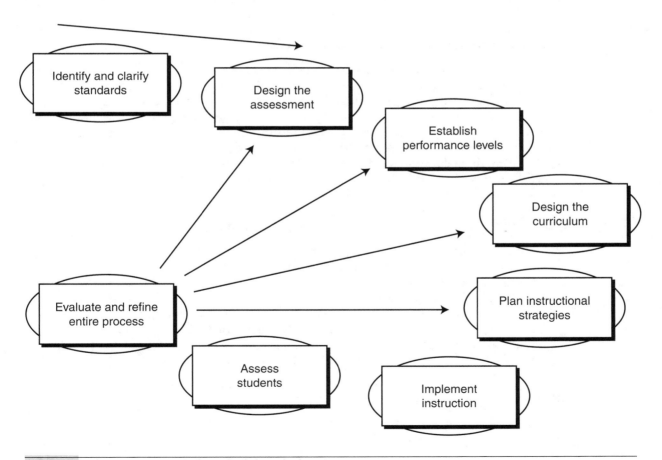

Figure 1.1 Planning sequence of standards-based education.

3. Limit the valued attributes included in grades to individual achievement (i.e., demonstration of knowledge and skill components of the standards). Effort, participation, attitude, and other behaviors should be reported separately.

4. Sample student performance—do not include all scores in grades. Provide feedback on formative performance (feedback and intervention to alter and improve students' learning while instruction is going on), but include information only from summative assessments (final judgments about students' learning at the end of instruction) in grades.

5. Keep records so they can be updated easily (e.g., grade in pencil). Use the most consistent level of achievement with special consideration of recent information and provide several assessment opportunities (i.e., vary methods and number).

6. Crunch numbers carefully—if at all. Avoid using the mean; consider using the median or mode. Weight components to match the intent of grades.

7. Use quality assessments and properly record evidence of achievement. Meet standards for quality assessment (i.e., clear targets, clear purpose, appropriate target–method match, appropriate sampling, and avoidance of bias and distortion). Maintain evidence of achievement (e.g., database, portfolio, tracking system).

8. Discuss and involve students in assessment, including grading, throughout the teaching and learning process (e.g., self-assessment and reflection, goal setting, record keeping, student-led conferences).

These guidelines are dealt with in greater detail in chapter 3 relative to student portfolios (pages 185-194). Grading in standards-based education is analyzed and procedures for converting rubric scores to grades are outlined in that chapter, and suggestions for grading portfolios are also provided.

Learning and Teaching Standards

The significance of standards-based education at all levels has been established. Clearly, student learning and teaching practices of the past are not adequate to meet the demands of the 21st century. Standards are the cornerstone of ongoing educational reform. That raises several questions about learning and teaching. For K-12 students, the question is, What should physically educated people know and be able to do as a result of their physical education program? For teacher candidates, the question is, What knowledge, skills, attitudes, and beliefs should the beginning physical education teacher possess? And, for practicing teachers, the question is, What knowledge, skills, dispositions, and commitments are essential for accomplished, effective teaching? The following sections explore some answers to these questions.

Content Standards for K-12 Physical Education Students

What should physically educated students know and be able to do? The answer to this question has evolved through a series of projects sponsored by the National Association for Sport and Physical Education (NASPE), leading to explicit standards for physical education programs. Initially, the NASPE "outcomes project" produced a definition of a physically educated person. The definition, consisting of five major focus areas, was expanded to 20 outcome statements. This was followed by a set of attendant benchmark statements for grades K, 2, 4, 6, 8, 10, and 12 in the publication *Outcomes of Quality Physical Education Programs* (NASPE, 1992, p. 7).

To pursue a lifetime of healthful physical activity, a physically educated person:

- *Has* learned skills necessary to perform a variety of physical activities
- *Knows* the implications of and the benefits from involvement in physical activities
- *Does* participate regularly in physical activity
- *Is* physically fit
- *Values* physical activity and its contributions to a healthful lifestyle

The national redesign of education provided the impetus for the continued development of physical education content. In 1993 NASPE appointed a standards and assessment task force to develop content standards and assessment material based on the *Outcomes* publication. Work of the task force was published in *Moving Into the Future: National Standards for Physical Education* (NASPE, 1995a). The document established seven content standards for the physical education school program and teacher-friendly guidelines for assessment. It was designed to expand and complement, not replace, the *Outcomes* publication.

In 2002, to ensure that materials were up-to-date and reflected current knowledge, research, and practice, NASPE appointed a K-12 national standards review committee. Following an extensive review and revision process, a second edition of *Moving Into the Future: National Standards for Physical Education* (NASPE, 2004) was published. The document was developed around six content standards for grades K-12 describing what students should know and be able to do. For each standard, student expectations and sample performance outcomes are indicated for grade-level ranges representing kindergarten through 2nd grade, 3rd grade through 5th grade, 6th grade through 8th grade, and 9th grade through 12th grade. These ranges are consistent with developmental patterns, reflect organizational levels in school settings, and align with other subject areas. Student expectations reflect what students should know and be able to do at the end of each grade-level range. Performance outcomes provide examples of student behavior at each grade-level range that demonstrate progress toward achieving the standards. The six physical education content standards and their general descriptions appear in table 1.1. The corresponding student expectations and performance outcomes across each grade-level range are presented in chapter 3 to facilitate the organization of student portfolios (see table 3.2 on pages 141-142).

Table 1.1 Content Standards for Physical Education

A physically educated person:	General description
Standard 1: Demonstrates competency in motor skills and movement patterns needed to perform a variety of physical activities.	Development of the physical skills needed to enjoy participation in physical activities, including: movement fundamentals as a foundation to facilitate continued motor skill acquisition; maturity and versatility in the use of fundamental motor skills (e.g., running, skipping, throwing, striking); specialized skills (e.g., a specific dance step, chest pass, catching with a glove, use of a specific tactic); selected regular participation of a few activities by high school students; and skills to participate in a wide variety of leisure and work-related physical activities.
Standard 2: Demonstrates understanding of movement concepts, principles, strategies, and tactics as they apply to the learning and performance of physical activities.	Facilitate learners' ability to use cognitive information to understand and enhance motor skill acquisition and performance, including: use the mind to control or direct one's performance including the application of concepts from the subdisciplines; establish a movement vocabulary and apply introductory concepts; apply and generalize concepts to real-life physical activity situations; independent and routine use of a wide variety of increasingly complex concepts; and sufficient knowledge and ability to independently use knowledge to acquire new skills while continuing to refine existing ones.
Standard 3: Participates regularly in physical activity.	Establishment of patterns of regular participation in meaningful physical activity, including: connect what is done in class with lives outside class; develop an active, healthy lifestyle outside of class; demonstrate effective self-management skill for participation in physical activity; develop voluntary participation from initial enjoyment derived from activity and requisite skills; enjoy physical activity recognizing that a certain level of personal commitment and earnest work is required; developmentally appropriate activities help develop movement competence for moderate to vigorous physical activity and unstructured play; increase structure of activity and opportunities for participation in activity outside class; and participation commensurate with contemporary recommendations regarding type of activity and frequency, duration, and intensity of participation.

(continued)

Table 1.1 *(continued)*

A physically educated person:	General description
Standard 4: Achieves and maintains a health-enhancing level of physical fitness.	Development of knowledge, skills, and willingness to accept responsibility for personal fitness, leading to an active, healthy lifestyle, including: higher levels of basic fitness and physical competence; health-related fitness components; improvement of fitness levels on a personal basis; progress from moderate to vigorous physical activities that address health-related fitness components and skill; awareness of fitness components and fun while participating in health-enhancing activities; gradually acquire a greater understanding of fitness components and the ways each is maintained; and develop an appropriate personal fitness program to achieve health-related levels of fitness.
Standard 5: Exhibits responsible personal and social behavior that respects self and others in physical activity settings.	Achievement of self-initiated behaviors that promote personal and group success in activity settings including safe practices, adherence to rules and procedures, etiquette, cooperation and teamwork, ethical behavior, and positive social interaction, including: develop respect for individual similarities and differences, including characteristics of culture, ethnicity, motor performance, disabilities, physical characteristics, gender, age, race, and socioeconomic status; recognition of classroom rules, procedures, and safety; working independently, with a partner, and in small groups; begin to recognize individual similarities and differences and participate cooperatively; identify purpose of rules and procedures, become involved in decision-making processes to establish rules and procedures, and participate cooperatively in physical activity with persons of diverse characteristics and backgrounds; initiate responsible behavior, function independently, and positively influence the behavior of others; participate with all people, avoid and resolve conflicts, recognize the value of diversity; and develop strategies for inclusion of others; and understand how adult work and family roles and responsibilities affect their decisions about physical activity and how physical activity, preferences, and opportunities change over time.
Standard 6: Values physical activity for health, enjoyment, challenge, self-expression, and/or social interaction.	Development of an awareness of the intrinsic values and benefits of participation in physical activity that provides personal meaning, including: opportunities for self-expression and social interaction as well as enjoyment, challenge, and fun; develop self-confidence and promote a positive self-image, enticing people to continue participation; derive pleasure from movement sensations and experience challenge and joy as students sense a growing competence in movement ability; opportunities for challenge, social interaction, and group membership, as well as opportunities for continued personal growth in physical skills; continues to provide enjoyment and challenge as well as opportunities for self-expression and social interaction; and intrinsic benefits of participation leads to the active pursuit of life-long physical activities to meet own needs.

Standards for Teacher Candidates

Efforts to establish standards and policies that affect the quality of teachers in training (preservice) have been noteworthy. For beginning teacher licensing, performance standards were developed by the Interstate New Teacher Assessment and Support Consortium (INTASC), a group of more than 30 state and professional organizations formed under the auspices of the Council of Chief State School Officers. The consortium's model standards present teacher candidates as reflective, inquiry-oriented professionals who are cognizant of equity and diversity issues, competent in their subject matter, and able to select instructional strategies best suited to the varying needs of their students (Darling-Hammond, 1992). The designated headings for the 10 standards are (Campbell, Cignetti, Melenyzer, Nettles, & Wyman, 2003, pp. 4-6)

1. knowledge of subject matter,
2. knowledge of human development and learning,
3. adapting instruction for individual needs,
4. multiple instructional strategies,
5. classroom motivation and management skills,
6. communication skills,
7. instructional planning skills,
8. assessment of student learning,
9. professional commitment and responsibility, and
10. partnerships.

What knowledge and skills are essential for effective teaching in physical education? The standards-based reform of physical education teacher education can help answer this question. The National Association for Sport and Physical Education (NASPE) was one of the first specialty professional associations to use the INTASC model for developing teacher standards. NASPE formed a beginning teacher standards task force to provide focus and direction for teacher education and teaching practice. The task force published *National Standards for Beginning Physical Education Teachers* (NASPE, 1995b), consisting of nine standards reflecting the knowledge, performances (skills), and dispositions (attitudes, beliefs) needed to teach physical education. The standards also served as the basis for the review and accreditation of initial physical education licensure programs in collaboration with the National Council for the Accreditation of Teacher Education (NCATE).

In 2001 the beginning physical education teacher task force sought to revise and update the knowledge, skills, and dispositions that the teacher candidate should possess upon entering the teaching ranks. The second edition of *National Standards for Beginning Physical Education Teachers* (NASPE, 2003) presents 10 standards that define competent and exemplary physical education teaching. The document provides a description of each standard along with "acceptable" and "target" outcomes. For each standard, the knowledge, performances, and dispositions a beginning teacher must demonstrate are also detailed. The 10 standards are described and the associated outcomes are identified in table 1.2. The dispositions, knowledge, and performances associated with each standard will be presented in chapter 2 to facilitate the organization of professional portfolios for teacher candidates (see pages 55-59).

Standards for Practicing Teachers

Originally, the wave of reform initiatives that engulfed school programs and teacher education left out a critical element of the education equation—the practicing teacher. The knowledge and skills of many accomplished teachers were often unacknowledged and underused. Delineating outstanding practice and recognizing those who achieve it was critical to defining the kind of teachers needed. In 1987 this challenge was embraced with the establishment of the National Board for Professional Teaching Standards (NBPTS). The vision of advancing the quality of teaching and learning through continuing professional development (in-service) was born. The National Board's mission is to

1. establish and maintain high and rigorous standards for what accomplished teachers should know and be able to do,
2. develop and operate a national voluntary system certifying teachers who meet the standards, and
3. advance related education reforms for the purpose of improving student learning.

What knowledge and skills are essential for effective teaching? The National Board has led the vanguard effort to develop professional standards for school teaching. Certification is a symbol of

Table 1.2 Standards for Beginning Physical Education Teachers With Outcomes

A beginning physical education teacher should:	Outcomes of the standard
1. Content knowledge Understand physical education content and disciplinary concepts related to the development of a physically educated person.	• Identify critical elements of motor skill performance; combine motor skills into appropriate sequences. • Demonstrate competent motor skill performance. • Describe performance concepts and strategies. • Describe and apply bioscience and psychological concepts. • Understand and debate current physical activity issues. • Know approved state and national content standards, and local program goals.
2. Growth and development Understand how individuals learn and develop, and provide opportunities that support physical, cognitive, social, and emotional development.	• Monitor individual and group performance for safe instruction. • Implement appropriate learning/practice opportunities based on expected progressions and levels of readiness. • Implement appropriate learning/practice opportunities based on understanding the student, the learning environment, and the task.
3. Diverse learners Understand how individuals differ in their approaches to learning and create appropriate instruction adapted to these differences.	• Implement appropriate instruction that is sensitive to students' strengths and weaknesses, multiple needs, learning styles, and prior experiences. • Use appropriate strategies, services, and resources to meet diverse learning needs.
4. Management and motivation Use and have an understanding of individual and group motivations and behavior to create a safe learning environment that encourages positive social interaction, active engagement in learning, and self-motivation.	• Use managerial routines that create smoothly functioning learning experiences. • Organize, allocate, and manage resources to provide active and equitable learning experiences. • Use a variety of developmentally appropriate practices to motivate school age students. • Use strategies to help students demonstrate responsible personal and social behaviors. • Develop an effective behavior management plan.
5. Communication Use knowledge of effective verbal, nonverbal, and media communication techniques to enhance learning and engagement in physical education settings.	• Describe and demonstrate effective communication skills. • Communicate managerial and instructional information in a variety of ways. • Communicate in ways that demonstrate sensitivity to all students. • Describe and implement strategies to enhance communication among students.
6. Planning and instruction Understand the importance of planning developmentally appropriate instructional units to foster the development of a physically educated person.	• Implement appropriate program and instructional goals. • Develop short- and long-term plans that are linked to goals and student needs. • Implement instructional strategies, based on selected content, student needs, and safety issues, to facilitate learning. • Implement learning experiences that are safe, appropriate, relevant, and based on principles of effective instruction. • Apply disciplinary and pedagogical knowledge. • Provide learning experiences that allow students to integrate knowledge and skills from multiple subjects. • Implement appropriate teaching resources and curriculum materials. • Use effective demonstrations and explanations. • Use appropriate instructional cues and prompts. • Develop a repertoire of direct and indirect instructional formats.

A beginning physical education teacher should:	Outcomes of the standard
7. <u>Student assessment</u> Understand and use the varied types of assessment and their contribution to overall program continuity and the development of the physical, cognitive, social, and emotional domains.	• Identify key components of various types of assessment, describe their appropriate and inappropriate use, and address issues of validity, reliability, and bias. • Use a variety of appropriate authentic and traditional assessment techniques, provide feedback, and communicate student progress. • Interpret and use learning and performance data to inform curricular and instructional decisions.
8. <u>Reflection</u> Understand the importance of being a reflective practitioner and its contribution to overall professional development and actively seek opportunities to sustain professional growth.	• Use a reflective cycle (describe, justify, and critique teaching, set teaching goals, and implement change). • Use available resources to develop as a reflective professional. • Construct a plan for continued professional growth.
9. <u>Technology</u> Use information technology to enhance learning and personal and professional productivity.	• Know current technologies and their application. • Implement student-learning activities that integrate information technology. • Use technologies to communicate, network, locate resources, and enhance continuing professional development.
10. <u>Collaboration</u> Understand the necessity of fostering collaborative relationships with colleagues, parents/guardians, and community agencies to support the development of a physically educated person.	• Identify strategies to become an advocate in the school and community to promote physical activity. • Actively participate in the professional physical education community and within the broader field of education. • Identify and seek community resources to enhance physical activity opportunities. • Establish productive relationships with parent/guardians and school colleagues to support student growth and well-being.

Reprinted from *National Standards for Beginning Physical Education Teachers,* 2nd edition (2003) with permission from the National Association for Sport and Physical Education (NASPE), 1900 Association Drive, Reston, VA 20191-1599.

professional teaching excellence. Offered voluntarily, it complements, not replaces, entry-level state licensing for beginning teachers. The advanced standards for experienced teachers seek to identify and recognize teachers who effectively enhance student learning and demonstrate the high level of knowledge, skills, dispositions, and commitments reflected in five core propositions advanced by the National Board for Professional Teaching Standards (1999). Teachers who display these abilities and traits are considered accomplished teachers, regardless of their subject field. The core propositions; supporting standards; and corresponding knowledge, skills, dispositions, and beliefs appear in table 1.3. They will be used in chapter 4 to facilitate the organization of professional portfolios for practicing teachers (see table 4.1 on page 242).

National Board Certification for physical education teachers was created in 2000. Two certificates are available covering two age ranges of students—early and middle childhood physical education (student ages 3 through 12) and early adolescence through young adulthood physical education (student ages 11 through 18+). Standards of accomplished practice for physical education teachers were also developed in support of the certification review and assessment process (NBPTS, 2001). These 13 standards will also be presented in chapter 4 to facilitate the organization of professional portfolios for practicing teachers (see table 4.1 on page 242). Additional information is accessible through the NBPTS Web site (www.npbts.org).

Table 1.3 Professional Teaching Standards

What accomplished teachers should know and be able to do:	Supporting standards: knowledge, skills, dispositions, and beliefs
Core proposition 1: Teachers are committed to students and their learning.	Teachers act on the belief that all students can learn. Accomplished teachers are dedicated to and skilled at making knowledge, skills, and values accessible to all students, even as they acknowledge their distinctive traits and talents. Success depends on teachers' belief in the dignity, worth, and potential that exists within each child. Teachers are attentive to human variability and its influence on learning. • Teachers recognize individual differences in their students and adjust their practice accordingly. • Teachers have an understanding of how students develop and learn. • Teachers treat students equitably. • Teachers' mission extends beyond developing the [motor] capacity of their students.
Core proposition 2: Teachers know the subjects they teach and how to teach those subjects to students.	Accomplished teachers are dedicated to exposing students to the social, cultural, ethical, and physical worlds in which they live, and they use the subject as an entree into those worlds. • Teachers appreciate how knowledge [and skill] in their subjects is created, organized, and linked to other disciplines. • Teachers command specialized knowledge of how to convey a subject to students. • Teachers generate multiple paths to [learning].
Core proposition 3: Teachers are responsible for managing and monitoring student learning.	Professional teachers hold high expectations for all students and see themselves as facilitators of student learning. Teachers must create, enrich, and alter the organizational structures in which they work with young people. They also find ways to capture and sustain the interest of their students and they attempt to make the most efficient use of time. To accomplish these tasks, teachers seek to master the body of generic pedagogical knowledge. • Teachers call on multiple methods to meet their goals. • Teachers orchestrate learning in group settings. • Teachers place a premium on student engagement. • Teachers regularly assess student progress. • Teachers are mindful of their principal objectives.
Core proposition 4: Teachers think systematically about their practice and learn from experience.	Teaching requires an open-ended capacity that is not acquired once and for all. Teachers have a professional obligation to be lifelong students of their craft, seeking to expand their repertoire, deepen their knowledge and skill, and become wiser in rendering judgments. Accomplished teachers are inventive in their teaching and stand ready to incorporate ideas and methods developed by others that fit their aims and their students. Excellence is a reverence for the craft, a recognition of its complexities, and a commitment to lifelong professional development. • Teachers are continually making difficult choices that test their judgment. • Teachers seek the advice of others and draw on education research and scholarship to improve their practice.
Core proposition 5: Teachers are members of learning communities.	Teaching reaches beyond the boundaries of individual classrooms to wider communities of learning. Accomplished teachers have a range of duties and tasks outside the direct instruction of students that contribute importantly to the quality of the school and to student learning. One responsibility involves participation in collaborative efforts to improve the effectiveness of the school. The second entails engaging parents and others in the community in the education of young people. • Teachers contribute to school effectiveness by collaborating with other professionals. • Teachers work collaboratively with parents. • Teachers take advantage of community resources.

Assessment Literacy

The national attention on achieving excellence in education has resulted in school accountability models that transform high standards and expectations into rigorous assessments such as on-demand, standardized achievement tests. Our nation—particularly legislators, parents, and many educators—is obsessed with the belief that increased student learning, and therefore, school improvement, comes from frequent, intense, high-stakes testing. Although such tests provide important information for program and policy decision making, they are limited in meeting the information needs of teachers and students at the classroom level. If teachers are to respond to the various roles suggested by the trends in education previously outlined, quality assessments are a must. The keys to quality assessment practices are built on five dimensions (Stiggins, Arter, Chappuis, & Chappuis, 2004). For each of the following dimensions, which are italicized, questions are posed to facilitate quality assessment. Assessments should

1. arise from and be designed to serve the *specific information needs of intended users* (Why do we assess? What's the purpose? Who will use the results?);

2. arise from clearly articulated and appropriate *achievement targets* (What are we assessing? Are the achievement targets clear? Are they good?);

3. *accurately reflect* student achievement (How do we assess? What method do we use? How do we sample? How do we avoid bias?);

4. yield results that are *effectively communicated* to their intended users (How do we communicate? How do we manage information? How do we report results?); and

5. *involve students* in classroom-level assessment, record keeping, and communication (How do we involve students? What recording tools do we use? How do we disseminate information? What decisions can students make?).

The assessment contexts—intended users and uses (dimension 1) and learning targets (dimension 2)—are combined to help determine a proper assessment design (dimension 3), from which the best mode of communication is derived (dimension 4). Students are involved during all phases (dimension 5). High-quality classroom assessment means accurate information (i.e., clear purposes, clear targets, appropriate design) used effectively to help students learn. To apply these standards of assessment quality, teachers must develop assessment literacy. Assessment-literate teachers are able to determine what to assess (learning targets) and how to assess (methods), and then to match the proper method of assessment with the intended target.

The following sections provide a foundation for developing assessment literacy. A crucial distinction is made between assessment *of* learning (achievement status at a point in time, usually at the end of the learning process) and assessment *for* learning (student-involved assessment to promote achievement during the learning process). Also, the meaning of authentic assessment is presented relative to measuring student achievement and documenting effective teaching in physical education.

Assessment *for* Learning

The premise for this section is that teaching, learning, and assessment must be integrated. But, this notion seems to conflict with the realities of proficiency or achievement testing. For example, the No Child Left Behind Act of 2001 (NCLB Act) reflects a consensus on how to improve the performance of U.S. elementary and secondary schools while at the same time ensuring that no child is trapped in a failing school. The NCLB Act (www.NoChildLeftBehind.gov) was built on a set of accountability and assessment requirements. These requirements, which mandate the overall direction of states' education policy initiatives, are as follows:

1. Setting standards
2. Measuring students' progress against standards
3. Providing help for struggling students
4. Holding schools accountable for results

The NCLB Act redefined the federal role in K-12 education to help close the achievement gap between disadvantaged and minority students and their peers. School districts and schools that fail to make adequate yearly progress (AYP) toward statewide proficiency goals will, over time, be subject to improvement, corrective action, and restructuring measures aimed at getting them back on course to meet state standards.

As a result of the NCLB Act, national, state, and district standards have been widely established; continuous improvement planning and management has been implemented; accountability for student achievement has been accepted among educators; and rigorous testing systems are in place and growing. Instead of using minimum competencies, we have "raised the bar" by setting world-class standards for student achievement. To determine accountability, we rely on high-stakes assessment *of* learning that measures achievement status at a point in time. Supposedly, this summative assessment tells us how much students have learned, the degree to which standards are being met, and whether schools are effective. To further intensify the impact of standards and assessments, there is the promise of rewards for schools that produce high scores and sanctions for those that do not. At the classroom level, assessment of learning is grading. This is not to suggest that assessment of learning is inappropriate. Rather, it is simply insufficient to maximize learning for all students. Some students respond favorably to the intimidation and the rewards or punishments associated with testing, but this model does not work for an increasing number of students (Stiggins, 2002).

The focus on standards, accountability, and testing has resulted in an assessment crisis in the form of a failure to connect classroom-level assessment to school improvement. Amid the wave of reform movements in education, assessment is often viewed as separate from teaching. Rather, it should be fully integrated into the teaching–learning process. The problem with layer upon layer of large-scale summative assessments is the lack of a compelling case showing that the uses of tests for student and school accountability have improved education and student learning in dramatic ways (Linn, 2000). There is increasing evidence, however, that student achievement improves through assessment *for* learning—assessment that promotes student achievement during the learning process. Such formative assessment is used to adapt teaching to meet student needs.

In a comprehensive review of research, Black and Wiliam (1998) found that strengthening the practice of formative assessment produces significant and often substantial learning gains. Another conclusion was that improved formative assessment helps low achievers more than other students, thus reducing the range of achievement while raising achievement overall. This finding has practical implications at the classroom level for students who lack motivation to learn, perform poorly on summative tests, or see themselves as unable to learn. Follow-up projects confirmed that improving formative assessment raises student achievement. A change in teacher practice and a change in student behavior means that everyone shares responsibility for the students' learning (Black, Harrison, Lee, Marshall, & Wiliam, 2004). The crucial distinctions between assessment *of* learning and assessment *for* learning are summarized in table 1.4.

Assessment *for* learning is dependent on the interplay between student and teacher. Students engage in and take active responsibility for their learning while teachers can help by answering three questions and taking specific steps (seven strategies) associated with each question (Stiggins, Arter, Chappuis, & Chappuis, 2004, p. 42):

- Where am I going?
    1. Provide a clear and understandable vision of the learning target.
    2. Use examples and models of strong and weak work.
- Where am I now?
    1. Offer regular descriptive feedback.
    2. Teach students to self-assess and set goals.
- How can I close the gap?
    1. Design lessons to focus on one aspect of quality at a time.
    2. Teach students focused revision.
    3. Engage students in self-reflection, and let them keep track of and share their learning.

Table 1.4 Distinctions Between Assessment *for* Learning and Assessment *of* Learning

Aspect	Assessment *for* learning	Assessment *of* learning
Reasons	Promotes increases in achievement; helps students meet more standards; supports ongoing student growth; improvement	Documents individual or group achievement or mastery of standards; achievement status at a point in time for purposes of reporting; accountability
Audience	Students about themselves	Others about student
Focus	Specific achievement targets selected by teachers that enable students to build toward standards	Achievement standards for which schools, teachers, and students are held accountable
Timing	A process during the learning	An event after learning
Users	Students, teachers, parents and guardians in partnership	Policy makers, program planners, supervisors, teachers, students, parents and guardians
Uses	Provides students with insight to improve achievement; helps teachers diagnose and respond to student needs; helps parents and guardians see progress over time and support learning	Certifies student competence; sorts students according to achievement; promotion and graduation decisions; grading
Motivation	Belief that success in learning is achievable	Promise of rewards; threat of punishment
Teacher's role	Transform standards into classroom targets; inform students of targets; build assessments; adjust instruction based on results; offer descriptive feedback to students; involve students in assessment	Administer tests carefully to ensure accuracy and comparability of results; use results to help students meet standards; interpret results for parents and guardians; build assessments for report card grading
Student's role	Self-assess and keep track of progress; contribute to setting goals; understand success; act on classroom assessment results to be able to do better next time	Study or practice to meet standards; take tests; strive for the highest possible score; avoid failure
Examples	Using rubrics with students; student self-assessment; descriptive feedback to students	Achievement tests; final exams; placement tests; short cycle assessments

From Stiggins, R.J., Arter, J.A., Chappuis, J., & Chappuis, S., 2004, *Classroom Assessment for Student Learning: Doing It Right—Using It Well.* (Portland, OR: Assessment Training Institute), 33. By permission of Stephen Chappuis.

Formative assessment is more than testing frequently; it is even more than using student information to plan next steps. Formative assessment in the context of assessment for learning also means that students are involved in their own assessment and goal setting, record keeping, and communication. Student-involved assessment includes anything that helps students understand learning targets, engage in self-assessment, watch themselves grow, talk about their learning growth, and plan next steps for learning. In physical education, student-involved assessment is evidenced, for example, when students do the following:

1. Engage in regular self-assessment, with movement standards held constant so that they can track their growth over time

2. Communicate with the teacher, other students, and family members about their achievement status and improvements (e.g., student-led conferences, reflections)

3. Assist in developing scoring criteria for various sports skills

4. Create assessment rubrics including criteria and descriptive indicators for each level of excellence

5. Plan their own next steps for learning based on a comprehensive skill analysis (i.e., goal setting)

6. Maintain fitness records relative to learning targets

Student portfolios reflect many of the characteristics of assessment *for* learning such as goal setting, self-assessment, record keeping, and communication. The underlying principles and concepts of assessment *for* learning will be applied in chapter 3.

Authentic Assessment

One result of the educational reform movement is the focus on clearly developed, publicly stated standards that are linked to assessment. This redesign of learning and teaching, however, has exposed the dissatisfaction with traditional forms of assessment—multiple-choice tests, group-administered achievement tests, and standardized skill tests. These kinds of assessment make it nearly impossible to measure the broad range of skills and competencies represented by established standards.

Although society has been oriented toward standardized achievement tests, the readiness for change is apparent toward a broader array of assessment methods. Alternatives have centered on more naturalistic, performance-based approaches. They measure not only knowledge and skills, but other outcomes such as attitudes, motivation, social conduct, and values. Evaluation that scans this full spectrum of learning reflects the trend toward authentic assessment. Actual exhibits and work samples of student performance serve as the measure of learning instead of the highly inferential estimates provided by the objectively scored and normative interpretation of tests.

Authentic assessment is usually thought to be the process of gathering evidence about students' levels of achievement. However, collecting authentic information about teachers' performance is just as valuable. Clearly, the concept applies to both students and teachers where assessment is structured around real-life samples of learning and actual classroom performance, respectively. In physical education, multiple-choice, machine-scored tests, or standardized sport skill or fitness tests, do not seem to be good indicators of what students really learn. Likewise, multiple-choice tests of basic skills and general knowledge seem woefully inadequate to measure teaching skill. Thus, authentic techniques are needed to assess the degree to which student and teacher meet established standards specific to physical education. That is the purpose of the following sections.

Measuring Student Achievement

An assessment is considered authentic if the student demonstrates the desired behavior in real-life situations rather than in artificial or contrived settings. Teachers want more practical, relevant assessment tools to measure what students really know and are able to do. With traditional testing, teachers may know that students are learning, but that is often not what is being measured, nor do the tests seem to facilitate learning. Instead, students respond to prompts or perform tasks that have no worthwhile, real-life, or authentic counterparts. Standardized measures of motor ability, fitness parameters, sports skills, knowledge, and psychosocial traits may be objective and reliable, but they may fail to measure authentic outcomes of interest to the teacher and students.

Probably the most difficult challenge of authentic assessment is determining an appropriate real-life context in which to conduct learning tasks. An example might be helpful. One outcome of a physical fitness unit could be that students are able to develop a personalized program. Traditional assessment might involve written tests of understanding, summaries of articles about fitness programs, and an essay about a case study. These measures are not wrong, but there is a question of whether students are moving toward broader outcomes. In contrast, a group project could be structured to (1) evaluate the fitness needs of teachers and staff at the school, (2) design custom fitness programs for these people, (3) provide training on how to safely and effectively engage in fitness activities, and (4) monitor the people as they progress through their programs. The teacher serves as a facilitator. Students present oral synopses and reflections of their challenges and successes at each stage of the process. Feedback from the teacher or peers or through self-analysis is received by students during the process so that learning takes place during the assessment (NASPE, 1995a).

Traditional testing also focuses too much on whether students get right answers. When students take a multiple-choice test on offensive strategies in soccer, you don't know who selects the right answer because they truly understand the principle of switching, who understands the principle but makes a careless recording mistake, or who has no idea and guesses correctly. In addition, multiple-choice tests lead to multiple-choice teaching—an emphasis on the acquisition of facts and predetermined answers.

Using authentic assessment and allowing performance in naturalistic settings require students to actually demonstrate knowledge or skills. Students in math, for example, could show their understanding of interest rates by comparison shopping for a used car loan and identifying the best deal. The teacher would know whether a student really understands the concept of interest, can calculate it, and can perform mathematical operations accurately. To illustrate further, students could demonstrate their understanding of English grammar by editing a poorly written passage (Rudner & Boston, 1994). In physical education, performance in naturalistic game settings (e.g., volleyball bump pass when returning a "real" serve) could be assessed using an observation rating sheet instead of performing at a testing station (e.g., volleyball bump pass from a partner toss).

Authentic assessment provides other benefits over conventional, norm-based measures. It is nonstigmatizing, it enhances motivation, it assists teachers with decision making, and it is effective for reporting accomplishments and progress to families. Traditional grades may be replaced with anecdotal records, performance samples, and student profiles. Despite new attempts to restructure report cards that emphasize performance standards, social skills, higher-order thinking, and other meaningful outcomes, traditional As, Bs, Cs, Ds, and Fs still dominate as the "weapon of choice." Teachers can pass judgment with the stroke of a pen or the "bubble" of a scantron computer sheet (Burke, 2000).

The common goals of authentic assessment are to capitalize on students' actual work, enhance teacher and student involvement, and satisfy accountability needs. Furthermore, these performance-based assessments can be longitudinal (across grade levels), multidimensional (physical, intellectual, social, emotional), and individually modifiable (wide range of student variability). This broadened view of assessment coincides with holistic approaches to teaching, including

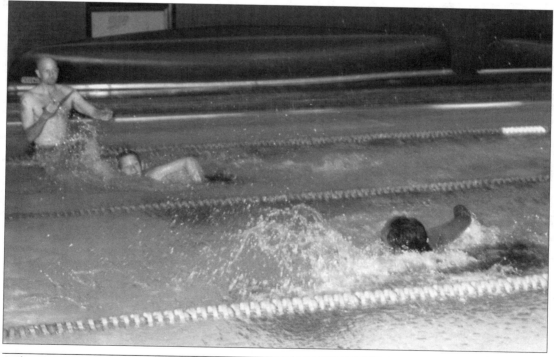

Authentic assessment of swim strokes is determined during a real, in-class swimming competition using a performance checklist.

recommended practice in physical education. Developmentally appropriate practice in physical education means that teacher decisions are based primarily on ongoing, formative assessments of individual students as they participate in physical education class activities and not on the basis of single, summative test scores.

Although these approaches are intended to promote a better alignment of instruction and assessment, they entail new roles for teachers and students in the evaluation process (Melograno, 1997). However, in physical education, these roles may not be entirely new because a performance-based approach is used for what is typically evaluated (e.g., motor abilities, sports skills, game strategies, fair play). Performance assessment is based on the observation of an actual performance or product and a judgment as to its quality. For example, a complex performance might be a floor exercise routine, whereas a product might be a personal health-related fitness plan. A variety of techniques is available for conducting authentic assessment. Although some of the techniques are not new, an authentic context is needed for their use in the teaching–learning process. It is not simply tacked on to the end of a learning segment. Therefore, selected options are described and illustrated in table 1.5. The activity or product examples show how authentic assessment serves as a measure of real student learning.

Table 1.5 Authentic Assessment Options for Physical Education

Options	Descriptions	Activity and product examples
Reflection	Students engage in the thoughtful examination of the learning process in order to plan, monitor, assess, and improve their own performance and their own thinking.	Small groups design and perform a movement sequence that uses matching and mirroring movements; students respond in writing to the questions: What was easy about working together? What was difficult? What should be changed about working together? How was your performance affected?
Log	Performance of specific behaviors over a certain time period is recorded by individual students, small groups, or the whole class to show changes, sequences, choices, feelings, progress, or participation.	Fitness calendar is maintained for three months showing aerobic and strength training workout schedules, weekly changes from baseline data, and the status of target goals at the midpoint and end point.
Worksheet	Students complete a written task or exercise that usually consists of selected response (select correct or best response from a list provided) or extended written response questions (construct answer in response to a question or task).	Second-graders are given a sheet that has movement pictures of children with body parts labeled. Students color with crayon those body parts at a low level, medium level, and high level in red, blue, and yellow, respectively.
Self-evaluation	Students make critical and valid assessments of their own abilities by rating their performance for comparison with individual target goals, peer standards, teacher-established criteria, or all of these.	Following a segment on throwing different objects (e.g., Frisbees, sponge balls, deck tennis rings, footballs), students identify the different objects thrown, describe the types of throwing patterns used, and complete a self-check skill performance rating scale.
Individual project	With the guidance of a teacher, a student pursues an area of interest and takes responsibility for completing the following tasks: building a scenario, determining goals, planning a program of participation to achieve outcomes, and implementing the plan until the goals are achieved.	With "discovering my roots" as the theme, a student presents a game, dance, or other physical activity associated with his or her origins; project includes reading activities, interviews, written or art expressions, and demonstration of selected activities complete with costumes, equipment, and music.
Peer review	One student observes another student's performance, compares and contrasts the performance against teacher's criteria (critical elements), draws conclusions, and communicates results (verbal, nonverbal, or written feedback).	Student A watches student B during a tennis game; using a criteria task sheet, five forehand strokes are observed; six "points to look for" are rated +, ✓, or – for each stroke.

Options	Descriptions	Activity and product examples
Group project	Several students work cooperatively to solve a problem; learn a skill, concept, or generalization; engage in shared discovery; or carry out a series of performance tasks in an atmosphere of interdependence and accountability.	In groups of five or six, students design an obstacle course of straight, curved, and zigzag pathways using wands, ropes, and other manipulative objects. The pathways must connect. Students must decide what locomotor movements to use in traveling the various pathways.
Role playing	Students pretend they are a particular person in order to solve a problem or act out a real-world situation; allows students to re-create (simulate) or act out issues in interpersonal relations such as social events, personal concerns, values, problem behaviors, or social skills.	Students are given this scenario: You are at a basketball game where your best friend's sister plays for the opposing team. Another friend from your school makes disruptive noises when the other team shoots free throws, boos the officials, and makes derogatory remarks to the other team. What would you say to this friend? Create a dialogue.
Event task	A performance task is written broadly enough (loosely structured) so that many solutions or answers are possible, it captures the interest of students, and it replicates or simulates a real-world experience.	Students watch a tape of an athletic performance and discuss, in writing, the space awareness concepts athletes used during their performances. They answer these questions: What did the athletes do at a high, medium, or low level? What kinds of pathways did they use? Directions? What kind of space did they move in? Give examples of how athletes use these concepts.
Observation	The teacher uses different tools to record information about students' performance or behavior (live observation or video analysis) such as anecdotal notes, narrative descriptions, rating scales, checklists, frequency index scales, or scoring rubrics.	Students choreograph their own dance routines. Using a scoring rubric, the teacher watches each routine and rates the following criteria on a scale of 1 to 5: rhythm with music, creativity, fluidity, and diversity. Critical elements for each criterion are built into the rubric.

Note: Information for this table was derived from the following sources: *Moving Into the Future: National Standards for Physical Education: A Guide to Content and Assessment* (NASPE, 1995a), *Developing the Physical Education Curriculum* (Kelly & Melograno, 2004), and *Teaching for Outcomes in Elementary Physical Education: A Guide for Curriculum and Assessment* (Hopple, 1995).

When information is gathered in reference to established student standards, and serves as a guide to teaching, it can enhance learning as well as measure it. Teachers have known that the time spent on assessment does not always yield the desired educational benefits. How often have we heard from a student, "That test didn't really show what I can do!" The inadequacy of standardized, group-based assessment begs for an alternative. Authentic assessment offers an approach that is context responsive—real learning that is found in naturalistic settings.

Documenting Effective Teaching

Traditional assessment of teaching has many of the same challenges as traditional testing of students does. For example, goals conferences with supervisors or principals; formal observations by peers, supervisors, or principals; or self-evaluation of goals do not seem to be good measures of a teacher's knowledge and skills. Like student testing, more naturalistic, performance-based approaches are needed that document real teaching effectiveness. Knowledge tests for an initial teaching license also lack an authentic quality. Most tests rely on selected response or recognition kinds of items such as multiple-choice questions. Although such tests may provide some measure of knowledge, the validity of a paper-and-pencil test as a measure of teaching ability is doubtful. And, there is little agreement as to acceptable minimum passing scores for entry into teaching.

Authentic systems for assessing the skills of teachers in their own settings should be linked to established teacher standards. As discussed earlier, a distinction is made between beginning teacher candidates (initial license) and experienced teachers (advanced certification), although nearly all of the standards overlap in some manner. For example, the management standards may differ in degree, but beginning and experienced teachers are expected nonetheless to create a teaching environment conducive to learning. Also, both beginning and experienced teachers are expected to engage in reflection, but are likely to draw on different sources to improve their practice.

In the case of beginning teachers, the Educational Testing Service (ETS) developed assessments ranging from entry into teacher education to actual classroom teaching. *The Praxis Series: Professional Assessments for Beginning Teachers* (ETS, 1992) offers measures of academic skills, subject knowledge, and classroom performance. Of particular significance is *Praxis III: Classroom Performance Assessments* (ETS, 2001), a system for assessing the skills of beginning teachers in their own classroom settings. Its framework of knowledge and skills includes assessment criteria (standards), scoring rules, and the assessment process. *Praxis III* uses three assessment methods: (1) direct observation of a lesson or instructional event, (2) review of written documentation by the teacher that conveys a sense of the general classroom context and the students as well as information about the lesson, and (3) semistructured interviews before and after the observation to explore the teacher's decisions and practices.

Four interrelated domains comprise the framework of knowledge and skills: (A) organizing content knowledge for student learning, (B) creating an environment for student learning, (C) teaching for student learning, and (D) teacher professionalism. Criteria for each domain are used to assess teaching performance, and each criterion represents a critical aspect of teaching. The 19 criteria covering the domains are listed in the following box. The results of *Praxis III* are considered to yield an authentic assessment of teaching effectiveness.

For experienced teachers, the National Board for Professional Teaching Standards (NBPTS) developed and operates a national voluntary system to assess and certify teachers who meet its standards. The standards (NBPTS, 1999) presented earlier establish what accomplished teachers should know and be able to do. Like *Praxis III*, advanced certification by NBPTS requires the assessment of teachers' competencies in real classroom settings. In addition, common standards were developed for the two physical education certificates covering two age ranges of students, early and middle childhood (ages 3 through 12) and early adolescence through young adulthood (ages 11 through 18+). The 13 standards will be presented in chapter 4 to facilitate the organization of professional portfolios for practicing teachers (see table 4.1 on page 242).

The two-part assessment process is authentic in nature. First, teachers complete a portfolio in their classroom composed of student work, teaching videos, and other teaching artifacts. The student work samples and videos are supported by commentaries on the goals and purposes of instruction, the effectiveness of the practice, reflections on what occurred, and the rationale for professional judgments. Second, exercises conducted at an assessment center are designed to complement the portfolio and are organized around challenging teaching issues. Teachers are given an opportunity to demonstrate knowledge, skills, and abilities in situations across the age range and topics of the certificate field (NBPTS, 1996).

Formal involvement in the *Praxis III* and NBPTS teacher assessment systems may not be feasible for all teachers. However, the information presented in this chapter should be sufficient for determining teacher effectiveness based on practical and relevant measures. This information should motivate beginning and practicing physical education teachers to seek the best way to document their real knowledge and skills.

Role of Portfolios in Standards-Based Assessment

Given the national focus on learning and teaching in standards-based education, it follows that attempts to assess students and teachers should correspond to any established standards. A strong case has been made that such assessments reflect two broad concepts, (1) assessment *for* learning (student-involved assessment through goal setting, self-assessment, reflecting on work, tracking progress, record keeping, and communication) and (2) authentic assessment (performance-based, naturalistic, real-life approaches). Therefore, assessment systems are needed that merge learning and teaching standards with the characteristics of assessment *for* learning and the qualities of authentic assessment.

Teacher Performance Assessment Criteria

Domain A: Organizing Content Knowledge for Student Learning

A1: Becoming familiar with relevant aspects of students' background knowledge and experiences

A2: Articulating clear learning goals for the lesson that are appropriate for the students

A3: Demonstrating an understanding of the connections between the content that was learned previously, the current content, and the content that remains to be learned in the future

A4: Creating or selecting teaching methods, learning activities, and instructional materials or other resources that are appropriate for the students and that are aligned with the goals of the lesson

A5: Creating or selecting evaluation strategies that are appropriate for the students and that are aligned with the goals of the lesson

Domain B: Creating an Environment for Student Learning

B1: Creating a climate that promotes fairness

B2: Establishing and maintaining rapport with students

B3: Communicating challenging learning expectations to each student

B4: Establishing and maintaining consistent standards of classroom behavior

B5: Making the physical environment as safe and conducive to learning as possible

Domain C: Teaching for Student Learning

C1: Making learning goals and instructional procedures clear to students

C2: Making content comprehensible to students

C3: Encouraging students to extend their thinking

C4: Monitoring students' understanding of content through a variety of means, providing feedback to students to assist learning, and adjusting learning activities as the situation demands

C5: Using instructional time effectively

Domain D: Teacher Professionalism

D1: Reflecting on the extent to which the learning goals were met

D2: Demonstrating a sense of efficacy

D3: Building professional relationships with colleagues to share teaching insights and to coordinate learning activities for students

D4: Communicating with parents or guardians about student learning

Adapted PRAXIS materials from *Praxis III: Classroom Performance Assessments—Orientation Guide*, Educational Testing Service, 2001. Used by permission of Educational Testing Service, the copyright owner. Permission to adapt/reproduce PRAXIS materials does not constitute review or endorsement by Educational Testing Service of this publication as a whole or of any other testing information it may contain.

The pendulum of alternative educational assessment has swung toward a portfolio format (Kelly & Melograno, 2004; Melograno, 1994). Although relatively new to education, portfolios have been used for a long time by commercial artists, journalists, architects, photographers, models, and other professionals to showcase talent, skills, style, and range of work. For education, it should be clear that *portfolios are not an assessment method, but a device for collecting and communicating about student learning and teaching competence*. Although a portfolio can be assessed as a whole, its true purpose is to enrich the ability to learn, the desire to learn, and the learning itself. Thus, portfolios can play a significant role in keeping track of and celebrating standards-based learning and creating assessment *for* learning and authentic assessment.

In general, a portfolio is a purposeful, integrated collection of actual exhibits and work samples showing effort, progress, or achievement in one or more aspects. It presents a broad, genuine picture of student learning or teacher performance and allows all concerned to have input (ongoing, formative feedback). Portfolios are not made up of anything and everything. Establishing targets, selecting artifacts, judging quality, and communicating results are key phases of the portfolio creation process.

The type of portfolio used depends on the needs that the portfolio serves. Portfolios feature artifacts collected over time, so they are well suited for demonstrating student growth and achievement of standards. For example, an array of artifacts could be used to indicate the extent to which students *understand how to monitor and maintain a health-enhancing level of physical fitness* by using such tools as exercise logs, nutrition journals, self-check rating scales, workout schedules, and charts showing the diagnosis and prescription of weight training routines. Likewise, portfolios can be used by teacher candidates and practicing teachers to document teaching effectiveness in reference to standards. Any number of products could reveal, for example, that teachers truly *recognize individual differences in their students and adjust their practices accordingly,* such as lesson plans that outline multiple outcomes, individualized class materials, samples of student work, videos depicting alternative strategies, and written teacher behavior analyses and reflections.

Student Portfolios

Portfolios offer a dynamic, visual presentation of a student's abilities, strengths, and areas of needed improvement over time. Students must be involved in selecting and judging the quality of their own work including self-reflection. With portfolios, traditional teaching roles may not work. Teachers need to facilitate, guide, and offer choices rather than inform, direct, and predetermine priorities. Partnerships are established among teacher, students, and parents.

Some teachers look at portfolios and say, "I have too many students and not enough time." However, portfolios demand a high level of student responsibility in terms of self-management, self-assessment, and peer conferencing and evaluation. If students are guided toward a system of portfolios, restrictions of time and too many students are minimized. Use of partners, small groups, and self-directed tasks can go a long way in compensating for high student–teacher ratios. Obviously, the system needs to be well planned and organized.

As they collect portfolio data, teachers should report progress at regular intervals to parents, administrators, and others. They should gather information using multiple methods (e.g., observations, performance samples, testlike procedures). The following guidelines and strategies create the framework for a student portfolio system. In chapter 3 these aspects are developed in greater detail, specific to K-12 physical education programming.

Purposes and Types

Some general purposes for creating portfolios are to keep track of students' progress, have students assess their own accomplishments, determine the extent to which standards have been achieved, and help parents understand their child's effort and progress. Purposes specific to physical education might be to help students practice a healthy lifestyle, determine personal growth in an adventure-outdoor program, and communicate students' strengths and areas of needed improvement in gross and fine motor skills. Different types of portfolios can be used that correspond to the identified purpose. For example, some general types of portfolios could be focused on a particular project, growth or progress, achievement, or celebration.

Organization and Management

Strategies are needed for making decisions about portfolio construction (e.g., file folders inside an accordion file, pocket folders, hanging files, boxes), storage (e.g., plastic crates, file cabinets, shelves, drawers, covered cereal boxes, computer program), who should have access to the portfolios (e.g., peers, parents, other teachers), and how the portfolios will be set up and reviewed to avoid a large accumulation of materials.

Artifacts Selection

Usually, students' first items are *baseline* samples collected through preassessment. Selection criteria should reflect the purpose of the portfolios and possibly include something that shows improvement, something that was hard to do, and the best or most representative skill. Item variety provides students with selection options, thus enabling them to establish standards by which their work can be evaluated. In addition to student decisions, some teacher and administrator selections may become part of the total portfolio picture, including preinstruction inventories, journals, task sheets, student reflections, self-assessment checklists, projects, logs, independent study contracts, rating scales, videos, peer reviews, teachers' anecdotal statements, parent observations and comments, skill tests, and written tests.

Assessment and Communication

Portfolios should be assessed relative to student standards. Some teachers have abandoned conventional symbols (grades, scores) in favor of ways that describe, analyze, discuss, annotate, and confer. Other aspects of judging quality include reflection on portfolios (self, peers, parents), conferences (individual student-led, small group of peers, parents), and progress reports (rubrics, narrative statements, descriptive labels).

Professional Portfolios

To demonstrate teaching competence, teachers need creative ways to present themselves to others. For teacher candidates, these people might include education professors, field supervisors, cooperating teachers, school principals, or state departments of education personnel. For practicing teachers, these people might include teaching peers, department heads, subject matter supervisors, school principals, and parents. Regardless of whether teachers are beginners or have experience, they have a common goal of becoming effective professionals.

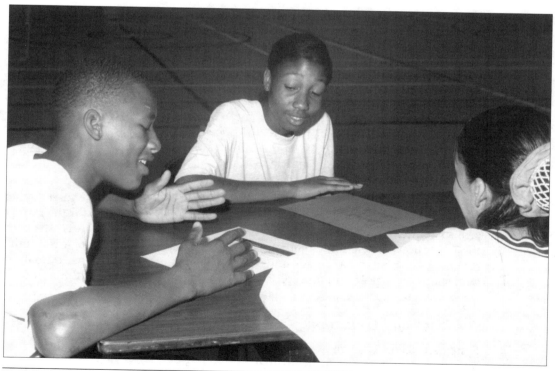

Portfolio feedback can be obtained through conferences with a small group of peers.

Most professionals want all of their knowledge and experiences to count when they are evaluated. Excellent teachers are characteristically similar in that they seek ongoing professional training; remain current about educational research; read professional writings; attend workshops; ask questions of others; refine their practice; and try out new ideas, reflect on the results, and discard or adapt the ideas. However, the same teachers often have difficulty demonstrating how these various experiences fit into their pattern of professional competency.

The professional portfolio can be a convincing, empowering tool that brings sense to a wealth of experiences. It is not just a scrapbook of teaching memorabilia, but an authentic representation of teaching performance. The professional portfolio is an organized, standards-based, goal-driven documentation of a teacher's professional growth and achieved competence in the complex act of teaching. Although it is a collection of documents, the professional portfolio is tangible evidence of the wide range of knowledge, dispositions, and skills that the teacher possesses as a growing professional. The strategies and guidelines that create the framework for a professional portfolio system follow. In chapters 2 and 4, these aspects are developed in greater detail for physical education teacher candidates and practicing teachers, respectively.

Purposes and Types

There are several different types of professional portfolios. The introductory portfolio introduces the teacher as a person and as a future or present teaching professional. It serves as a catalyst for self-reflection and continual sharing of ideas and insights. Although it is not technically a type of portfolio, the "working portfolio" is the ongoing systematic collection of professional exhibits that forms the basis for self-assessment and goal setting. The presentation portfolio offers artifacts that best reflect a teacher's achieved competence, individuality, and creativity as a professional physical educator. It is selective and streamlined. The employment portfolio focuses on artifacts to enhance job placement. The showcase portfolio includes a limited number of items to exhibit growth over time and to serve a particular professional purpose such as seeking national certification or state license renewal.

Organization and Management

Regardless of the type of portfolio, it should be organized around the set of standards being sought. Advanced organizers should be considered, depending on teaching status, that might serve as the primary goal of the portfolio, such as getting a job, contributing to the school's mission, creating a "symbol" of professional excellence, qualifying for merit, or achieving advanced certification. Storage options for working portfolios include a large file box, cardboard banker's boxes, several large notebooks divided into sections, file drawers in a cabinet, or a computer program. For presentation portfolios, notebooks, expanding files, folders, or portfolio satchels are common. Teachers assume responsibility for the storage of their own portfolios.

Artifacts Selection

Whenever possible, teachers should select exhibits that represent more than one standard. Each section of the portfolio should be labeled with an abbreviated title for the standard. For each artifact, a brief rationale should be included (e.g., reflection cover sheet). The type and goal of the portfolio will determine required and optional artifacts, including case studies, computer programs, lesson plans, thematic units, professional development plans, journals, meetings and workshops logs, peer critiques, projects, samples from student portfolios, student contracts, custom-made materials, and unit plans.

Feedback and Evaluation

Systematic feedback from peers or colleagues should be built into the portfolio process through reflection, conferences, or formal ratings. Portfolios should be evaluated relative to the established standards. Scoring rubrics are commonly used for assessing the whole portfolio in terms of completeness, creativity, diversity of selections, reflectiveness, and accuracy. Critical elements of each teacher standard should serve as the criteria against which individual artifacts are judged.

Technology Use in Portfolio Development

Technology advances were identified earlier as a major trend in education. The reality of our information-based, high-tech world has created an educational imperative to empower all students and teachers to function effectively with increasing change, information growth, and evolving technologies. Emerging technologies promise to have a significant impact on education. Another imperative is to keep abreast of the ever-changing landscape of technology and its uses in physical education, including student portfolios and professional portfolios for teacher candidates and practicing teachers.

Information in this section is generally applicable to the development of portfolio systems for teacher candidates in physical education teacher education (PETE) programs, K-12 students in physical education, and practicing physical education teachers. These systems are developed in chapters 2, 3, and 4, respectively. The information presented here is referenced in each chapter, as appropriate, where additional technology information is provided, specific to the intended user. Also, templates are available on the accompanying CD-ROM for creating electronic-based portfolios for teacher candidates, K-12 students, and practicing teachers.

Electronic-Based Portfolios

The terms *electronic portfolio* or *e-portfolio* are commonly used to describe a type of portfolio. However, because all types of portfolios (e.g., thematic, achievement, integrated, showcase, employment) can be constructed, stored, and managed electronically, the term *electronic-based portfolios* is used in comparison to commonly used paper-based portfolios. The distinctions between these two types of portfolios are clarified throughout the book.

Using technology for portfolio development enhances every aspect of portfolios including assembly, management, storage, reflection, self-reliance, goal setting, record keeping, self-assessment, communication, and feedback and assessment. Moving from paper-based portfolios to electronic-based portfolios maximizes efficiency, production, and quality. However, the use of electronic-based portfolios does require additional planning and certain hardware and software. At a minimum, one computer is required for input and storage along with software (see the software section on page 41) to assist with the organization of the material. In school settings, for example, in which students have access to computers only during class time, computers should be available for 10 percent of the class. In this case, students could rotate through a circuit that includes a computer station. Ideally, each student would have access to a computer during and after class. Although this may seem impossible, some schools provide every student with a notebook (laptop) or handheld computer.

Advantages

An electronic-based portfolio is simply an extension of a paper-based portfolio. It includes all the components of a paper-based portfolio, but in a digital format. Any original paper-based documents must be converted to digital formats, typically by scanning materials or keying the information into word processing software or a database. An electronic-based portfolio can take the form of any type of portfolio. Typically, each portfolio "author" would have an electronic storage device (e.g., folder on a local hard drive or server) that contains the portfolio. Electronic-based portfolios offer much more versatility and efficiency in documenting authentic learning and have several distinct advantages.

Storage

Electronic-based portfolios allow for the storage of large amounts of data in a small package. The information can be stored on a network or storage medium compared to the storage of paper-based portfolios in hanging files, boxes, plastic crates, or other kinds of containers. Access is an important aspect of storing portfolios of any kind. *Confidentiality and privacy must be protected.* Some folders and files on hard drives, for example, may be designated as public, whereas others are private. Password codes can be used for this purpose. Guidelines should be established from the beginning and strictly enforced thereafter by both teachers and students.

Media Variety

Paper-based portfolios are limited to text, hard copies of pictures, and videotapes, whereas electronic-based portfolios can store graphics, video clips, audio clips, and multimedia projects. For example, video is ideal for documenting growth in physical education, but it can be cumbersome to store videotapes and time consuming to access particular episodes. Electronic-based portfolios provide for easy storage of digital video clips that allow for quick access to any point in the clip.

Backup

Photocopying the contents of a folder or box along with reproducing videotapes is often impractical and time consuming, not to mention space consuming. However, making one or more copies of an entire electronic-based portfolio might take only seconds and it results in an exact duplicate in terms of both content and organization. With technology, the need to back up (copy) work cannot be overemphasized. This topic of backup is discussed again in the later section on storage (see page 40).

Distribution

In addition to making copies of a portfolio for backup purposes, copies can be made on a compact disc (CD), for example, for distribution to parents, students, school personnel, and other appropriate people. Teachers and students may also post electronic-based portfolios on the Internet where they are easily accessible by teachers, other students, family members, or potential employers. Web-based portfolios represent another way to distribute or make portfolios more easily accessible.

Assembly, Management, and Assessment

The electronic-based portfolio allows for easier assembly and management, especially when dealing with a large amount of data. Hypertext links may be used to organize portfolios by linking standards to actual examples of students' work. Electronic-based portfolios may also be linked to electronic grade books so that teachers can assess portfolio work and have the score automatically recorded in a grade book.

Array of Learning

The sets of learning and teaching standards outlined previously will be the basis around which portfolios are organized for students, teacher candidates, and practicing teachers. Paper-based portfolios provide documentation of student achievement and teacher competency specific to physical education standards (i.e., NASPE content standards, NASPE beginning teacher standards, NBPTS standards). Electronic-based portfolios can also focus on learning and teaching standards, but have the added benefit of developing specific technology skills. Through the production of electronic-based portfolios, students and teachers display technology abilities such as the following:

- Transferring graphics and video images to a computer
- Using cameras, camcorders, and scanners
- Using software selected for organizing the portfolio
- Developing multimedia projects

The ISTE *National Educational Technology Standards for Students* (NETS-S) and the ISTE *National Educational Technology Standards for Teachers* (NETS-T) identify the technology skills that students, teacher candidates, and practicing teachers should know and be able to demonstrate (International Society for Technology in Education, 2000, 2002). The summary standards are listed here, but complete sets appear in table 3.3 (pages 151-152) for students, table 2.2 (page 67) for teacher candidates, and table 4.2 (page 245) for practicing teachers. Additional information is available at the ISTE Web site (www.iste.org).

Technology Standards for Students

1. Basic operations and concepts
2. Social, ethical, and human issues
3. Technology productivity tools
4. Technology communication tools
5. Technology research tools
6. Technology problem-solving and decision-making tools

Technology Standards for Teachers

1. Technology operations and concepts
2. Planning and designing learning environments and experiences
3. Teaching, learning, and the curriculum
4. Assessment and evaluation
5. Productivity and professional practice
6. Social, ethical, legal, and human issues

Hardware

At a minimum, a computer is required for electronic-based portfolios. In addition, equipment such as printers, scanners, digital cameras, digital camcorders, and microphones are desirable to derive the full benefits of technology in the production of portfolio systems for students and teachers. Information is needed about how to select each of these devices for use in the electronic-based portfolio process.

Computers

Computers are available in three sizes—desktop, notebook (2 to 10 pounds), and handheld. The term *desktop* refers to a stationary computer used at a desk or workstation. The advantages of the desktop computer are the number and variety of ports, the lower cost, and the amenities (e.g., large monitor). However, its lack of portability makes it the last choice for maintaining electronic-based portfolios.

Notebook computers are lightweight mobile alternatives to desktop computers. Although the number and variety of ports may be limited and the screen may be smaller; these computers are more ideal for electronic-based portfolio development in physical education settings (i.e., gymnasiums, outdoors) because of their portability and battery power. In addition, most notebook computers can be attached to a larger monitor for student and teacher use in the classroom or office. There are two choices for desktop and notebook operating systems—Macintosh and Windows®. When making this decision, consider the following questions (Mohnsen, 2004):

- Which platform is predominant at your site? It helps to stay consistent with other users at your school.

- Are the applications you want to use supported by Macintosh, Windows, or both? The applications and hardware must match. It is actually better to select your applications first and then match the hardware.

- Do you have a personal preference? Users tend to be more comfortable with the type of computer on which they learned.

On desktop and notebook computers, the ports provide access points for interfacing with peripherals. For example, the ethernet port connects to networks, the video port connects to external monitors and projection systems, and the sound port connects to external speakers. The other external devices connect through Universal Serial Bus (USB) and IEEE1394 (FireWire) ports. These ports are faster and can connect to digital cameras and camcorders for electronic-based portfolio use. The connection of a camcorder to a notebook computer USB port is shown in figure 1.2.

There are other considerations for selecting the appropriate desktop or notebook computers in support of electronic-based portfolios. Three important variables should be explored when purchasing a computer: speed, random access memory, and internal hard drive capacity.

- *Speed.* The speed of a new "minimum-level" computer (measured in mega- or gigahertz) will suffice to meet the needs of electronic-based portfolios, unless there are plans for video editing. Video editing is one component that requires the fastest computer possible.

- *Memory.* Random access memory (RAM) is where programs and data are stored temporarily when the computer is in use. Each program requires a certain amount of RAM (measured in mega- or gigabytes) to load and run. The amount of memory that an application needs is shown on its packaging. Probably, more than one program will be loaded at a time so that users can move quickly from program to program. Therefore, the computer will need to have enough RAM to collectively hold all the programs that are needed for use at one time. Additional RAM can be purchased and installed as needed, but it is more expensive than purchasing it with a new computer. As is the case with speed, working with video requires more RAM. A minimum of one gigabyte of RAM is recommended for electronic-based portfolio work.

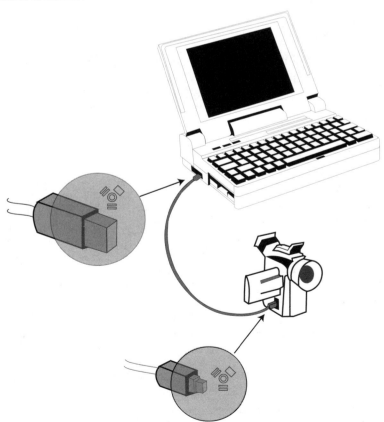

Figure 1.2   Computer ports provide access points for connecting external devices.

- *Hard drive capacity.* The primary storage device used by virtually all computer users is the internal hard drive (measured in gigabytes), regardless of whether it is a stand-alone computer or a server. This is the location where electronic-based portfolios are initially written for easy access, updating, and storage. The hard drive must hold all applications (see the software section on page 41) as well as all electronic-based portfolios. The amount of storage required for each program is identified on the packaging when purchasing the program. To determine the amount of storage required for each electronic-based portfolio, one must consider the size of the portfolio file plus any additional elements (files) such as video clips, audio clips, and multimedia projects. Secondary devices are used for archiving files, transferring data, and making backup copies (see the storage section on page 40). The following formula can be used to calculate the storage space needed for electronic-based portfolios:

Total storage space needed = application size[1] + (portfolio size[2] × number of portfolios) + (video clip size[3] × number of video clips) + (audio clip size[4] × number of audio clips) + (multimedia project size[5] × number of multimedia projects) + (images size[6] × number of images)

[1] For example, Microsoft Word® is approximately 15 MB (all applications list the hard drive requirements on the packaging).
[2] For example, Physical Education Portfolio (Bonnie's Fitware) is 50 MB.
[3] For example, a five-second video clip is 0.5 MB (depending on size and compression).
[4] For example, a 20-second audio clip is 0.5 MB (depending on quality and compression).
[5] For example, a 10-screen HyperStudio project is 1 MB.
[6] For example, a low-resolution (72 dpi) image is 200 k.

Handheld computers are battery operated, fit in one hand, and normally weigh less than a pound as shown in figure 1.3. A stylus is typically used for input, but minikeyboards are also available. The stylus allows for tapping on various buttons on the screen, tapping on a small keyboard image, or actually writing on the screen. Many handheld computers come with slots for memory cards, which allows for external storage. Some come with cameras capable of shooting still and video images. The handheld computer can be kept in a shirt or jacket or a protective case or fanny pack and is convenient for on-the-field use. In addition, the low price (as low as $100 per device) makes it reasonable for each student and teacher to have one.

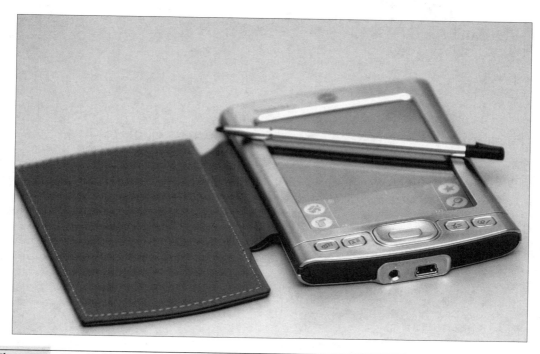

Figure 1.3 Handheld computers are practical for collecting student data.

Numerous operating systems are available for handheld computers. The two most popular systems are the Palm Operating System and the Windows Mobile Software for Pocket PC. Macintosh users should go with the Palm OS. Windows users may choose either operating system using the criteria for selecting a desktop or notebook operating system. Currently, there are more software applications for the Palm OS, but the most important variable when selecting a handheld computer is choosing one with a transflective display so that it can be used outdoors when collecting data for the electronic-based portfolio.

Memory works differently on handheld computers. The random access memory (RAM) and storage memory are the same on a handheld computer. Determining the amount of memory needed is much like determining the amount of RAM on a desktop computer: Add up the amount of memory needed by the programs that will be installed and allow room for data. Notice that the memory on a handheld computer is much less than that of a notebook or desktop computer because data are stored differently. Taking pictures or video clips using the handheld computer requires much more memory. This storage can be in the form of one or more external memory cards such as the ones shown in figure 1.4. Be sure to purchase the external memory card that works with your handheld computer.

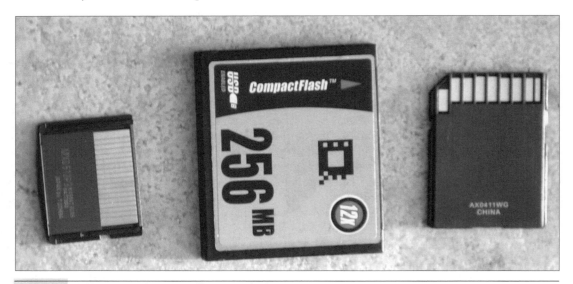

Figure 1.4   Memory cards are small storage devices.

Printers

Printers are only necessary for the electronic-based portfolio process if there are plans to print out the material. Although this is one way of distributing the information to students, parents, and teachers for assessment purposes, it is the least effective method. If all or part of an electronic-based portfolio is to be printed, either an ink jet or laser printer should be selected. An ink jet printer prints characters in the form of tiny dots clustered together. The quality of the printing is not quite laser-crisp, and the printed image can smear if the paper gets damp. However the cost and ability to print color make ink jet printers the first choice of many educators.

Laser printers create photocopy-quality documents. They can print any text, in any style, in any size, and at any angle—and everything looks perfect. PostScript laser printers can also print graphics that look phenomenal. Laser printers are the best choice for fast, cheap, top-quality text. Color laser printers are more expensive, both for the initial purchase and for the cost of the toner.

Scanners

Scanners work like copy machines, except that the image (graphic or text) is copied into a computer and stored as digital data. A scanner, as shown in figure 1.5, is needed if paper-based materials are to be included in an electronic-based portfolio. When looking for a scanner, consider the resolution (the fineness of the image). The lower the resolution is, the grainier the image will be. Resolutions of 1200 × 1200 dots per inch (dpi) or higher with 48-bit recognition are recommended. Scanners come in three basic types—flatbed, sheet-fed, and handheld. The flatbed is recommended for electronic-based portfolio work because it is the easiest to use and produces the sharpest image.

The scanning process is controlled by the application that comes with the scanner. The image to be scanned is placed on the bed of the scanner and a button is clicked in the application, typically labeled Preview, to begin the process. Once the preview scan has been completed, there is a prompt to designate a location in which to save the image. The image should be stored in the student's or teacher's folder or directly into an individual electronic-based portfolio.

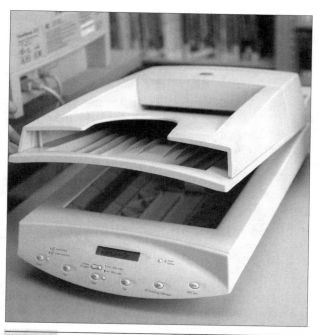

Figure 1.5 Scanners copy an image (graphic or text) into a computer as digital data.

The format in which to save the image must also be selected based on how the image will be used. For example, for posting on the Internet, users should choose .gif for graphics and .jpg for photos. For inclusion in authoring and presentation programs, .tif is the best choice. The process is completed by clicking on a button in the software program, typically labeled Scan. The basic types of graphics formats are as follows:

- .gif: Used for bitmapped pictures that are transmitted over the Internet
- .jpg: Used to create a standard for color or grayscale image compression; effective on continuous tone color spaces; best used on the Internet and for monitor presentations
- .png: Designed to replace the older and simpler gif format and to some extent the much more complex TIFF format
- .eps: Used for storing vector graphics and bitmapped artwork
- .wmf: Common vector graphics file format
- .tif: Very versatile; commonly used method for storing bitmapped or picture images in various resolutions, gray levels, and colors; created specifically for storing grayscale images; standard format for scanned images such as photos
- .pict: Oldest generic file format for Mac
- .bmp: Bitmap storage on the Windows platform

Digital Cameras

Digital cameras create digital images that are stored in digital files. If a "film-based" camera is used, a scanner is definitely needed to convert images to digital format. Resolution and storage are the important features to consider when selecting a digital camera for electronic-based portfolios. If images will not be printed, then the camera using the lowest number of megapixels is sufficient. Digital camera resolution determines the maximum size of a high-quality printed photo as follows:

- Two-megapixel cameras provide excellent 4 × 6- or 5 × 7-inch prints
- Three-megapixel cameras provide excellent 8 × 10-inch prints
- Four-megapixel cameras provide excellent 11×14-inch prints
- Five-megapixel cameras provide excellent 16 × 20-inch prints

Most digital cameras use memory cards for storage, including CompactFlash, MemoryStick, SecureDigital (SD), SmartMedia, and xD. It is important to have a memory card reader that matches the camera's memory card. Most card readers have a USB connection, although some have a FireWire connection. Also, be aware that most cameras come with cards that have a small amount of memory space (e.g., 64 MB). It will probably be desirable to purchase one or more additional memory cards. Some memory cards can hold one to two gigabytes of information. Following are some other considerations when selecting a digital camera:

- Ease of use
- An LCD (liquid crystal display) that can be viewed outside in the sun
- A glass lens instead of a plastic lens, because it will produce clearer images
- An optimal zoom lens of 3X for general-purpose use; ignore the digital zoom
- Nickel metal hydride (NiMH) or lithium ion (Li-Ion) batteries

Users new to photography will want a camera with programmed screen modes. These modes provide preset settings for specific situations, such as night exposure, landscape shots, portrait shots, close-ups, and athletic shots. This feature takes the guesswork out of proper camera exposure. Also, users should be sure to include a tripod with the purchase of either a digital camera or camcorder.

Once pictures have been taken, they need to be transferred to the computer. Because most cameras have memory cards, these can be ejected from the camera and inserted into an adapter for the computer. Then it becomes a simple matter of copying the images off the memory cards onto the computer's hard drive. As noted in the earlier software section, all students and teachers should have their own folders on the hard drive so that they can copy pictures into the appropriate folder.

Sometimes it is desirable to edit the pictures that have been taken. Adobe Photoshop is the premier program for editing pictures and drawings. However, it may be too expensive for some. Fortunately, most digital cameras come with digital imaging software (e.g., Adobe Photoshop Elements). Imaging software can greatly improve digital photos by changing colors, increasing sharpness, and replacing unwanted items in a photo. A few keystrokes can crop a photo, remove the red flash spots from someone's eyes, change the brightness, or switch a picture from left to right. The imaging software also can reduce the resolution and color depth for smaller images when posting to the Web. Finally, digital imaging software often can export or save to different formats, which may be necessary for importing into different programs.

Digital Camcorders

Digital camcorders offer superior audio and video quality while storing the data in a digital format. Digital camcorders come in two basic models. The first, the DV camcorder, uses cassettes (digital video cassettes) that are slightly larger than a matchbox. These cassette tapes hold up to 60 minutes of video and audio. These cameras typically come with an IEEE1394 (i.link/FireWire) connection that can send a digital signal (the video) directly to the computer. The second digital option is the DVD-CAM. It writes MPEG-2 video directly to DVD rewritable or recordable discs. These discs may then be played in the computer.

The normal shutter speed on a camcorder is 30 frames (60 fields) per second. However, cameras can be purchased with variable shutter speeds. High-speed shutters from 2,000 to 10,000 frames per second are great for shooting sporting events and analyzing motor skills because even small changes in movement can be captured. However, users should be sure there is extra light when using high-speed shutters, because exposure times are very small. Following are several other features to include when selecting a digital video camera:

- Lithium-ion or NiMH batteries
- LCD (liquid crystal display) that can be viewed outside in the sun
- Automatic white balance
- Automatic focus
- Electronic image stabilization feature
- Motorized, variable-speed optical zoom feature; ignore the digital zoom ratios
- Lux rating of three to five unless the gym or indoor facility has exceptionally poor lighting, in which case a lower lux rating is recommended

Combination cameras can take both still and video images. When selecting a combination camera, users should be sure that it provides true digital still frames because these images are of much higher quality when compared to camcorders with just a freeze frame feature. The freeze frame image is simply recorded on the tape. With true digital still frame capability, a JPEG or TIFF image is captured on a separate memory module, such as a MemoryStick. Many combination cameras, as well as some still cameras and some camcorders, have a burst or continuous shoot mode that allows the option of taking 30 shots at three frames per second (fps).

Once the video is recorded, the next step is to transfer the data to a file on the hard drive and store it in the respective student's or teacher's folder. Numerous video programs are available for capturing and editing. Adobe Premiere is the flagship program. However, programs that come with the operating system (e.g., Windows' MovieMaker, Macintosh's iMovie) allow for video transfer (capturing) as well as simple editing (e.g., cut out pieces, add transitions). Users should carefully follow the step-by-step instructions provided with these products.

If a digital camcorder is not accessible, digital video clips can still be created. A video capture device is necessary to convert the analog video into digital video. The input source for digitized video is any analog medium, such as an analog video camera or videocassette player. A cable connects the video source to the video capture device, which in turn is connected to the computer via a FireWire or USB cable. A second cable connects the audio port on the video source to the audio port on the computer. Software distributed with the video card controls the computer display and saving options.

Microphones

Most camcorders come with a built-in omnidirectional microphone. Although microphones that are built into the front of the camera are better than the ones on the top, neither provide optimal sound. This is especially true in gymnasiums and indoor swimming areas where there are echoes. The addition of a wireless camcorder microphone system, such as the one shown in figure 1.6, allows for cable-free audio recording at distances of up to 200 feet. There are three parts to the wireless microphone system: receiver, transmitter, and microphone. The receiver is mounted on the camcorder's accessory shoe and plugged into the microphone input jack. An earphone or headphone jack on the receiver lets the user monitor the input. A single directional lapel microphone, headset microphone, or handheld microphone is attached to the transmitter and used by the person who is being videotaped. An in-use indicator light tells the user when the transmitter and receiver are turned on and ready to go. In addition, a wireless microphone with multiple channels is recommended because, at times, two microphones may be used in the gymnasium, and one camera may pick up the other microphone unless they are on separate channels. Microphones also may be used without a video camera for the recording of audio only.

Audio digitizing is the process of converting a sound from analog to digital format so that it can be manipulated, saved, and available through electronic-based portfolios. Digitizing sound requires a sound source (e.g., CD, tape cassette), a microphone attached to the computer (audio card), or a line port so that a cable can connect the sound source to the computer. Video digitizing software can be used for digitizing sound. Sampling rates determine how often an analog audio signal is cut up to make a digital audio clip. The higher the number of samples per second (5 kHz, 7 kHz, 11 kHz, or 22 kHz), the more lifelike the digitized sound and the more memory it will require. Whenever possible, digitize sound at 22 kHz to maximize the quality. You can always reduce the sampling rate when you compress the sound for storage. Sound editing programs, such as Adobe Audition, allow for more sophisticated sound editing.

Storage

Computer internal hard drives serve as the primary storage device for electronic-based portfolios as well as other programs and data. However, be aware that data on hard drives are never permanent. All hard drives will crash (fail) eventually as a result of disk failure, static electricity, or other ambient factors, which is why it is important to back up data. Additional storage devices are available for maintaining and distributing electronic-based portfolios.

External Hard Drive

An external hard drive, like an internal hard drive, is a device that uses a magnetic medium to store large amounts of data. Although all hard drives will fail eventually, external hard drives are still the most reliable storage system because they are closed. They do not allow dirt to enter and harm the read/write mechanism that allows the user to read, add, or delete

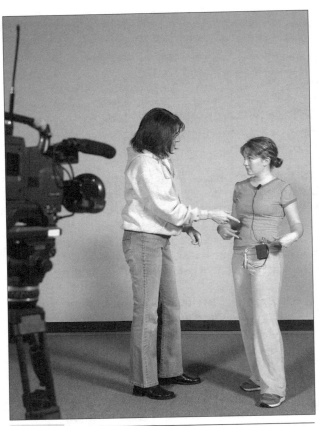

Figure 1.6 A wireless microphone system is needed for physical education settings.

information. This durability, along with size (measured in gigabytes) and speed options, makes an external hard drive a good choice for backing up material. External hard drives are available in capacities up to 500 gigabytes, and this capacity will continue to increase. Using FireWire 800, transfer rates of approximately 80 megabytes per second are available using external hard drives.

CDs

Another storage device is the optical disc that stores and retrieves data using laser technology. Optical discs can hold hundreds of megabytes of data. There are two types of compact discs—compact disc-recordable (CD-R) and compact disc-rewritable (CD-RW). CD-R discs let the user record information on the compact disc. However, once recorded, it cannot be erased. CD-RW discs let the user record over and over again on the compact disc. To use CD-RWs, the CD drive must be designed to write to the RW format. Historically, special software was necessary to write to any CD. However, Windows XP and Macintosh OSX come with the capability of copying files to a CD. Because virtually every computer now comes with a CD drive, this is an excellent option for distributing electronic-based portfolios.

USB Memory Devices

USB memory devices are small and come in a variety of shapes as shown in figure 1.7. They connect directly to the USB port that is available on most computers. Storage capacity for these devices has reached two gigabytes. A USB memory device, sometimes referred to as a "thumb drive," works much like a floppy disk. Files are simply dragged onto the device's icon for easy copying. These attributes make for a convenient and fast method for backing up and transporting data.

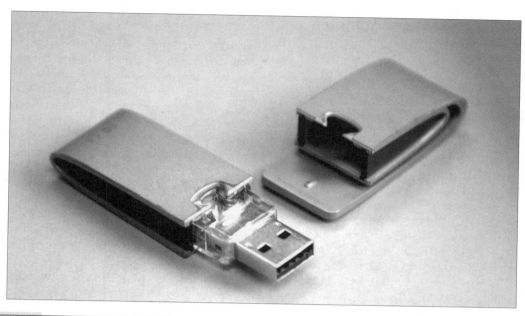

Figure 1.7 USB memory devices are convenient for backing up and transporting data.

Software

Once decisions are made regarding hardware and storage equipment, software is needed to assist with the organization and management of electronic-based portfolios. Options to consider include word processing software, presentation software, Web development software, authoring software, and database software. Each option should be explored carefully so that informed decisions can be made. Organizational ideas for setting up and managing electronic-based portfolios should also be considered.

Word Processing

Word processing allows the computer to replace the typewriter. Anything that could be accomplished previously using a typewriter can now be done on a computer. Word processing applications such as Microsoft Word allow the user to set margins, spacing, justification, tabs, headers, footers, font size and style, and character spacing for the entire document or to change the specifications for every word, line, or paragraph. Pictures and images also may be embedded in documents. These features greatly facilitate the creating of electronic-based portfolio files.

Each file in a word processing system, for example, could contain one assessment piece (e.g., fitness plan, motor skill rubric). A folder must be created for each student, normally on a hard drive or disc. It is best to name the folder using the student's name. Each file should contain the name of the physical education standard being met by the material contained in the file (e.g., standard1, stand1, s1, motor) and the name of the assignment. For example, the file that contains the fitness plan for standard 4 could be named s4fitplan. Information is typed or scanned into the document, along with images if appropriate.

The advantage of using word processing programs is that they are readily available at home and school and most students know how to use them. In addition, because each file simply represents an assignment, there is no need to create a template for the entire portfolio. The disadvantages of using word processing are (1) the inability to create links between the files, (2) the need to find each folder and open each file to grade its content, and (3) its limitation to text and still images.

Presentation Software

The market for presentation applications has been dominated by PowerPoint (Microsoft). Apple has released presentation software called Keynote that it hopes will compete with PowerPoint. Presentation software allows for the easy creation of slide shows. It can also be used to create electronic-based portfolios. Advantages of using presentation software, like word processing software, are that it is readily available at most school sites and most students and teachers know how to use it. Minimum lag time should be needed while students get familiar with the program. In addition, presentation software can store video clips and audio clips. It also has the feature of buttons that allow linking between screens and external documents. One disadvantage is that teachers or reviewers need to find the folder for each student and open the file in order to grade it. Also, a template needs to be created for the layout, at least for younger users, so that they know where information should be stored.

An example of a template for PowerPoint appears in figure 1.8. The title screen notes the user's name, and a table of contents screen lists the physical education content standards with links to the list of assessment pieces for each standard. These assessment listings then link to specific assessment artifacts. The actual assessment pieces must either fit on one screen or buttons must be created linking one screen to the next for the duration of the assessment piece. In addition, all video clips, audio clips, or multimedia projects must be copied into the student's or teacher's folder along with the PowerPoint file.

The CD-ROM that accompanies this text contains portfolio builders that are developed in PowerPoint. The three templates—one each for teacher candidates, K-12 students, and practicing teachers—are organized around a set of appropriate standards. Buttons, or links, have been created to access slides and files that contain, for example, documents, spreadsheets, photos, and video clips. Creating buttons or links in PowerPoint involves the following steps:

Linking to Slides

1. Select Slide Show from the menu bar, then Action Buttons.
2. Select the preferred button, drag the button to the desired location on the slide, and click Action Settings.
3. Select Hyperlink to: and select the slide that you want to link to from the menu.
4. Click OK.

Linking to External Documents

1. Select Slide Show from the menu bar, then Action Buttons.
2. Select the preferred button, drag the button to the desired location on the slide, and click Action Settings.
3. Select Hyperlink to: and select Other File.
4. Browse to the slide you want to link and click OK.

Web Development Software

Certain types of portfolios for students, teacher candidates, and practicing teachers make Web-based formats desirable. These portfolios are discussed in the following chapters. For example, selected pages from a Web-based portfolio for teacher candidates are shown in figure 2.2 (page 69).

Web development software includes programs such as DreamWeaver (Macromedia), GoLive (Adobe), FrontPage (Microsoft), and Composer (Netscape). These programs make it very easy to create Web pages. Each program functions much like a word processing program. However, the output is in the form of a code known as html (hypertext markup language) that allows a variety of Internet users, regardless of their operating systems, to view Web pages. Web development programs also allow the user to embed links to other Web pages, as well as sounds, pictures, and video clips. This makes the software also ideal for organizing and accessing Web-based portfolios.

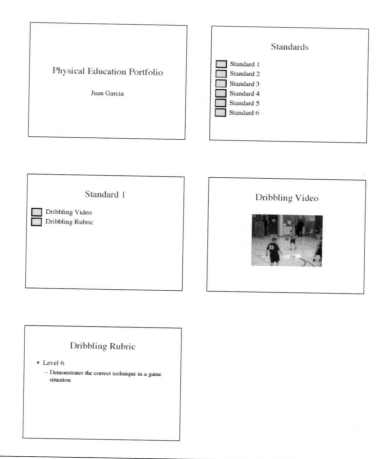

Figure 1.8 Example of a template for PowerPoint.
Courtesy of Bonnie S. Mohnsen, Bonnie's Fitware Inc., Cerritos, CA; www.pesoftware.com.

Web development software has several advantages and some disadvantages.

Advantages

- Availability at most schools
- Accessibility for viewing by anyone, any time, once it is loaded onto an Internet server
- Access for the user to update pages at anytime from anywhere
- Ability to include images, video clips, and audio clips
- Ability to link each Web page to other pages

Disadvantages

- Need to store images, video clips, and audio clips separate from the Web pages in the student's or teacher's folder
- Need to create separate Web pages for each element (e.g., each standard, if not each artifact)
- Difficult to include multimedia projects
- Web site must be accessed for each student or teacher and then linked to individual pages to view the entire Web-based portfolio or specific items

Using Web development software to create Web-based portfolios is best done by those who know how to create Web pages, including how to upload files; insert images, video, and audio; and link pages. There are two options for organizing Web pages into portfolios:

1. Create a home page with links to a separate page for each portfolio element (e.g., standard, artifact, photo or video clip gallery). On a "standard" Web page, for example, include all the artifacts that align with the standard. Each artifact can be marked with an anchor. Then, using a table of contents at the top of each standard's Web page, users can quickly jump to each individual assignment.

2. Create a home page with links to a separate page for each portfolio element (e.g., standard, artifact, photo or video clip gallery). On the Standards Web page, for example, include a list of all the related artifacts and links to each artifact's Web page. This means that there is a separate Web page for each artifact.

Regardless of the approach taken, users should be sure to include links back to the organizing element (e.g., standards, home page). For example, the student portfolio home page shown in figure 1.9 includes links to the six NASPE content standards.

Following are instructions for linking one page to another and for linking to specific locations on the page. The instructions are provided for Netscape Composer because it is a free program. However, the instructions are similar for all Web development programs.

Linking to Other Pages

1. Highlight the word or image that will serve as the link.

2. Select the link icon in the menu bar.

3. Type in the Web address for the linked page.

4. Click OK.

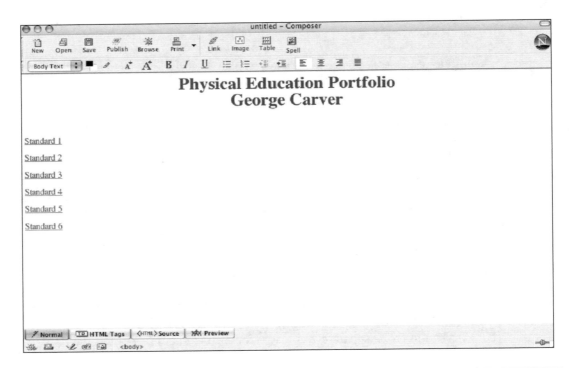

Figure 1.9 Home page for a Web-based portfolio organized around physical education content standards.

Courtesy of Bonnie S. Mohnsen, Bonnie's Fitware Inc., Cerritos, CA; www.pesoftware.com.

Linking to Specific Locations on a Page

This is a two-step process. First, an anchor needs to be placed on the page containing the link. Then, a link needs to be created that directs the user to the anchor.

1. Create the anchor.
   a. Go to the point in the page where the anchor should be placed.
   b. Select Insert-Named anchor; type a name for the anchor (e.g., first).
2. Link to the anchor.
   a. Highlight the word or image that will serve as the link.
   b. Select the link icon in the menu bar.
   c. Type in the Web address for the linked page.
   d. After the Web address, add the symbol # followed by the name of the anchor (e.g., www.pesoftware.com/index.html#first).
   e. Click OK.

Multimedia Authoring Software

Authoring software such as HyperStudio (Knowledge Adventure) and Director (Macromedia) brings together in one package text, still images, animation, sound, analog video, and digital video. Like Web development software, authoring software uses buttons ("hot spots") or links that let the user create a variety of pathways (known as hypermedia) to move through the program. Buttons are most commonly used to link one screen to another, but they can provide for other actions as well. The action is determined by the designer and might include playing sounds, displaying images, playing video clips, or displaying animations—almost anything imaginable. These programs are typically used to create multimedia projects, but they may also be used to organize electronic-based and Web-based portfolios.

Of the many multimedia authoring software programs, only HyperStudio allows the user to create and edit text, sound, video, graphics, digital images from a camera, and animations from within the program. Without this capability, users must purchase additional software and undergo additional training. Templates can be designed within HyperStudio to structure the use of portfolios including tasks, rubrics, reflection, and assessment components. This allows users to customize the portfolio to meet targeted standards as well as the specific needs of their classrooms or programs. Students or teachers then need only complete the individual screens. The basic format, similar to the second option for Web development software, is to create one screen for the title page and one screen for listing, for example, all the standards with links to individual screens for each standard, then with links to screens for each supporting artifact. Multimedia authoring software has several advantages and some disadvantages.

Advantages

- Images, video clips, and audio clips can be stored as part of the program.
- Screens can be linked (e.g., creating relationships between standards and artifacts).
- Easily links to complete multimedia projects.

Disadvantages

- Cannot be viewed by others without special software.
- Must access each student's or teacher's portfolio to view the entire portfolio or specific artifacts.

Database Programs

Database software is used to organize information such as lockers, events, student records, schedules, and anything else that would normally be maintained on file cards or in folders. Popular databases include Microsoft Access and FileMaker Pro along with FileMaker Mobile, HanDBase and ThinkDB for the Palm OS. The key benefits of a database are to reduce data redundancy, save time locating and updating information, and allow for comparisons of information across files. Databases also allow for the creation of a wide variety of reports (Mohnsen, 2004). The information in this section considers the use of FileMaker Pro. The following general abilities of databases also apply to their use as an electronic-based portfolio. Users of database programs are able to

- store all student or teacher portfolios in one file;
- input data on a handheld computer;
- quickly view all elements for one student or teacher, or one artifact for all students or teachers;
- quickly interface the grades given to a portfolio to a grading program;
- easily post material on the Internet;
- store all types of data (e.g., video clips, audio clips, pdf documents, text, graphics) as well as links to multimedia projects; and
- link one layout to another so that one layout can include a list of all the elements (e.g., standards) with buttons taking the user to a layout with artifacts.

A database consists of fields (spaces in which to insert information) and records (complete sets of fields). The consistency of fields across all records is what allows databases to quickly arrange (sort) records by one or more fields. The record selection feature permits the user to specify which records to view. For example, a teacher can view all records (student portfolios) in which a particular artifact has not been assessed. Then, the teacher can select the layout in which the artifact is visible and quickly view and assess the artifact, and then move on to the next student. An example is shown in figure 1.10.

The steps in creating links to layouts in FileMaker Pro are as follows:

1. Select View in the menu bar and choose Layout.
2. Select text or image.
3. Select Format in the menu bar and choose Button.
4. Select Navigation, go to Layout, and then select the layout for linking.

Technology Resources

The growing field of technology changes daily in terms of products and capabilities. Obviously, the need to update information and remain current is important to designing and maintaining student and teacher portfolio systems. The following Web sites should be particularly helpful in meeting this need. Suggested readings are also provided.

Web Sites

National Educational Technology Standards: http://cnets.iste.org

International Society for Technology in Education: www.iste.org

Bonnie's Fitware Inc.: www.pesoftware.com

Electronic portfolios: http://eduscapes.com/tap/topic82.htm

Web portfolios: www.webportfolio.info

Electronic portfolio resources: www.uvm.edu/~jmorris/portresources.html

Electronic Portfolios.com: http://electronicportfolios.com

Electronic portfolios plus mentoring: www.nebo.edu/e_portfolio

Creating electronic portfolios: www.hyperstudio.com/showcase/portfolio.html

Gateway to Professional and Student Portfolios

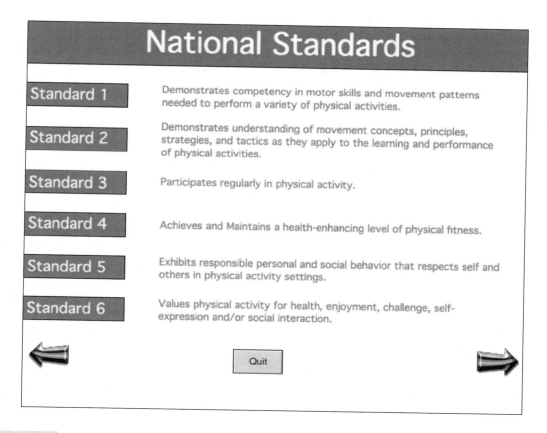

Figure 1.10 This database provides links to standards data that can be used as portfolio artifacts.

Courtesy of Bonnie S. Mohnsen, Bonnie's Fitware Inc., Cerritos, CA; www.pesoftware.com.

Suggested Readings

Barrett, H. (1998). Strategic questions: What to consider when planning for electronic portfolios. *Learning and Leading with Technology, 26* (2), 6-13.

Barrett, H. (2000). Create your own electronic portfolio. *Learning and Leading with Technology, 27* (7), 14-21.

Horton, M.L. (2004). Digital portfolios in physical education teacher preparation. *Journal of Physical Education & Recreation, 75* (9), 35-38.

McKinney, M. (1998). Preservice teachers' electronic portfolios: Integrating technology, self-assessment, and reflection. *Teacher Education Quarterly, 25* (1), 85-103.

Mitchell, M., & McKethan, R. (2003). *Integrating technology and pedagogy in physical education.* Cerritos, CA: Bonnie's Fitware Inc.

Mitchell, M., McKethan, R., & Mohnsen, B.S. (2004). *Integrating technology and physical education.* Cerritos, CA: Bonnie's Fitware Inc.

Mohnsen, B.S. (2004). *Using technology in physical education* (4th ed.). Cerritos, CA: Bonnie's Fitware Inc.

Wiedmer, L.T. (1998). Digital portfolios: Capturing and demonstrating skills and levels of performance. *Phi Delta Kappan, 79* (8), 586-589.

Summary

Have you achieved the expected outcomes (see page 2) for this chapter? You should have acquired the foundation needed for developing professional and student portfolios in physical education. The contemporary contexts for educational change are grouped within two broad dimensions. One dimension, the redesign of learning and teaching, focuses on what students and teachers should know and be able to do, high-stakes testing for students and teachers, and school accountability. The other dimension involves the impact of some highly significant, complex trends and issues in education (i.e., culturally responsive teaching, student diversity, inclusive education, developmentally appropriate practices, emphasis on standards, quality assessment, and advances in technology).

The national standards movement has resulted in standards-based education practices that are guided by widely accepted sets of learning and teaching standards. Content standards and corresponding student expectations serve as the framework for K-12 physical education programs, and the knowledge, skills, and dispositions essential for effective teaching in physical education are organized in a standards-based format for teacher candidates and practicing teachers. To apply the standards of assessment quality, teachers must develop assessment literacy. Assessment-literate teachers are able to determine what to assess (learning targets) and how to assess (methods), and then to match the proper method of assessment with the intended target. Formative assessment, in the context of assessment *for* learning, means that students are involved in their own assessment through goal setting, record keeping, and communication. Student-involved assessment includes anything that helps students understand learning targets, engage in self-assessment, watch themselves grow, talk about their learning growth, and plan next steps for learning. In addition, authentic assessment applied to students and teachers is centered on real-life work samples and actual classroom performance, respectively. Such approaches focus on more naturalistic, performance-based situations.

Portfolios are justified as devices for collecting evidence and communicating about student learning and teaching competence. Although a portfolio can be assessed as a whole, its true purpose is to enrich the ability to learn, the desire to learn, and the learning itself. Thus, portfolios are particularly useful in keeping track of and celebrating standards-based learning and creating assessment *for* learning and authentic assessment.

Technology plays an important role in the development and implementation of portfolio systems for teacher candidates, K-12 students, and practicing teachers. Portfolio construction, management, storage, and communication are enhanced significantly through electronic-based and Web-based protocols.

Professional Portfolios for Teacher Candidates

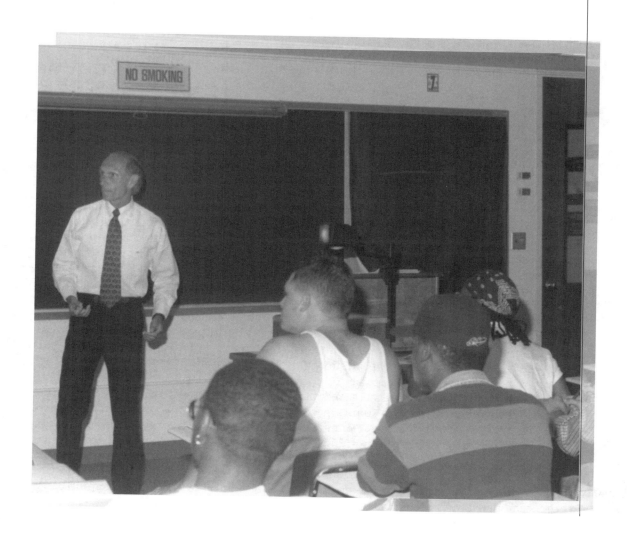

The public demand for school and teacher accountability has never been greater; even though the art and science of teaching is so complex, effective teaching is difficult to define. However, there is general agreement about what teacher candidates should know and be able to do. Once acquired and verified, presumably, these beginning teacher standards lead to the ultimate criterion of success—student achievement. Licensure and accreditation standards emphasize these essential knowledge, skills, and dispositions (attitudes and values), and performance assessment is now a mandate for teacher education programs. Therefore, a comprehensive, standards-based system is needed to document the growth and achievement of prospective teachers. A transcript of grades, the number of hours spent in field experiences, and scores on written exams seem woefully inadequate as measures of teaching ability. Teacher candidates need more authentic, broad-based ways to show their professional competence. So, what is the best way to verify the achievement of professional education outcomes?

EXPECTED OUTCOMES

This chapter will help teacher candidates in physical education and those who educate them develop professional portfolios and systems for professional portfolios, respectively. After reading this chapter, you will be able to do the following:

1. Determine the uses of portfolios based on the various purposes and types of professional portfolios for teacher candidates.
2. Use standards for beginning physical education teachers as the organizing framework for professional portfolios.
3. Decide what implementation strategy and processes for involvement will be used for a physical education teacher education (PETE) portfolio system.
4. Develop portfolio assembly, management, and storage options including the use of technology.
5. Establish guidelines for selecting artifacts for the teacher candidate portfolio.
6. Design assessment tools and procedures for the formative and summative review of professional portfolios for teacher candidates.

Teacher education programs face a dilemma in this era of standards-based assessment. Fully competent graduates are confronted with a highly competitive job market, and they must convey to others the knowledge and skills acquired in something as complex as teaching. This chapter proposes a scheme—the teacher candidate professional portfolio—that can integrate, interrelate, and communicate the knowledge and skills acquired in a physical education teacher education (PETE) program.

First, to help determine the uses of portfolios, various purposes and types of portfolios are outlined. Then, standards are recommended as the basis for organizing these portfolios. Alternative sets of standards are presented including general standards for teachers and specific standards for physical education. In addition, processes for implementation are provided that usually involves some combination of advisers, course instructors, committees, and mentors representing program phases. Next, for each type of portfolio, guidelines in portfolio assembly and structure are offered. Management techniques, storage options, and practical considerations for maintaining portfolios electronically and for creating Web-based portfolios are provided. In addition, training concerns are identified along with some aspects of assessment including reflection, self-assessment, presentations, and conferences. Required and optional artifacts for the different types of portfolios are also suggested. Lastly, portfolio evaluation tools and procedures that serve formative and summative purposes are described and illustrated. To synthesize this information, a sample PETE portfolio system is provided at the end of the chapter. In addition, the CD-ROM accompanying the book provides a template (portfolio builder) to create an electronic-based teacher candidate professional portfolio.

Designing an integrated, professional portfolio system for teacher candidates is a complex process involving many decisions. The following nine steps, which are also identified throughout the chapter, can help with this process (Melograno, 1999):

1. Determine the primary and secondary purposes of the teacher candidate portfolio.
2. Select the types of teacher candidate portfolios that will be included in the system.
3. Identify the standards around which the teacher candidate portfolio will be organized.
4. Choose an implementation strategy that matches the advising philosophy and commitment of the PETE program.
5. Determine how various processes of involvement will be included in the teacher candidate portfolio system.
6. Identify options for organizing, maintaining, and storing the teacher candidate portfolio.
7. Decide *what, how, who,* and *when* relative to the selection of required and optional artifacts for the teacher candidate portfolio.
8. Develop checkpoints and feedback procedures that will provide a formative review of the teacher candidate portfolio.
9. Establish the approaches to be used for conducting a summative review of the teacher candidate portfolio.

Purposes and Types of PETE Portfolios

Any successful program of study includes a systematic way to determine the progress of individual students and the effect of the program across the broad spectrum of student development. Before introducing portfolios into an evaluation system, educators should determine the primary and secondary purposes of portfolios. Some hard questions need to be answered. Why involve teacher candidates in the ongoing process of gathering artifacts of their work throughout a semester, year, or entire teacher education program? How are the portfolios going to be used? What is the real purpose of this data collection and communication tool? What are the potential uses, overuses, and abuses of portfolios for assessment purposes and beyond (Burke, Fogarty, & Belgrad, 2001)?

Purposes of Portfolios

Imagine the difficulty of selecting items for a portfolio with no sense of what the portfolio is to represent. The first consideration in any portfolio system is its purpose (step 1 of the portfolio-designing process). There needs to be a reason for creating portfolios. The professional portfolio is a flexible and powerful tool that can serve multiple purposes. The primary purpose of the portfolio developed by teacher candidates is to verify the wide range of knowledge, skills, and dispositions acquired through coursework, clinical and field experiences, community involvements, and student teaching. This primary purpose is supported by the following secondary purposes:

- *To help teachers grow professionally.* Teacher candidates can learn to assess their own progress as teachers. When they review and reflect on their accomplishments, they engage in a self-assessment process that fosters lifelong professional development. Strengths and weaknesses are revealed so that teacher candidates can monitor their own growth. They also learn that this cumulative process is just as valuable as the product (exhibits and work samples).

- *To provide for program review.* Teacher education faculty can keep track of individual teacher development and determine the overall success of their teacher training program. Feedback is needed about the goals and objectives of the teacher education program. Gathering various work samples in a sequential manner yields valuable information that serves as the basis for making curriculum improvement decisions.

- *To satisfy licensing and accreditation requirements.* Compelling evidence of teacher competence is becoming more necessary to meet licensing and accreditation requirements. The authentic, broad-based, and impartial assessments found in a professional portfolio demonstrate teacher candidates' range of abilities and knowledge.

- *To enhance employment opportunities.* Employers require that prospective teachers demonstrate teaching competence in concrete ways. The information derived from actual exhibits and work samples can be used during the job interview process, in which reviews by superintendents, supervisors, principals, department heads, teachers, and even school board members are likely.

Types of Portfolios

Once the primary and secondary purposes for implementing a teacher candidate professional portfolio system are determined, then consideration should be given to the type of portfolio that can best achieve these purposes (step 2 of the portfolio-designing process). The different types (i.e., introductory, presentation, employment) can be used in any combination to fulfill the purposes of the portfolio. Additional information about each type is covered again in subsequent sections of this chapter that deal with portfolio assembly, management, and storage; selection of portfolio items; and assessment of the portfolio. Before the types of portfolios are described, it is necessary to clarify some misconceptions.

- *Working portfolio.* The so-called "working portfolio" is not really a portfolio. It is a working repository or holding folder for selected work samples compiled from courses and evidence (exhibits) of school and community activities. This process is a continual "work in progress" and serves as the repository for everything associated with the standards underlying the PETE program. The collection of artifacts and work products forms the framework for reflection, self-assessment, and goal setting, and it provides all possible artifacts from which to make selections for the other types of portfolios. The teacher candidate manages and keeps this "working repository"—the term used throughout this book. The working repository also provides a basis for formative review throughout the PETE program at planned intervals.

- *Electronic portfolio.* Another misconception arises from the terms *electronic portfolio* or *e-portfolio*. Because each type of portfolio can be constructed, managed, and stored electronically, including on the Internet, "electronic portfolios" are not included as a type of portfolio. Technological advances have made electronic management, storage, and portfolio-related processes a reality. However, if portfolios are simply software databases—storage for pictures, sound, or words—they are really no different from hanging files or containers. The content of portfolios and the process of creating them are the most important concerns. Multimedia writing tools, scanners, digital cameras, and recordable CD-ROM drives have all helped in the creation of true portfolios. Self-reflection, data sharing, and assessment can be built in. Information about and guidelines for constructing, managing, and storing portfolios electronically, and uploading them to the Web, are covered later in this chapter (pages 64-69).

Introductory Portfolio

The introductory portfolio presents the individual as a person and as a future teaching professional in physical education. It serves as a catalyst for self-reflection and continual sharing of ideas and insights throughout the PETE program. Introductory portfolios help teacher candidates begin the process of collecting, analyzing, and communicating about their knowledge and performance skills as well as their attitudes and values.

Presentation Portfolio

The presentation portfolio includes samples of work that best reflect the teacher candidate's achieved competence, individuality, and creativity as a professional physical educator. The presentation portfolio should be selective and streamlined. It is used during the PETE program to satisfy different purposes (e.g., field course requirement, clinical experiences, posterlike show-cases, student-led conferences) and audiences (e.g., faculty members, mentors, teachers, peers). In addition, depending on how and when it is used, it may help in the formative evaluation process. Portfolio materials and artifacts should be converted to electronic formats to facilitate organization, maintenance, storage, and review.

Employment Portfolio

The employment portfolio provides a rich overview of the personality and abilities of the teacher candidate. It focuses on selected artifacts to enhance job placement, and it may be customized to a particular school. After streamlining and adding materials of special interest to prospective employers, the job seeker should present this portfolio as part of the job inquiry, application, and interview process. At this point, the portfolio should be produced electronically, preferably in a Web-based version. The employment portfolio offers a basis for summative evaluation.

Organization Around Standards

Regardless of purpose or type, professional portfolios need an organizational scheme that is clear and meaningful. The art and science of teaching is complex and cannot be easily reduced to a universal set of behavioral categories. Yet the goals, competencies, and outcome statements established by professional organizations attempt to determine the knowledge, skills, and dispositions that define excellent teachers. Dispositions refer to one's fundamental attitudes, beliefs, and assumptions about teaching and learning. Charting and demonstrating professional competence through a portfolio requires some system of organization. Therefore, everything collected for teacher candidate professional portfolios—except possibly the introductory portfolio—should be organized around the chosen standards (step 3 of the portfolio-designing process). Some sources of standards are provided in the following sections.

General Standards

Portfolios could be organized around the knowledge, performance abilities, competencies, or outcomes available through professional societies, state departments of education, and college teacher education programs. For example, the INTASC standards (see pages 14-15 in chapter 1), developed by a consortium of state and professional organizations, and the *Praxis* (Educational Testing Service, 1992) teaching domains and supporting knowledge and skills criteria (see page 27) are generally applicable for teachers of all disciplines and all levels. Although the core propositions and supporting standards of the National Board for Professional Teaching Standards (see table 1.3 on page 18) were developed for experienced teachers, they could also serve as the basis for organizing the teacher candidate portfolio.

PETE Program Standards

The teacher education curriculum models developed for accreditation purposes are useful frameworks. Teacher candidate portfolios could be organized logically around the set of themes, goals, and competencies normally contained in these models. To illustrate, the teacher education program at Cleveland State University was designed to produce beginning teachers who can demonstrate certain knowledge and skills within the theme, "The teacher as a responsive, reflective professional—a partner in learning" (Cleveland State University College of Education and Human Services, 2005). Specific outcome statements reflect the professional, instructive, and managerial skills that teachers are expected to demonstrate. These outcomes were also used to design the professional portfolio system and to help teacher candidates organize their portfolios. The 12 outcomes (standards) are applied to the PETE program as described in table 2.1.

Table 2.1 PETE Program Standards

PHYSICAL EDUCATION TEACHER AS A RESPONSIVE, REFLECTIVE PROFESSIONAL—A PARTNER IN LEARNING	
Standards	**Descriptions**
1. Personal philosophy	The teacher candidate articulates a personal philosophy of physical education, teaching, and learning that is grounded in theory and practice.
2. Social foundations	The teacher candidate possesses knowledge and understanding of the social, political, and economic factors that influence education in general and physical education, and shape the world in which we live.
3. Knowledge of subject matter and inquiry	The teacher candidate understands physical education content, disciplinary concepts, and tools of inquiry related to the development of a physically educated person.
4. Knowledge of development and learning	The teacher candidate understands how individuals learn and develop and that students enter the learning setting with prior experiences that give meaning to the construction of new skills and knowledge.
5. Diversity	The teacher candidate understands how individuals differ in their backgrounds and approaches to learning and incorporates and accounts for such diversity in teaching and learning.
6. Learning environment	The teacher candidate uses an understanding of individual and group motivation to promote positive social interaction, active engagement in learning, and self-motivation.
7. Communication	The teacher candidate uses knowledge of effective verbal, nonverbal, and media communication techniques to foster inquiry, collaboration, and engagement in learning environments.
8. Instructional strategies	The teacher candidate plans and implements a variety of developmentally appropriate instructional strategies to develop performance skills, critical thinking, and problem solving, as well to foster social, emotional, creative, and motor development.
9. Assessment	The teacher candidate understands, selects, and uses a range of assessment strategies to foster motor, cognitive, social, and emotional development of students and gives accounts of students' learning to the outside world.
10. Technology	The teacher candidate understands and uses up-to-date technology to enhance the learning environment across the full range of student needs.
11. Professional development	The teacher candidate is a reflective practitioner who evaluates his or her interactions with others (e.g., students, parents and guardians, colleagues, and professionals in the community) and seeks opportunities to grow professionally.
12. Collaboration and professionalism	The teacher candidate fosters relationships with colleagues, parents and guardians, community agencies, and colleges and universities to support students' growth and well-being.

Reprinted, by permission, from College of Education and Human Services, 2005, *Student Portfolio Handbook* (Cleveland, OH: Cleveland State University), 4.

Standards for Beginning Physical Education Teachers

Because of their widespread acceptance, the *National Standards for Beginning Physical Education Teachers* (National Association for Sport and Physical Education, 2003) are recommended for organizing the teacher candidate professional portfolio. The standards and corresponding outcomes were identified and described in table 1.2 (pages 16-17). The artifacts selected should provide tangible evidence that each standard has been met. They should document the knowledge that has been gained, skills that have been mastered, and dispositions that are characteristic of the teacher candidate. Although artifacts cannot conclusively prove the attainment of knowledge, skills, and dispositions, they can indicate competence. The dispositions, knowledge, and performances (skills) that support each standard are outlined on pages 55-59. They will be used in subsequent sections of this chapter that deal with portfolio management and assembly, selection of items, and assessment.

Dispositions, Knowledge, and Performances for Teacher Standards

Standard 1: Content Knowledge

Understand physical education content and disciplinary concepts related to the development of a physically educated person.

Dispositions

Believes physical activity and fitness are important; has enthusiasm for the importance of physical education; seeks to keep abreast of new ideas and understandings; believes that physical activity can foster self expression, development, and learning.

Knowledge

Critical elements and sequencing of basic motor skills; concepts and strategies related to physical activity and fitness; the relationship among physical activity, fitness, and health; historical, philosophical, sociological, and psychological factors associated with diverse physical activities; the organic, skeletal, and neuromuscular structures, how these systems adapt, and how they contribute to motor performance, fitness, and wellness; concepts, assumptions, debates, and processes of inquiry; appropriate instructional cues and prompts.

Performances

Demonstrates basic motor skills and physical activities with competence; applies disciplinary concepts and principles to skillful movement; incorporates interdisciplinary learning experiences; supports and encourages learner expression through movement.

Standard 2: Growth and Development

Understand how individuals learn and develop, and provide opportunities that support physical, cognitive, social, and emotional development.

Dispositions

Appreciates and promotes physical activity in the overall growth and development of learners; appreciates individual variations in growth and development; is committed to helping learners become competent and self-confident.

Knowledge

How learning and development occur; physical, cognitive, social, and emotional development and their influence on learning and instructional decisions; expected developmental progressions and ranges of individual variation; the value of practice opportunities for growth and development.

Performances

Assesses individual and group performance to meet learner developmental needs; stimulates learner reflection on prior knowledge, experiences, and skills, and encourages them to assume responsibility for their own learning.

Standard 3: Diverse Learners

Understand how individuals differ in their approaches to learning and create appropriate instruction adapted to these differences.

Dispositions

Believes that all learners can develop motor skills, feel successful, and enjoy physical activity; appreciates and values human diversity and shows respect for varied talents and perspectives; is committed to helping learners become physically educated; seeks to understand and is sensitive to learners' families, communities, cultural values, and experiences.

(continued)

(continued)

Knowledge

Differences in approaches to learning and physical performance and can design instruction that uses learners' strengths; areas of special need including physical and emotional challenges, learning disabilities, sensory difficulties, and language barriers; how learning is influenced by individual experiences, talents, and prior learning, as well as culture, family, and community values.

Performances

Selects and implements developmentally appropriate instruction that is sensitive to the multiple needs, learning styles, and experiences of learners; uses appropriate strategies, services, and resources to meet special and diverse learning needs; creates a learning environment which respects and incorporates learners' personal, family, cultural, and community experiences.

Standard 4: Management and Motivation

Use and have an understanding of individual and group motivation and behavior to create a safe learning environment that encourages positive social interaction, active engagement in learning, and self-motivation.

Dispositions

Accepts responsibility for establishing a positive climate; believes that providing opportunities for learners' input into instructional decisions increases their commitment to learning; recognizes the importance of positive peer relationships; recognizes the value of intrinsic motivation to lifelong physical activity; is committed to using appropriate motivational strategies to meet the needs of individuals.

Knowledge

Developmentally appropriate practices to motivate learners; strategies to teach learners to use behavior change techniques; strategies to help learners demonstrate responsible personal and social behavior; the principles of effective management and a variety of strategies to promote equitable and meaningful learning; factors related to intrinsic motivation and strategies to help learners become self-motivated.

Performances

Uses a variety of developmentally appropriate practices to motivate learners; uses strategies to promote mutual respect, support, safety, and cooperative participation; uses managerial and instructional routines which create smoothly functioning learning experiences; organizes, allocates, and manages resources to provide active and equitable learning experiences.

Standard 5: Communication

Use knowledge of effective verbal, nonverbal, and media communication techniques to enhance learning and engagement in physical education settings.

Dispositions

Recognizes the importance of communication skills and being informed of technological advances; appreciates the cultural dimensions of communication; seeks to foster sensitive interactions with and among learners; is committed to communicating with school colleagues, parents/guardians, and the community; is committed to serving as a role model.

Knowledge

Communication techniques; appropriate use of verbal and nonverbal cues; how ethnic, cultural, economic, ability, gender, and environmental differences affect communication; how to use computers and other technologies to communicate and network; strategies for building a community of learners; strategies for communicating with school colleagues, parents, and the community.

Performances

Communicates in ways that demonstrate sensitivity to ethnic, cultural, economic, ability, gender, and environmental differences; communicates managerial and instructional information in a variety of ways; communicates with school colleagues, parents/guardians, and the community through open houses, faculty meetings, newsletters, and conferences; models communication strategies.

Standard 6: Planning and Instruction

Understand the importance of planning developmentally appropriate instructional units to foster the development of a physically educated person.

Dispositions

Values short- and long-term planning to reach goals; values the use of multiple instructional strategies; believes that plans must be open to revision; is committed to using learner strengths as a basis for planning instruction; is committed to continuous learning about pedagogical content knowledge; believes that the safety of students is the first priority in any movement setting.

Knowledge

Learning theory and current curricular models; contextual issues to consider when planning instruction; how to design instructional sequences and learning experiences that maximize learner participation and success; the uses of a variety of equipment, materials, human, and technological resources; principles, techniques, advantages, and limitations of various instructional strategies; safety issues to consider when planning and implementing instruction.

Performances

Can identify program goals; selects instructional strategies based on developmental levels, learning styles, program goals, and safety issues; applies disciplinary and pedagogical knowledge; selects teaching resources and curriculum materials for their comprehensiveness, accuracy, usefulness, and safety; uses curricula that encourage learners to see, question, and interpret physical activity from diverse perspectives; designs and implements learning experiences that are safe, appropriate, realistic, and relevant based on principles of effective instruction; uses demonstration and explanations to capture key components and link them to learners' experiences; helps learners incorporate problem solving and critical thinking strategies in the process of becoming a physically educated person; chooses varied roles in the instructional process based on the content, purpose of instruction, and the needs of learners; creates short- and long-term plans that are linked to learner needs and performance, and adapts plans; models instructional strategies that facilitate learning in physical activity settings; asks questions and poses scenarios to stimulate interactive learning opportunities.

Standard 7: Student Assessment

Understand and use the varied types of assessment and their contribution to overall program continuity and the development of the physical, cognitive, social, and emotional domains.

Dispositions

Values ongoing assessment to identify learner needs and ability; recognizes that a variety of assessment strategies are necessary.

Knowledge

Characteristics, uses, advantages, and limitations of different types of assessment; how to select and use developmentally appropriate assessment strategies and instruments; measurement issues, such as validity, reliability, and bias; the use of assessment as an integral part of instruction to provide feedback to learners; how to use and interpret learner performance data to inform instructional decisions and report progress.

(continued)

(continued)

Performances

Uses a variety of formal and informal assessment techniques to assess learner progress; uses assessment strategies to involve learners in self-assessment; maintains records of learner performance and communicates learner progress based on appropriate indicators.

Standard 8: Reflection

Understand the importance of being a reflective practitioner and its contribution to overall professional development and actively seek opportunities to sustain professional growth.

Dispositions

Is committed to ongoing self-reflection, assessment, and learning; values critical thinking and self-directed learning; is committed to seeking, developing, and refining practices to address individual needs of learners; recognizes responsibility for engaging in and supporting appropriate professional practices.

Knowledge

A variety of self-assessment and problem-solving strategies for reflecting on practice and its influences on learning; literature on teaching physical education and resources available for professional physical educators.

Performances

Reflects upon and revises practice based on observation of learners; consults professional literature, colleagues, and other resources; participates in the professional physical education community and within the broader educational field; reflects on the appropriateness of program design on the development of physically educated individuals.

Standard 9: Technology

Use information technology to enhance learning and personal and professional productivity.

Dispositions

Recognizes the contribution of technology toward the design, development, and implementation of effective teaching; recognizes the varied use of technology toward both knowledge acquisition and knowledge transmission; values ongoing use of technology to enhance the learning and teaching environment.

Knowledge

Current technology available and its use; the different types of data gathered from different types of technology; the varied methods by which technology can be incorporated in the physical education setting; instructional strategies to present the appropriate use of technology to the student.

Performances

Uses technology to regularly collect data for curricular and student assessment; uses technology on a regular basis to communicate, network, and locate resources; encourages students to explore the varied uses of technology as it relates to developing and leading physically active lifestyles.

Standard 10: Collaboration

Understand the necessity of fostering collaborative relationships with colleagues, parents/guardians, and community agencies to support the development of a physically educated person.

Dispositions

Values collaborating with teachers of other subject matters; is willing to consult with others regarding the total well-being and education of learners; respects learners' privacy and the confidentiality of information; is willing to work with others to improve the overall working environment.

Knowledge

How schools and organizations function within the larger community; the influence of nonschool factors on learning and engagement in physical activity; laws related to learner rights and teacher responsibilities; issues related to the functions of schools.

Performances

Acts as an advocate in the school and community to promote physical activity; consults with counselors and other professionals in community agencies; identifies and uses community resources; establishes productive partnerships with parents/guardians; is sensitive and responsive to signs of distress and seeks help as needed and appropriate; participates in collegial activities to make the school a productive learning environment.

Reprinted from *National Standards for Beginning Physical Education Teachers,* 2nd edition (2003) with permission from the National Association for Sport and Physical Education (NASPE), 1900 Association Drive, Reston, VA 20191-1599.

Implementation Strategy

The teacher candidate professional portfolio should be a cumulative record of professional growth and achieved competence. It is the thread running throughout the entire teacher education program. Therefore, a systematic process for collecting, selecting, communicating, and evaluating appropriate portfolio entries is needed. Various checkpoints and periodic reviews are possible to (1) determine whether expectations have been approximated or achieved at key intervals, (2) decide whether teacher candidates can continue, and (3) plan future directions within the remaining program elements. The system should also include some way to introduce the portfolio model and a means for bringing closure to the process.

The teacher candidate portfolio model will vary from one institution to another depending on philosophy, program structure, faculty commitment, advising procedures, and prospective teachers' attitudes. The implementation strategy is usually based on some combination of advisers, courses, committees, and program phases (step 4 of the portfolio-designing process). Each of these strategies is described briefly in the following sections.

Adviser Directed Model

Teacher candidates are normally assigned an academic adviser who could also serve as portfolio adviser. Advisers guide their advisees through the various stages of portfolio development. When the adviser is assigned, portfolio guidelines (e.g., portfolio handbook) could be given to the teacher candidate at that time. To begin the process, the teacher candidate might be required to submit an introductory portfolio at an early advising session. During the teacher education program, the adviser might be expected to (1) confer with the candidate about the portfolio system, (2) discuss criteria for earning satisfactory ratings, (3) help select portfolio entries, and (4) evaluate portfolios at predetermined checkpoints, including the employment portfolio.

Course Affiliated Model

Development of the various types of professional portfolios (i.e., introductory, presentation, employment) could be linked with selected key courses in the teacher education program. Factors to consider are the nature of the course, the timing of the course in the program, and the instructor. Stages of the teacher candidate professional portfolio could become part of the individual courses and be graded by the instructor as part of course requirements. For example, a sophomore-level course such as Introduction to Physical Education, Exercise Science, and Sport could include the distribution of and an orientation to the entire portfolio model (e.g., a portfolio handbook). Teacher candidates could develop and present their introductory portfolios. Other late sophomore, junior, and early senior year courses could be affiliated with the cumulative development of the working repository and presentation portfolio. Finally, the employment (exit) portfolio could be required as part of a course that is completed along with student teaching, such as Gateway to the Profession or Senior Seminar.

Committee Oversight Model

A group of faculty members, school personnel, or teacher candidates could assume ultimate responsibility for overseeing the portfolio system. Upon application to the teacher education program, teacher candidates could receive portfolio guidelines (e.g., a portfolio handbook). As part of the screening process, teacher candidates might be required to submit an introductory portfolio. One criterion for admittance could be a satisfactory review of the introductory portfolio by a portfolio committee. Periodic feedback could also be provided by the committee throughout the teacher education program, including feedback on the employment portfolio.

Program Phases Model

Teacher education programs are often structured around various segments such as (1) blocks (e.g., preprofessional, I, II, III), (2) course groupings (e.g., professional core, forms of movement, major field theory or content, planned electives), (3) practical experiences (e.g., clinical or field experiences, practicums or internships, student teaching), or (4) knowledge bases (e.g., organizing content knowledge, creating a learning environment, teaching for learning, professionalism). The collection, selection, reflection, presentation, and evaluation of portfolio documents could be associated with any of these program segments. However, deciding whether an adviser, course instructor, or committee would direct the portfolio development within each program segment would still be necessary.

Processes for Involvement

Whether the portfolio implementation strategy involves advisers, courses, committees, or program phases, there are other considerations. Certain processes for involvement should be built into the system including training, reflection, self-assessment, presentations, and conferences (step 5 of the portfolio-designing process). These aspects are described briefly here; additional details are provided in subsequent sections of this chapter.

Training

Those directing the portfolio process (i.e., advisers, course instructors, committee members) *and* teacher candidates should receive formal portfolio training. Teacher candidates could be trained at the time the portfolio system is introduced (e.g., in a required general advising session or a selected introductory course). Training should include a set of guidelines, illustrative artifacts, and sample portfolios. In addition, the basic skills of self-management, reflection, self-assessment, peer review, and conferences should be developed during the training. Comprehensive training could be conducted for those who are new to the system, and a training update could be held for those who are experienced.

Reflection

At a minimum, teacher candidates should thoughtfully examine each artifact selected for the working repository and for the introductory, presentation, and employment portfolios. Each piece should be labeled to reveal its meaning and value to the entire portfolio with reference to the teacher standards being used. Teacher candidates need to express why an artifact was chosen for a particular standard; they should not merely summarize the contents of the artifact. The teacher candidate should try to answer the following questions: What is the artifact? Why is it filed under this standard? What does it say about my growing competence? A sample cover sheet for reflecting on individual artifacts selected for the teacher candidate portfolio appears on page 61. Other kinds of reflections will be described in the subsequent section of this chapter, Selection of Artifacts.

Reflection Cover Sheet

Name: _____ Date: _____

Standard #: _____ Name of standard: _____

Name of artifact: _____

Course/activity: _____

Rationale statement (Why is this artifact filed under this standard? What does the artifact say about my growing competence?):

_____

_____

_____

_____

_____

_____

_____

_____

_____

_____

From *Professional and Student Portfolios for Physical Education, Second Edition,* by Vincent J. Melograno, 2006, Champaign, IL: Human Kinetics.

Self-Assessment

In contrast to piece-by-piece reflection, teacher candidates need to review the entire collection of artifacts with reference to their short- and long-term goals and how the portfolio adheres to the teacher standards. This phase can be an informal self-check to make sure they are on the right track and to determine what changes might be needed. Teacher candidates should look for "holes"—standards that are not well documented by artifacts—and keep these in mind as they complete courses and professional activities. Consideration should be given to how an assignment, article critique, personal journal, or any number of school or community activities could help a standard that needs work. The Artifacts Self-Assessment Checklist shown on page 63 can help teacher candidates identify standards that are well documented (Good), standards that are satisfactorily evidenced (OK), and standards for which goals and artifacts are needed along with a target completion date (Artifacts needed). Other forms of self-assessment will be covered in the subsequent section of this chapter, Selection of Artifacts.

Presentations

Teacher candidates should be afforded several opportunities to present their portfolios to different kinds of audiences, in a variety of forums, and at key stages of the teacher education program. For example, the different types of portfolios could be presented orally in a one-on-one situation with an adviser, instructor, or peer; to a small group of peers; or to an entire class. They could also be presented in a posterlike session at which faculty and peer feedback is provided. Toward the end of the teacher education program, the portfolio could be presented in a job interview simulation conducted by a team playing the role of employers.

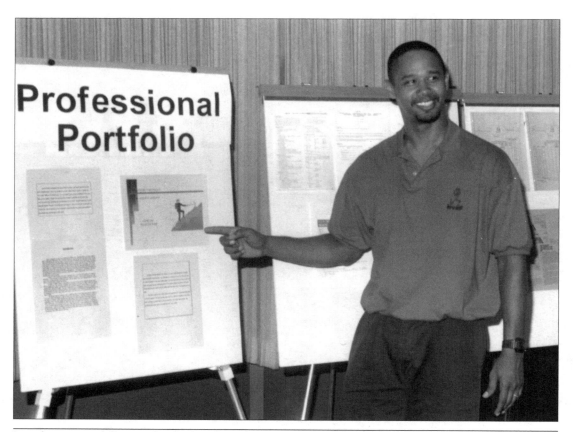

Introductory portfolios can be displayed in a beginning course for teacher candidates.

Artifacts Self-Assessment Checklist

Name: _____ Date: _____

Standard	Good	OK	Artifacts needed
1. Content knowledge			Goal: Target date:
2. Growth and development			Goal: Target date:
3. Diverse learners			Goal: Target date:
4. Management and motivation			Goal: Target date:
5. Communication			Goal: Target date:
6. Planning and instruction			Goal: Target date:
7. Student assessment			Goal: Target date:
8. Reflection			Goal: Target date:
9. Technology			Goal: Target date:
10. Collaboration			Goal: Target date:

From *Professional and Student Portfolios for Physical Education, Second Edition,* by Vincent J. Melograno, 2006, Champaign, IL: Human Kinetics.

Conferences

A natural progression in the portfolio process is to share the finished product with others. A portfolio conference offers a chance to "connect" with others using the portfolio as the basis for discussion. Whereas presentations are portfolio exhibitions, conferences provide a chance for meaningful dialogue with other teacher candidates, advisers, instructors, and school personnel. In planning for conferences, the following questions should be answered: What will the goals be? What reflections do teacher candidates need to engage in? What questions should be prepared for the conference? When will it be held? Following are some basic questions for a teacher candidate to answer at a portfolio conference:

- What have you learned about yourself by putting together your portfolio?
- What artifacts are you particularly proud of and why?
- If you could publish one thing in your portfolio, what would it be and why?
- What areas of your teaching performance need further improvement?
- How do you feel about your role as a professional teacher?

Assembly and Structure

Ultimately, the teacher candidate assumes responsibility for organizing, maintaining, and storing the professional portfolio throughout the assessment process (step 6 of the portfolio-designing process). Decisions about the method of construction, how often to "manage" portfolios, and how and where to store portfolios depend on the type of portfolio. Clearly, teacher candidates need a plan to handle the logistics of the portfolio process. Although there are many ways to assemble and structure portfolios, several specific techniques and options can help in developing the management and storage plan.

Management Techniques

Teacher candidates may be good at collecting work samples and exhibits, but they may not be able to organize all the materials. Several management tools have proved to be effective. Although many of these ideas may seem like common sense, not everyone is good at managing loose ends, particularly something as comprehensive as a professional portfolio. These people should benefit from some of these simple management suggestions.

- *Dividers.* Whatever kind of container is used, divided notebook folders or divider pages can be used to separate artifacts according to the teacher standards or any other category that makes sense (e.g., courses, program phases, incomplete works, finished works). A filing system should be created so that the standards are easily identified. Each section could be labeled with a shortened version of the standard.

- *Color codes.* To facilitate management, colored dots or colored files could be used to code entries in the portfolio. Artifacts could also be coded using different color markers. A code for the colors needs to be included.

- *Artifact registry.* Using a sheet for each standard, teacher candidates could record the date, item, and reason for either adding or removing an item. Because the registry chronicles when and why items are removed or replaced, it can become a dynamic tool for reflection.

- *Work log.* A biography of work could show the evolution of a long-term project such as a portfolio. This would help in making necessary changes or shifting direction. The log could be as simple as dated entries that trace all activities and decisions associated with the portfolio.

- *Index.* An alphabetical index of items could be compiled as the portfolio evolves. Such an organizational tool would help in the cross-referencing of artifacts that represent more than one standard and vice versa. The index could be placed in the front of the portfolio like a table of contents.

- *Self-stick notes.* Artifacts need to be cataloged so that ideas are not lost over time. A self-stick note or index card could be attached to each artifact to identify the standard and could include a brief statement explaining why the artifact was collected. Specific descriptors from the standard statement may help later in connecting the artifact to the standard. Using a self-stick note or index card also protects the original works.

Storage Options

Because teacher candidates are responsible for storing their own portfolios, the "container" for collecting artifacts is a matter of personal preference. For hard copies, possibilities include notebooks, expanding and accordion files, large file boxes, folders, satchels, pockets for electronic documents, large notebooks divided into sections, and file drawers in a cabinet. Ultimately, materials can be scanned for storage on computer disks or stored on computer internal hard drives. Refer to chapter 1 for additional information about the use of technology for storage (page 40).

The type of portfolio will likely determine the most practical way to store portfolio items. For example, the introductory portfolio is a scaled-down version of a complete portfolio. Because the number of artifacts is relatively small, an accordion file or cardboard box may be all that is needed. By contrast, the working repository may require considerable space to accommodate a maximum number of artifacts. The presentation portfolio should not be cumbersome or unwieldy. Sample pages from a large project might replace the entire project. A large notebook or accordion file may be all that is needed. Finally, the employment portfolio should be a succinct representation of one's teaching competence. A limited number of carefully selected items should be included in a "professional" container, such as a portfolio satchel, which can provide easy access to prospective employers.

Portfolio Type

Just as the various types of portfolio can be stored differently, so can each type of portfolio be assembled differently. In the introductory portfolio, teacher candidates should introduce themselves to the profession by revealing personal characteristics and professional goals. These aspects serve as the basis for managing the portfolio. Artifacts could be assembled that are keyed to the following topics: (1) relationships with family, friends, and professionals; (2) personal interests or hobbies; (3) teaching and professional experiences; and (4) reasons for wanting to be a physical education teacher.

Although the other types of portfolios should be organized around the teacher standards, they are assembled and managed quite differently. Even the required and optional artifacts for each type of portfolio will vary, as shown in the next chapter section on artifact selection. For the working repository, anything should be collected that relates to a standard, even if not required or eventually selected as an optional piece. Teacher candidates should continually look for ways to document how they have met standards, particularly those they are having trouble documenting.

For the presentation portfolio, less is more. Artifacts could represent more than one standard. Artifacts should be selected from both those that were required for the working repository and those that were optional. Each section should be labeled with an abbreviated title for the standard so that someone viewing the portfolio will know what it means. A rationale for choosing the artifact should be included. The reflection cover sheet on page 61 could be used for this purpose.

The employment portfolio may be the first impression an employer has of the teacher candidate. Spelling, grammar, and neatness should be carefully checked. Because employers do not have a great deal of time to peruse portfolios, the overall presentation should be consistent and artifacts should be easy to follow. In addition to the teacher standards, artifacts should exemplify the kind of position being sought (e.g., elementary school, high school). As a supplement to the employment portfolio, a brochure could be produced that reflects the teacher candidate's "theme" along with a biographical sketch, summary of the teacher standards, and outline of portfolio contents. A "business card" with the same theme could accompany the brochure. A sample brochure and business card are shown in figure 2.1.

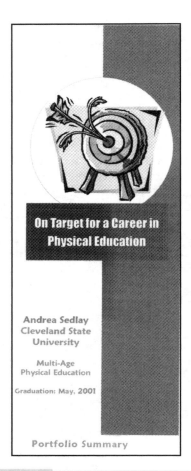

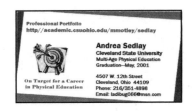

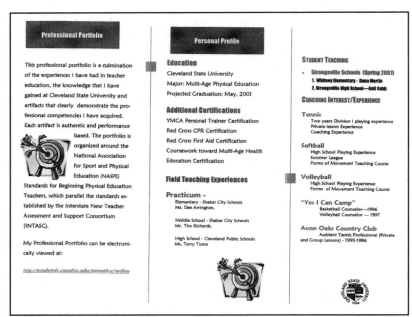

Figure 2.1 A brochure and "business card" can accompany the employment portfolio.

Courtesy of Andrea Horba.

Using Technology

The section in chapter 1 titled Technology Use in Portfolio Development (pages 31-48) is a useful introduction to the subject of technology. The information about hardware, storage, and software has general applicability to developing electronic-based professional portfolios for teacher candidates. Because electronic-based portfolios are an extension of paper-based portfolios, the earlier information in this chapter on management techniques and storage options is also applicable (pages 64-65). However, some additional information regarding the development of portfolios for physical education teacher education (PETE) programs is important.

Technology Standards

The International Society for Technology in Education (ISTE) has developed national educational technology standards for teachers (NETS-T) that cover three stages of development for teacher candidates: general preparation, professional preparation, and student teaching/internship (ISTE, 2002). The standards and corresponding performance indicators are identified in table 2.2. In addition, standard 9 of the national standards for beginning physical education teachers (see page 58) addresses the dispositions, knowledge, and performance in support of technology. Competence related to these standards can be addressed by requiring teacher candidates to create an electronic-based or Web-based portfolio.

Table 2.2 Educational Technology Standards and Performance Indicators for Teachers

Standards	Performance indicators
Standard I: Technology operations and concepts Teachers demonstrate a sound understanding of technology operations and concepts.	Teachers: • demonstrate introductory knowledge, skills, and understanding of concepts related to technology. • demonstrate continual growth in technology knowledge and skills to stay abreast of current and emerging technologies.
Standard II: Planning and designing learning environments and experiences Teachers plan and design effective learning environments and experiences supported by technology.	Teachers: • design developmentally appropriate learning opportunities that apply technology-enhanced instructional strategies to support the diverse needs of learners. • apply current research on teaching and learning with technology when planning learning environments and experiences. • identify and locate technology resources and evaluate them for accuracy and suitability. • plan for the management of technology resources within the context of learning activities. • plan strategies to manage student learning in a technology-enhanced environment.
Standard III: Teaching, learning, and the curriculum Teachers implement curriculum plans that include methods and strategies for applying technology to maximize student learning.	Teachers: • facilitate technology-enhanced experiences that address content standards and student technology standards. • use technology to support learner-centered strategies that address the diverse needs of students. • apply technology to develop students' higher-order skills and creativity. • manage student learning activities in a technology-enhanced environment.
Standard IV: Assessment and evaluation Teachers apply technology to facilitate a variety of effective assessment and evaluation strategies.	Teachers: • apply technology in assessing student learning of subject matter using a variety of assessment techniques. • use technology resources to collect and analyze data, interpret results, and communicate findings to improve instructional practice and maximize student learning. • apply multiple methods of evaluation to determine students' appropriate use of technology resources for learning, communication, and productivity.
Standard V: Productivity and professional practice Teachers use technology to enhance their productivity and professional practice.	Teachers: • use technology resources to engage in ongoing professional development and lifelong learning. • continually evaluate and reflect on professional practice to make informed decisions regarding the use of technology in support of student learning. • apply technology to increase productivity. • use technology to communicate and collaborate with peers, parents, and the larger community in order to nurture student learning.
Standard VI: Social, ethical, legal, and human issues Teachers understand the social, ethical, legal, and human issues surrounding the use of technology in PK-12 schools and apply those principles in practice.	Teachers: • model and teach legal and ethical practice related to technology use. • apply technology resources to enable and empower learners with diverse backgrounds, characteristics, and abilities. • identify and use technology resources that affirm diversity. • promote safe and healthy use of technology resources. • facilitate equitable access to technology resources for all students.

Electronic-Based and Web-Based Portfolios

Teacher candidates typically work on their portfolios during all phases of the PETE program. Depending on the implementation strategy, assistance and feedback are provided at various intervals. For example, at Cleveland State University, a course-affiliated model is used. The different types of portfolios (i.e., introductory, presentation, employment) are reviewed and assessed during four checkpoint courses, beginning with a sophomore-level introductory course and ending with a senior-level seminar course during student teaching. Electronic-based portfolios are introduced in a junior-level methods course. Teacher candidates are supported through a dedicated Portfolio Computer Lab that houses desktop computers, printers, scanners, DVD camcorders, and digital cameras. Word processing, presentation, and multimedia software is also built into the system.

Teacher candidates store their electronic-based portfolios on a CD or USB drive. They assume complete responsibility for the portfolio including the maintenance of a backup copy. Note that if the campus is networked with access from off campus, students (teacher candidates) can simply access folders online at any time from anywhere. In this system, the institution assumes the responsibility for backing up all the files on the network.

After the junior year, teacher candidates then begin working on the development of a Web-based portfolio. The expectation is that the employment portfolio, finalized during student teaching, is Web based. This conversion is made easier because an electronic-based portfolio already exists. Again, the information provided in chapter 1 on hardware and software, including Web development software, should be helpful in constructing such a system. Examples of Web-based portfolios can be accessed from the World Wide Web (www.csuportfolio.com). The components of the Web-based portfolio are introductory home page, coursework, resume, standards (with links to artifacts), gallery (with photos and video clips), and references. Sample pages from a Web-based teacher candidate portfolio appear in figure 2.2.

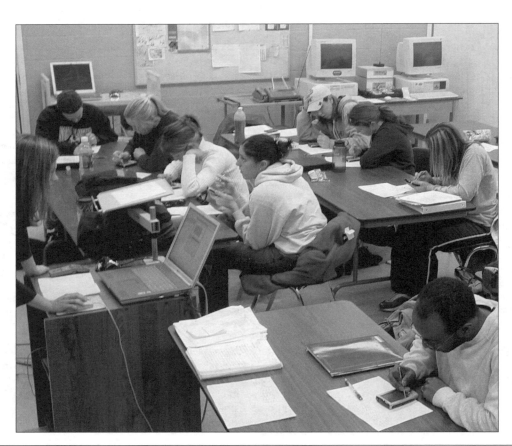

Teacher candidates use handheld computers to analyze assessment data.

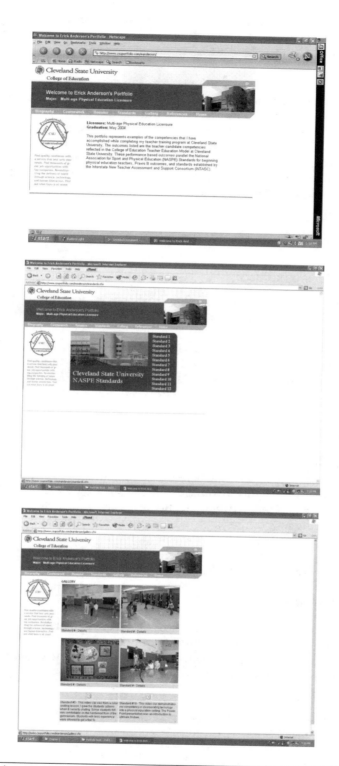

Figure 2.2 This Web site for a teacher candidate employment portfolio includes a home page, standards with links to artifacts, and a gallery of photos and video clips.

Selection of Artifacts

The selection of portfolio items is the next consideration for the teacher candidate portfolio system (step 7 of the portfolio-designing process). The actual selection process is closely linked to any established criteria (i.e., teacher standards) and the type of portfolio (i.e., introductory, presentation, employment). It also depends on the implementation strategy being used (i.e., advisers, course affiliations, oversight committees, program phases). As artifacts are created and selected, confidentiality should be maintained. Names or other identifying information should be avoided when referring to students or teachers.

Several key questions should be asked when selecting portfolio items:

- *What* items should be included?
- *How* will items be selected?
- *Who* will select items?
- *When* will items be selected?

The primary focus of this section is to outline the range of possibilities of artifacts to include in a portfolio. This section also describes the basic processes of reflection and self-assessment, offers suggestions for required and optional artifacts, and provides a design for analyzing artifacts. How items are selected relates directly to whether they demonstrate a teacher candidate's ability to meet the beginning teacher standards. Any combination of teacher candidate, adviser, course instructor, committee member, and school personnel may be involved in selecting items. When items are selected depends on where the types of portfolios are taught within the PETE program.

Basic Processes

Most required and optional artifacts will be derived from courses, clinical and field experiences, and school and community activities. Before looking at these kinds of artifacts, commonly referred to as work samples or exhibits, two basic processes are reviewed that can yield other kinds of artifacts—reflection and self-assessment. The information introduced previously (pages 60-62) is expanded here because of the value of developing reflection and self-assessment artifacts for the professional portfolio. Because of the emphasis on the process of portfolio development, not just its products, the teacher candidate must actively participate in selecting items *and* determine the merits of the items through reflection and self-assessment.

Reflection Artifacts

In addition to the reflection cover sheets (see page 61) that should accompany each work sample and exhibit, more extensive reflection artifacts would enhance the working repository and introductory, presentation, and employment portfolios. Such artifacts could include reflective stems for individual pieces, such as the following:

- This is my favorite piece because . . .
- If I could do this piece over again, I would . . .
- This piece will impress other teachers because . . .
- Other teacher candidates liked this piece because . . .
- This piece was my greatest challenge because . . .

Teacher candidates can also ask themselves questions to help "bridge" individual items into the entire portfolio as they contemplate their selections. Following are some bridging questions:

- Why should I choose this piece?
- What are its strengths and weaknesses?

- Why is it important?
- How does it fit into what I already have?
- What if I took it out?
- How will others react to it?

In addition, reflection artifacts should be related to the teacher standards. Artifacts could be generated representing an overall reflection on each standard. Reflective questions to consider for this kind of artifact, specific to each standard, are listed in table 2.3.

Table 2.3 Reflective Questions for Teacher Standards

Standards	Descriptions	Reflective questions
1. Content knowledge	Understand physical education content and disciplinary concepts related to the development of a physically educated person	• What special insights did I develop about the physical education discipline? • What area of physical education would I like to study in greater depth? • What special project (e.g., report, experiment, learning experience, unit plan) added to my knowledge of physical education? • What person (e.g., instructor, adviser, supervisor, teacher) made an indelible impression on me about physical education? • What aspects of physical education need the greatest emphasis in elementary schools? Middle or junior high schools? High schools?
2. Growth and development	Understand how individuals learn and develop, and provide opportunities that support physical, cognitive, social, and emotional development	• How do I help students in their physical, cognitive, social, and emotional development? • What developmentally appropriate practices do I rely on most in teaching physical education? • How do I know that students are developmentally ready to engage in physical education activities?
3. Diverse learners	Understand how individuals differ in their approaches to learning and create appropriate instruction adapted to these differences	• What do I understand about my own culture? • What are some ways that I have used to learn about the students I teach? • What experiences have I had that affect teaching and learning in diverse environments? • What are some characteristics of teachers who work effectively in diverse classrooms? • What skills do I need to develop to work effectively in diverse classrooms? • What experiences have I had in the role of a minority, and how did this help my understanding of diversity?
4. Management and motivation	Use and have an understanding of individual and group motivation and behavior to create a safe learning environment that encourages positive social interaction, active engagement in learning, and self-motivation	• How have I successfully motivated students to participate in physical activity? • What managerial and instructional routines create smoothly functioning learning experiences? • How do I establish a positive climate in the physical education setting and school environment? • What strategies are best for promoting mutual respect, support, safety, and cooperative participation in physical education?

(continued)

Table 2.3 *(continued)*

Standards	Descriptions	Reflective questions
5. Communication	Use knowledge of effective verbal, nonverbal, and media communication techniques to enhance learning and engagement in physical activity settings	• Is my communication clear, and how do I check for understanding? • What communication strategies do I model that have proven successful? • How do I communicate with school colleagues, parents and guardians, and the community? • How do ethnic, cultural, economic, ability, gender, and environmental differences affect the ways I communicate in the physical education setting?
6. Planning and instruction	Understand the importance of planning developmentally appropriate instructional units to foster the development of a physically educated person	• What are my primary program goals and desired outcomes in physical education? • What instructional strategies do I prefer to maximize student participation and success? • If a lesson is not successful, what do I do to improve my teaching the next time? • What principles of effective instruction do I try to build into my teaching routine? • How do I adapt plans to ensure student progress, motivation, and safety?
7. Student assessment	Understand and use the varied types of assessment and their contribution to overall program continuity and the development of the physical, cognitive, social, and emotional domains	• How do I integrate assessment into my physical education instruction? • What are my favorite formal and informal assessment techniques? • What assessment strategies would I like to really develop for my physical education setting? • What kinds of student performance data should be reported for physical education?
8. Reflection	Understand the importance of being a reflective practitioner and its contribution to overall professional development, and actively seek opportunities to sustain professional growth	• How has my philosophy of education and physical education changed during the teacher education program? • What have I read or heard that has influenced my ideas about teaching physical education? • What experiences have had a significant impact on my teaching philosophy? • What are my primary reasons for wanting to teach physical education?
9. Technology	Use information technology to enhance learning and personal and professional productivity	• What is my basic understanding of technology operations and concepts? • How do I stay abreast of current and emerging technologies? • How can I plan and design effective learning environments and experiences in physical education that are supported by technology? • What is my ability to facilitate technology-enhanced experiences that address physical education content standards and student technology standards? • How can I apply technology to facilitate a variety of effective assessment and evaluation strategies? • How do I use technology to enhance my productivity, professional practice, and communication? • What technology resources can be used to help students with diverse backgrounds, characteristics, and abilities in physical education?

Standards	Descriptions	Reflective questions
10. Collaboration	Understand the necessity of fostering collaborative relationships with colleagues, parents and guardians, and community agencies to support the development of a physically educated person	• What are my personal characteristics that make me an effective team member? • How do schools function within the larger community context relative to physical education? • What do I find difficult about working with other teachers? • How do I encourage students to work together in the physical education setting? • What partnership activities with parents and guardians do I think will be most effective? • What personal skills should I improve to make me a better advocate for physical education in the school and community?

Self-Assessment Artifacts

The sample checklist on page 63 for reviewing the teacher standards represents an informal self-check of the entire collection of items. It might appear in the working repository, but it would not likely be included in the presentation and employment portfolios. More formal self-assessment artifacts would provide additional insight into the collection of items. For example, teacher candidates could look at the whole portfolio and rate, on a scale of 1 to 3, whether they have met criteria for quality work. Criteria might include several of the following areas: accuracy of information, completeness, connection to standards, creativity, diversity of items, insightfulness, organization, and visual appeal. Teacher candidates should also assess their strengths and weaknesses with respect to the teacher standards and then set short-term and long-term goals accordingly. They should analyze their attributes in terms of the knowledge, performances, and dispositions detailed on pages 55-59. The Self-Assessment of Teacher Standards form on page 75 could be used to generate self-assessment artifacts for each teacher standard. In addition, teacher candidates could use any of the scoring rubrics presented in the subsequent section of this chapter on assessment to assess their own portfolios.

Required Artifacts

Theoretically, the number of required portfolio items could range from all to none. Requiring all items would stifle teacher candidates. Because the portfolio process promotes reflection, self-assessment, individual choice, initiative, and autonomy, teacher candidates should develop a sense of ownership and responsibility along with a "voice" in selecting portfolio items. On the other hand, requiring no items would leave too much to chance. Some items are absolutely essential for a properly constructed portfolio, particularly one that is organized around a set of teacher standards. For these reasons, some combination of required and optional artifacts is recommended. The actual ratio will vary according to the purposes, types, and processes of the portfolio system in place.

In determining what should be required, educators should consider the link between established teacher standards and the artifacts selected to represent these standards. For example, the presentation portfolio could not only require a set number of artifacts for each standard, but also prescribe the nature of these artifacts (e.g., unit plan to document planning and instruction). The employment portfolio would be limited further in terms of what kinds of and how many artifacts are required from the working repository. The following are possible artifacts that could be required for each standard. All of these artifacts could be used for the sample professional portfolio system at the end of this chapter and the teacher candidate portfolio builder on the accompanying CD-ROM.

Standard 1: Content Knowledge

- Project titled Contributions of Physical Activity from a foundations course dealing with the principles, history, and philosophy of physical education
- Readings list organized by the subdisciplines of human movement (e.g., exercise physiology; kinesiology and biomechanics; motor learning, control, and development; sport sociology; sport psychology; sport pedagogy; and the sport humanities)

Standard 2: Growth and Development

- Research paper on the developmental stages children follow in learning to throw, catch, and strike objects
- Criteria checklists showing task analyses and progressions for basic tennis skills (e.g., forehand, backhand, serve)

Standard 3: Diverse Learners

- Anecdotal notes that focus on different learning styles in physical education from a series of field experiences in multicultural school settings
- Learning contracts for three middle school students as part of a voluntary after-school tutoring program for children who are physically challenged

Standard 4: Management and Motivation

- Written rules and procedures for conducting a high school elective course titled Personalized Health-Related Fitness
- Videotape demonstrating ability to gain students' cooperation, help students solve problems with peers, and promote self-management among students

Standard 5: Communication

- Log of activities during student teaching documenting interactions with school colleagues, parents, and the community
- Photographs showing various communication techniques (e.g., posters, bulletin boards, newsletter, conferencing) used in the role of a part-time coach

Standard 6: Planning and Instruction

- Lesson plans (three) representing critical thinking (cognitive), cooperative learning (affective), and locomotor skills development (psychomotor) from a senior-level methods course
- Teacher-made materials (e.g., task cards, worksheets, rating scales) for a three-week thematic unit plan titled Learning to Move Through Discovery

Standard 7: Student Assessment

- Case study of a middle school student showing the characteristics, uses, advantages, and limitations of different kinds of assessment (e.g., proficiency tests, motor performance measures, health appraisal questionnaire)
- Summary and critique of an article on the advantages and disadvantages of criterion-referenced and norm-referenced assessment in physical education

Standard 8: Reflection

- Journal of observations from an elementary school field experience focusing on the development of physically educated students
- Copy of questions and answers used in a conference with a student and his or her parent to discuss the student's progress report

Standard 9: Technology

- Collection of spreadsheets reflecting fitness data collected using a handheld computer, transferred to a database, and analyzed using an appropriate software program
- Multimedia program for use at a computer station where the volleyball spike is demonstrated and analyzed

Self-Assessment of Teacher Standards

Name: _____ Date: _____

Standard #: _____ Title: _____

My strengths	Knowledge	
	Performances	
	Dispositions	
My problem areas	Knowledge	
	Performances	
	Dispositions	

Short-term goals	Target date
1.	
2.	
3.	

Long-term goals	Target date
1.	
2.	
3.	

From *Professional and Student Portfolios for Physical Education, Second Edition*, by Vincent J. Melograno, 2006, Champaign, IL: Human Kinetics.

Standard 10: Collaboration

- Letter and certificate of appreciation for conducting a lunch-hour intramural program during student teaching
- Essay from a senior seminar on the Influence of Nonschool Factors on Learning and Engagement in Physical Activity

Another important factor to consider when deciding what artifacts should be required is the type of teacher candidate portfolio. Introductory, presentation, and employment portfolios are characteristically different. They serve different purposes, and they are reviewed by different audiences. For example, the employment portfolio should be streamlined toward enhancing job placement, and it targets prospective employers. Although some work samples and exhibits may be selected for all the portfolios, different portfolio types may also require different kinds of items. Note that the working repository is all-inclusive documentation of knowledge and skills, and it is assembled primarily for adviser or instructor review. It is included here because of the certainty that some items will be required. The natural progression is from the introductory portfolio to the ongoing management of the working repository and then to the presentation portfolio followed by the employment portfolio. Following are lists of items that could be required for each type of portfolio:

Introductory Portfolio

- Relationships with family, friends, and professionals (e.g., photographs, cards or letters, mementos, keepsakes, meaningful gifts)
- Personal interests or hobbies (e.g., tapes or CDs, ticket stubs, items from a collection, list of favorite books, leisure sport statistics)
- Teaching and professional experiences (e.g., custom-made materials, coaching handbook, journal entries, note or letter from parent or former employer evaluations)
- Reasons for wanting to be a physical education teacher (e.g., reflections, statement of philosophy, list of professional goals, essay on a controversial topic)

Working Repository

- Index
- Artifacts representing each teacher standard
- Reflection cover sheets for each artifact (see page 61)
- Artifacts self-assessment checklist (see page 63)
- Reflection artifacts on teacher standards (see table 2.3, pages 71-73)
- Artifacts analysis chart (see page 78)

Presentation Portfolio

- Creative cover (e.g., Traveling on a Journey Toward Teaching or On Target for a Career in Physical Education)
- Table of contents
- Artifacts representing each teacher standard selected from the working repository
- Reflection cover sheets for each artifact (see page 61) selected from the working repository
- Self-assessment of teacher standards (see page 75)

Employment Portfolio

- Table of contents
- Cover letter (i.e., introduce yourself, tell why you are a good job candidate, describe some pertinent experiences, point out areas of the portfolio that are exemplary)
- Biographical sketch
- Resume
- Philosophy of education statement
- Certification or licensing documents (e.g., copy of certificate, teacher exam scores, transcripts)
- Letters of recommendation (e.g., adviser, faculty member, supervisors, employers)
- List of relevant courses (i.e., titles, credits, grades, teacher standards to which courses relate)
- Student teaching evaluations (i.e., supervisor, cooperating teacher)
- Reflection artifacts on teacher standards (see table 2.3, pages 71-73)
- Artifacts representing the teacher standards selected from the working repository and presentation portfolios
- Evaluations of the working repository and presentation portfolio by advisers, instructors, or committees

Optional Artifacts

Teacher candidates should be encouraged to collect optional artifacts as part of the working repository. Particular consideration should be given to school and community activities. Many of them may ultimately be selected for the presentation and employment portfolios in accordance with previous guidelines. Reference to the teacher standards should always be a factor in making selection decisions. Several kinds of artifacts are listed and explained in this section to show the range of options that exist. Each contains a brief definition and the teacher standards it may reflect (numbers in parentheses). These do not exhaust all the possibilities that exist as artifacts. All of these artifacts could be used for the sample professional portfolio system at the end of this chapter and the teacher candidate portfolio builder on the accompanying CD-ROM.

1. *Anecdotal records.* Notes taken during teaching or personal observation about students' cognitive, affective, or motor development; documents growth and development (2), planning and instruction (6), or student assessment (7).

2. *Article summary or critique.* Review of article from a professional journal in connection to a teacher standard; documents potentially any of the teacher standards.

3. *Case study.* In-depth examination of an anonymous student's development over a certain time period; documents growth and development (2), diverse learners (3), or student assessment (7).

4. *Computer programs.* Documentation of software used or incorporated into teaching; documents content knowledge (1), management and motivation (4), planning and instruction (6), or technology (9).

5. *Curriculum plans.* Comprehensive program designs reflecting what students are to learn, how learning is acquired, and how learning is verified; documents diverse learners (3), management and motivation (4), communication (5), planning and instruction (6), or student assessment (7).

6. *Essays.* Written papers on topics pertinent to relevant education topics; documents potentially any of the teacher standards.

Artifacts Analysis Chart

Kind of artifact (e.g., curriculum plan)	Name of artifact (e.g., thematic unit on teamwork)	Teacher standards									
		1	2	3	4	5	6	7	8	9	10

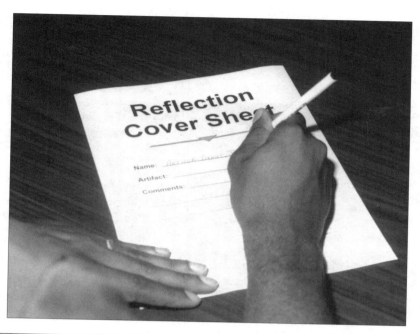

Reflection cover sheets are needed for each artifact in the working repository.

7. *Evaluations.* Performance assessments from clinical experiences, field experiences, student teaching, and jobs; documents potentially any of the teacher standards.

8. *Goal statements.* Provides information about the direction one wants to take professionally and the means for getting there; documents potentially any of the teacher standards.

9. *Honors.* Letters, awards, or certificates that verify outstanding contributions; documents communication (5) or collaboration (10).

10. *Instructional materials.* Custom-made teaching aids (e.g., transparencies, charts, videotapes, games, manipulations, multimedia programs); documents planning and instruction (6) or technology (9).

11. *Journals.* Ongoing record of experiences that includes dates, times, and reflections; documents potentially any of the teacher standards.

12. *Lesson plans.* Execution of instructional planning including objectives, activities, procedures, resources, time lines, and evaluation; documents growth and development (2), diverse learners (3), management and motivation (4), communication (5), planning and instruction (6), student assessment (7), or technology (9).

13. *Photographs.* Shows teacher competence and accomplishments that cannot be physically included in a portfolio; documents diverse learners (3), management and motivation (4), communication (5), planning and instruction (6), technology (9), or collaboration (10).

14. *Projects.* Products resulting from endeavors that involve problem solving or researching current topics; documents potentially any of the teacher standards.

15. *Readings list.* Identification of professional readings including reactions to issues and concepts; documents potentially any of the teacher standards.

16. *Technology resources.* Samples of materials representing how state-of-the-art technology is incorporated into teaching (e.g., information retrieval via the Internet, e-mail uses, interactive video, cable and electronic television); documents content knowledge (1), communication (5), planning and instruction (6), technology (9), or collaboration (10).

17. *Unit plans.* Integrated plan for instruction on a topic covering several days or weeks including goals, objectives, content outline, learning activities, and evaluation procedures; documents growth and development (2), diverse learners (3), management and motivation (4), communication (5), planning and instruction (6), student assessment (7), or technology (9).

18. *Videotapes or video clips.* Recording of actual teaching episodes in clinical, field, or work settings; documents diverse learners (3), management and motivation (4), communication (5), planning and instruction (6), student assessment (7), or technology (9).

Artifacts Analysis

In addition to the assembly and management guidelines offered previously in this chapter, teacher candidates need to "manage" their documentation of the teacher standards. Each artifact selected for the working repository and the presentation and employment portfolios should be analyzed to help determine (1) standards that need work, (2) an overreliance on some kinds of artifacts, and (3) the need to diversify artifacts. The artifacts analysis chart on page 78 can be used for this purpose. Check marks or dates could be entered to record the range of artifacts in support of the 10 teacher standards.

Assessment

Suggestions for self-reflection and self-assessment were previously outlined. The focus in this assessment section is on self-analysis. However, if teacher candidates are to become fully involved in evaluating their growth and competence, they also need to communicate the contents of their portfolio to others and receive assessment feedback. Whether portfolios are facilitated through advisers, courses, or oversight committees, results of formal and informal assessment should be provided at planned intervals.

The professional portfolio documents a teacher candidate's growth and competence throughout a physical education teacher education (PETE) program. If it truly represents an ongoing, cumulative development of knowledge, skills, and dispositions, then feedback and assessment should also be ongoing and cumulative. Continual review is fundamental to the portfolio process. Key checkpoints are also inherent to any teacher education program, such as admission, continuation decisions, entry to field experiences, and exit from student teaching. They represent the progressive stages of professional training. Normally, a process-level review is carried out at each stage that might include program course requirements and grade point average minimums. Therefore, it should be clear that periodic reviews are not only essential, but also natural to a portfolio system within a teacher education program.

Because the portfolio is tied to accountability and is itself an assessment tool, individual artifacts, the whole portfolio, or both should be evaluated according to established standards. Also, criteria should be referenced to the portfolio's *content* and *quality*. Guidelines for the formative and summative assessment of teacher candidate portfolios recognize these criteria.

Formative Assessment

When information is sought to help decide how to adjust or improve performance during a learning process, assessment serves a formative function (step 8 of the portfolio-designing process). The working repository and presentation portfolios are primarily associated with formative assessment. For example, if the working repository is linked to key courses, feedback and assessment could include peer reflection, peer conferences, instructor conferences, and grading by the instructor as part of course requirements. For the presentation portfolio, additional feedback and assessment could be received from peers, faculty members, and advisers during a posterlike session that is organized within a key course.

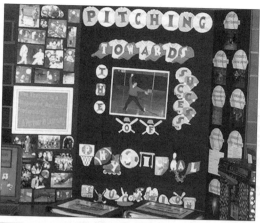

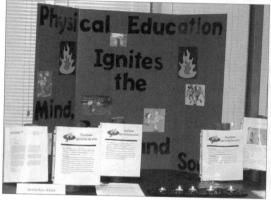
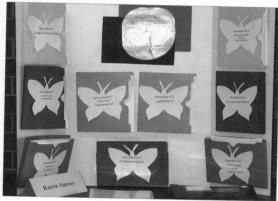

The presentation portfolio can be reviewed in a posterlike session.
Courtesy of Jilline R. Fuleki.

Various feedback and assessment constructs can serve a formative purpose, including peer reflection, candidate-led conferences, and performance assessment. They are applicable to both the working repository and presentation portfolios, and they can be used in systems guided by advisers, course instructors, or committees.

Peer Reflection

Because teacher candidates are deeply involved in their own portfolio development, they are qualified to review the work of other teacher candidates and provide feedback. In fact, they could even select items they feel should be included in another candidate's portfolio. However, it is important that teacher candidates who provide the feedback be trained in how to (1) offer constructive or encouraging words, (2) disagree with an idea rather than with the person, and (3) assess the quality of work based on the established standards. The sample peer reflection sheet that appears on page 86 could be used to provide a direct review of someone else's portfolio or to provide feedback in reaction to a portfolio presentation to a small group of peers, to an entire class, or through a posterlike session.

Candidate-Led Conferences

Previously, conferences were considered part of the general portfolio process in which teacher candidates shared their feelings about their portfolios. Conferences also serve a formative assessment purpose by giving teacher candidates an opportunity to discuss and receive information about their portfolios. The focus of conferences serving this function should be on the teacher standards and their documentation, regardless of who is providing the feedback. Some are reluctant to use direct personal communication as a legitimate form of assessment because it is considered too subjective. However, when structured properly and when led by the teacher candidate, conferences can yield important assessment data. If teacher candidates are responsible for handling the conference protocol, then autonomy and ownership are reinforced. Other benefits are increased communication and increased commitment to learning through responsible and self-directed behavior. Teacher candidates could organize the conference around the following bridging questions and reflective stems:

- Which teacher standards are documented most effectively? Why?
- Which teacher standards are documented least effectively? Why?
- What artifacts really made an impression on you? Why?
- What artifacts need the most work?
- The part(s) of my portfolio I am most proud of is . . .
- You will be impressed with . . .
- If I could do this over again, I would . . .

Conferences offer teacher candidates the opportunity to refine and clarify their abilities and to respond to others. As a result, they can become more thoughtful and truly reflective in assessing outcomes and setting goals. The portfolio would need to be available for review in advance of the scheduled conference. Upon review of the teacher candidate's working repository or presentation portfolio in preparation for the conference, peers, advisers, instructors, committee members, or school personnel could structure their feedback around the following reflective stems:

- The part of the portfolio I like best is _____ because . . .
- The part I'm not really clear about is _____ because . . .
- The part you need to tell me more about is . . .
- You could improve your portfolio by . . .
- My overall impression is . . .

Performance Assessment

During the formative assessment phase, the teacher candidate needs specific feedback about the teacher standards. Because the teacher standards serve as the basis for organizing the professional portfolio, they are central to any scheme that has meaningful feedback as its goal. Although many kinds of assessment tools are available, a rubric is recommended for judging the artifacts that are used to document individual standards. A rubric is a scoring guide designed to assess the quality of performance. It consists of a measurement scale of criteria that explains the possible levels of performance (achievement) for a learning goal. However, the purpose of the rubric is to define quality, not just to provide a scoring device. In this case, rubrics are used to provide feedback about the knowledge, skills, and dispositions that support each standard. For this reason, scoring rubrics have emerged as a popular assessment tool in conjunction with standards. Rubrics are illustrated in table 2.4 for two teacher standards—growth and development and student assessment. A judgment is made as to whether the set of artifacts demonstrates that the teacher candidate is at the exemplary, proficient, emerging, or unacceptable level for each of the standards. Additional information about rubric development that is applicable to the use of rubrics in PETE programs can be found in chapter 3 (pages 178-185).

The working repository represents the broadest view of the teacher candidate's growing competence and serves as the underlying framework for the presentation portfolio. As a result, advisers, course instructors, or committees should conduct a more formal rating of the presentation portfolio. If the portfolio system is linked to "checkpoint" courses, instructors may need to convert ratings to letter grades. The weighted rubric in the Teacher Candidate Portfolio Assessment form on page 88 could be used to make an overall judgment about the portfolio. A rating form such as the one on pages 89-91 is another tool for comprehensively analyzing the working repository or presentation portfolio.

Table 2.4 Rubrics to Assess Portfolio Artifacts: Documenting Growth and Development and Student Assessment Teacher Standards

STANDARD 2: GROWTH AND DEVELOPMENT

UNDERSTAND HOW INDIVIDUALS LEARN AND DEVELOP, AND PROVIDE OPPORTUNITIES THAT SUPPORT PHYSICAL, COGNITIVE, SOCIAL, AND EMOTIONAL DEVELOPMENT (NASPE, 2003).

Criteria	LEVELS OF ACHIEVEMENT			
	Unacceptable (0)	Emerging (1)	Proficient (2)	Exemplary (3)
<u>Knowledge and Understanding</u> Knows how learning and development occur—how students grow and develop, become physically fit, construct knowledge, and acquire skills; knows how to address development factors when making instructional decisions; understands progressions, ranges of individual variation, and levels of readiness; understands the value of practice opportunities for growth and development.	Lacks knowledge and understanding of major theories of cognitive, physical, emotional, and social development; of how students construct knowledge and acquire cognitive skills; and of motor developmental progressions.	Has limited knowledge and understanding of major theories of cognitive, physical, emotional, and social development; of how students construct knowledge and acquire cognitive skills; and of motor developmental progressions.	Has acceptable knowledge and understanding of major theories of cognitive, physical, emotional, and social development; of how students construct knowledge and acquire cognitive skills; and of motor developmental progressions.	Has extensive knowledge and understanding of major theories of cognitive, physical, emotional, and social development; of how students construct knowledge and acquire cognitive skills; and of motor developmental progressions.
<u>Skill and Performance</u> Assesses individual and group performance to design safe instruction that meets student developmental needs in the motor, cognitive, social, and emotional domains; stimulates student reflection on prior knowledge, experiences, and skills; encourages students to assume responsibility for their own learning.	Lacks ability to apply knowledge of educational theories and concepts, to build on prior knowledge in the development of students' thinking and moving and the implementation of appropriate instructional activities; lacks ability to integrate awareness of individual differences and similarities into practice.	Has limited ability to apply knowledge of educational theories and concepts, to build on prior knowledge in the development of students' thinking and moving and the implementation of appropriate instructional activities; has limited ability to integrate awareness of individual differences and similarities into practice.	Consistently applies knowledge of educational theories and concepts, to build on prior knowledge in the development of students' thinking and moving and the implementation of appropriate instructional activities; consistently integrates awareness of individual differences and similarities into practice.	Consistently and deliberately applies knowledge of educational theories and concepts; provides opportunities for students to discover connections between prior knowledge and movement and present learning; consistently and deliberately integrates awareness of individual differences and similarities into practice.

(continued)

Table 2.4 *(continued)*

STANDARD 2: GROWTH AND DEVELOPMENT
UNDERSTAND HOW INDIVIDUALS LEARN AND DEVELOP, AND PROVIDE OPPORTUNITIES THAT SUPPORT PHYSICAL, COGNITIVE, SOCIAL, AND EMOTIONAL DEVELOPMENT (NASPE, 2003)

Criteria	LEVELS OF ACHIEVEMENT			
	Unacceptable (0)	Emerging (1)	Proficient (2)	Exemplary (3)
<u>Dispositions</u> Appreciates and promotes physical activity in the overall growth and development of students; appreciates individual variations in growth and development and is committed to helping students become competent and self-confident.	Lacks appreciation and respect for developmental changes, individual differences, self-efficacy, the fact that all students are able to achieve, and the instructional opportunity of students' misconceptions.	Has limited appreciation and respect for developmental changes, individual differences, self-efficacy, the fact that all students are able to achieve, and the instructional opportunity of students' misconceptions.	Consistently appreciates and respects developmental changes, individual differences, self-efficacy, the fact that all students are able to achieve, and the instructional opportunity of students' misconceptions.	Consistently and deliberately appreciates and respects developmental changes, individual differences, self-efficacy, the fact that all students are able to achieve, and the instructional opportunity of students' misconceptions.

STANDARD 7: STUDENT ASSESSMENT
UNDERSTAND AND USE THE VARIED TYPES OF ASSESSMENT AND THEIR CONTRIBUTION TO OVERALL PROGRAM CONTINUITY AND THE DEVELOPMENT OF THE PHYSICAL, COGNITIVE, SOCIAL, AND EMOTIONAL DOMAINS (NASPE, 2003)

Criteria	LEVELS OF ACHIEVEMENT			
	Unacceptable (0)	Emerging (1)	Proficient (2)	Exemplary (3)
<u>Knowledge and Understanding</u> Knows characteristics, uses, advantages, and limitations of different types of assessment; knows how to select and use developmentally appropriate assessment strategies and instruments congruent with physical activity learning goals; understands measurement issues (e.g., validity, reliability, bias); understands the use of assessment as an integral part of instruction to provide feedback; understands how to use and interpret student performance data to inform instructional decisions and report progress.	Lacks understanding of rationale for adapting assessment procedures to meet students' individual needs; is familiar with a very limited range of formal and informal assessment strategies; lacks understanding of fundamental test statistics and constructs such as validity and reliability.	Is familiar with a limited range of formal and informal assessment strategies; possesses initial understanding of fundamental test statistics and constructs such as validity and reliability.	Is familiar with a variety of formal and informal assessment strategies; understands and can accurately calculate fundamental test statistics; possesses satisfactory knowledge of constructs such as reliability and validity.	Is very knowledgeable about a variety of formal and informal assessment strategies, including their inherent strengths and limitations; understands and can accurately calculate fundamental test statistics; knows different types of validity and reliability.

Skill and Performance Uses a variety of formal and informal assessment techniques to assess student progress (e.g., criterion- and norm-referenced, formative and summative, monitor performance and authentic assessments); uses assessment strategies to involve students in self-assessment; maintains records of student performance and communicates student progress based on appropriate indicators.	Selects and uses instruments for assessment that are incongruent with learning goals; lacks ability to develop, administer, and interpret a variety of formal and informal instruments to evaluate processes and products; is unable to devise and employ appropriate and reliable scoring procedures for evaluating student work; cannot adapt assessment procedures to meet students' individual needs or employs inappropriate adaptations; cannot explain, use, or report assessment strategies and results.	Selects and uses procedures and instruments for assessment that are congruent with learning goals, but lacks proficiency in designing and interpreting measures to assess complex tasks and higher-order knowledge and skills; is able to develop, administer, and interpret a limited range of formal and informal activities and instruments to evaluate products; has difficulty adapting assessment procedures to meet the individual needs of students; heavily relies on only one type of assessment; accurately explains and reports assessment strategies and results.	Selects and uses procedures and instruments for assessment that are congruent with learning goals and is somewhat proficient in designing and interpreting measures for assessing complex tasks and higher-order knowledge and skills; is able to develop, administer, and interpret a variety of formal and informal activities and instruments to evaluate products; usually employs reliable scoring procedures, clearly written items and prompts, and unambiguous directions to assess students; inconsistently adapts assessment procedures to meet the individual needs of students; clearly and accurately explains and reports assessment strategies and results.	Selects and uses procedures and instruments for assessment that are congruent with learning goals; is proficient in designing and interpreting measures for assessing complex tasks and higher-order knowledge and skills; is able to develop, administer, and interpret a variety of formal and informal activities and instruments to evaluate both products and processes; consistently employs reliable scoring procedures, clearly written items and prompts, and unambiguous directions to assess students; routinely adapts assessment procedures to meet the individual needs of students; uses multiple ways to clearly and accurately explain and report assessment strategies and results.
Dispositions Values ongoing assessment to identify student needs and abilities; recognizes that a variety of assessment strategies are necessary.	Does not perceive assessment as an integral part of instruction as evidenced by its lack of use in instructional planning; does not believe in adapting assessment procedures to meet students' individual needs.	Somewhat values the role of assessment in evaluating student progress, but generally fails to make use of the results of formative and summative measures to reflect on practice and improve instruction; believes in occasionally adapting assessment procedures to meet students' individual needs.	Values assessment as an integral part of instruction and endeavors to use the results of formative and summative assessments to reflect on practice and improve instruction; believes in adapting assessment procedures to meet individual needs but inconsistently uses adaptations.	Values assessment as an integral part of instruction; consistently uses the results of formative and summative assessments to reflect on practice and improve instruction; consistently demonstrates a belief in the adaptation of assessment procedures by using adaptations to meet individual needs.

Standards from *National Standards for Beginning Physical Education Teachers*, 2nd edition (2003) with permission from the National Association for Sport and Physical Education (NASPE), 1900 Association Drive, Reston, VA 20191-1599.

Peer Reflection Sheet

Date: _____

To: _____

From: _____

Please review the attached items that are included in my professional portfolio and provide feedback. Thanks!

1. What teacher standard is documented the most effectively? Why?

2. What teacher standard is documented the least effectively? Why?

3. What artifacts really made an impression on you? Why?

4. What artifacts do you feel need the most work? Why?

5. What is your overall impression of the organization and presentation of artifacts?

Signed: _____ Date: _____

Summative Assessment

Assessment of a summative nature is used to decide the extent to which teacher candidates have been successful in mastering final outcomes or standards (step 9 of the portfolio-designing process). Because the employment portfolio is viewed as the final or exit portfolio, it is subject to summative assessment protocols. However, any feedback and assessment format must recognize the purposes of the employment portfolio—to synthesize the knowledge, skills, and dispositions of the teacher candidate and enhance job placement. Feedback about the employment portfolio can be received from peers, but the primary feedback and assessment source should be experienced professionals (e.g., advisers, faculty members, committee members, school personnel).

Various feedback and assessment constructs can serve a summative purpose including conferences, simulation, and performance assessment. These constructs can be used in portfolio systems guided by advisers, course instructors, or committees.

Candidate-Led Conferences

The format of conferences for summative reviews is basically the same as the format described earlier for formative assessment. However, the focus is different because the employment portfolio is different from the working repository and presentation portfolio in terms of purpose, organization, and presentation. Regardless of who is involved in conferences, discussion should be centered on how effectively teacher candidates document their competence as fully qualified, professionally mature beginning physical education teachers. Upon review of the employment portfolio by peers, advisers, instructors, committee members, or school personnel, conferences could be structured around a comparison of the teacher candidate's perceptions and the conference participants' opinion regarding the following areas: (1) the candidate's overall strengths as a physical education teacher, (2) artifacts that represent "holistic" abilities and dispositions toward teaching, (3) how the portfolio verifies that the beginning teacher standards have been met, (4) what teacher standards the candidate will continue to move toward meeting as a practicing teacher, and (5) teacher standards that need work as revealed by the portfolio.

Simulation

The employment portfolio has an important practical use. It can be presented to prospective employers as documentation of teaching competence. So far, feedback and evaluation strategies have focused primarily on the "physical" qualities of portfolios. Certainly, the employment portfolio should be assessed in the same manner. But, it would also be beneficial to find out how well it serves the job search process.

A team playing the role of employers could conduct a job interview simulation. Peers can take on roles or school personnel can help create real-life interview situations. Participants and observers (e.g., peers, faculty members, advisers) could provide invaluable feedback, not only about the portfolio's contents and quality, but also about its use and effectiveness during a job interview. Feedback could be provided in answer to the following questions:

- How well does the portfolio portray teaching competence?
- Which teacher standards are clearly demonstrated?
- Which teacher standards are not clearly demonstrated?
- What changes in the portfolio would help the job interview?
- How could the portfolio be used more effectively during a job interview?

Performance Assessment

The importance of the employment portfolio cannot be overstated. Because this portfolio is a composite of the beginning physical education teacher, it deserves a more formal rating by advisers, course instructors, and committees. Although the teacher standards remain the foundation,

Teacher Candidate Portfolio Assessment

Name: _____

WEIGHTED SCORING RUBRIC					
PORTFOLIO CONTENTS					
Elements	**Not included** **0**	**Included, but incomplete** **1**	**Fully developed** **2**	**Weight**	**Score**
1. Cover design	❏	❏	❏	× 1	(2)
2. Table of contents/index	❏	❏	❏	× 1	(2)
3. Required/optional artifacts	❏	❏	❏	× 8	(16)
4. Reflective cover sheets for each artifact	❏	❏	❏	× 2	(4)
5. Artifacts self-assessment checklist	❏	❏	❏	× 2	(4)
6. Self-assessment of standards	❏	❏	❏	× 3	(6)
7. Artifacts analysis	❏	❏	❏	× 2	(4)
PORTFOLIO QUALITY					
Criteria	**Low quality; below expectations** **0**	**Satisfactory quality; meets expectations** **1**	**High quality; above expectations** **2**	**Weight**	**Score**
Organization	❏	❏	❏	× 2	(4)
Layout/visual appeal	❏	❏	❏	× 2	(4)
Creativity/expressiveness	❏	❏	❏	× 2	(4)

Comments: _____

Total score: _____
(50)

Grace: _____

Grade: _____

_____

_____

_____

Scale
A = 41-50

B = 31-40

C = 21-30

D = 11-20

F = 0-10

Signed: _____   Date: _____

From *Professional and Student Portfolios for Physical Education, Second Edition*, by Vincent J. Melograno, 2006, Champaign, IL: Human Kinetics.

Portfolio Rating Form

Name: _____ Date: _____

Instructions: Use the following scale to rate each portfolio item according to the following criteria.

$\quad$ 4 = Outstanding $\quad$ 3 = Good $\quad$ 2 = Satisfactory $\quad$ 1 = Fair $\quad$ 0 = Poor

Organization: Follows instructions; completeness of items; clear layout; overall creativity

Form and quality: Writing mechanics; expressiveness; visual appeal; spelling, punctuation, and grammar

Evidence of understanding: Explicit demonstration of standard's knowledge, skills, and dispositions; application of ideas

	Form and organization	Quality	Evidence of understanding
1. Content Knowledge			
Reflection artifact on standard	_____	_____	_____
Reflection cover sheets	_____	_____	_____
Required artifacts:			
Name: _____	_____	_____	_____
Name: _____	_____	_____	_____
Optional artifacts:			
Name: _____	_____		_____
Name: _____	_____	_____	_____
2. Growth and Development			
Reflection artifact on standard	_____	_____	_____
Reflection cover sheets	_____	_____	_____
Required artifacts:			
Name: _____	_____	_____	_____
Name: _____	_____	_____	_____
Optional artifacts:			
Name: _____	_____	_____	_____
Name: _____	_____	_____	_____
3. Diverse Learners			
Reflection artifact on standard	_____	_____	_____
Reflection cover sheets	_____	_____	_____
Required artifacts:			
Name: _____	_____	_____	_____
Name: _____	_____	_____	_____
Optional artifacts:			
Name: _____	_____	_____	_____
Name: _____	_____	_____	_____

(continued)

From *Professional and Student Portfolios for Physical Education, Second Edition*, by Vincent J. Melograno, 2006, Champaign, IL: Human Kinetics.

(continued)

	Form and organization	Quality	Evidence of understanding
4. Management and Motivation			
Reflection artifact on standard	————	————	————
Reflection cover sheets	————	————	————
Required artifacts:			
Name: _____	————	————	————
Name: _____	————	————	————
Optional artifacts:			
Name: _____	————	————	————
Name: _____	————	————	————
5. Communication			
Reflection artifact on standard	————	————	————
Reflection cover sheets	————	————	————
Required artifacts:			
Name: _____	————	————	————
Name: _____	————	————	————
Optional artifacts:			
Name: _____	————	————	————
Name: _____	————	————	————
6. Planning and Instruction			
Reflection artifact on standard	————	————	————
Reflection cover sheets	————	————	————
Required artifacts:			
Name: _____	————	————	————
Name: _____	————	————	————
Optional artifacts:			
Name: _____	————	————	————
Name: _____	————	————	————
7. Student Assessment			
Reflection artifact on standard	————	————	————
Reflection cover sheets	————	————	————
Required artifacts:			
Name: _____	————	————	————
Name: _____	————	————	————
Optional artifacts:			
Name: _____	————	————	————
Name: _____	————	————	————

	Form and organization	Quality	Evidence of understanding
8. Reflection			
Reflection artifact on standard	_____	_____	_____
Reflection cover sheets	_____	_____	_____
Required artifacts:			
Name: _____			
Name: _____	_____	_____	_____
Optional artifacts:	_____	_____	_____
Name: _____			
Name: _____	_____	_____	_____
	_____	_____	_____
9. Technology			
Reflection artifact on standard	_____	_____	_____
Reflection cover sheets	_____	_____	_____
Required artifacts:			
Name: _____			
Name: _____	_____	_____	_____
Optional artifacts:	_____	_____	_____
Name: _____			
Name: _____	_____	_____	_____
	_____	_____	_____
10. Collaboration			
Reflection artifact on standard	_____	_____	_____
Reflection cover sheets	_____	_____	_____
Required artifacts:			
Name: _____			
Name: _____	_____	_____	_____
Optional artifacts:	_____	_____	_____
Name: _____			
Name: _____	_____	_____	_____
	_____	_____	_____

Overall Evaluation

_____ This portfolio is *exemplary* in documenting the teacher standards at this point in the teacher candidate's program of study; *maintain progress*.

_____ This portfolio is *above expectation* in documenting the teacher standards at this point in the teacher candidate's program of study; *minor revisions are advised*.

_____ This portfolio is *marginal* in documenting the teacher standards at this point in the teacher candidate's program of study; *several revisions are advised*.

_____ This portfolio is *below expectations* in documenting the teacher standards at this point in the teacher candidate's program of study; *major revisions are advised*.

_____ This portfolio is *unacceptable* in documenting the teacher standards at this point in the teacher candidate's program of study; *reconsider role as teacher*.

Review by: _____ Date: _____

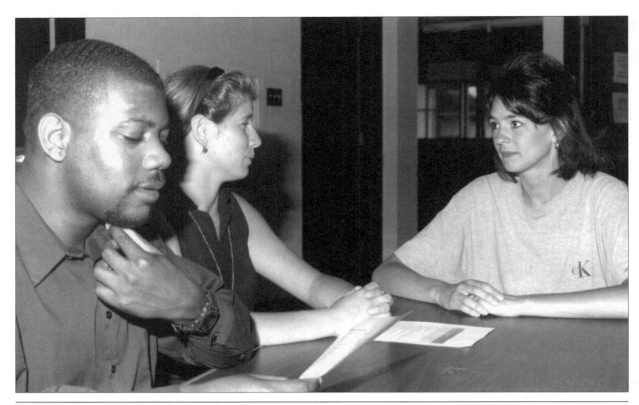

The employment portfolio is the focus for the simulated job interview.

any rating scheme should incorporate explicit content and quality criteria. As a supplement to the employment portfolio, a brochure could be produced that reflects the teacher candidate's "theme" along with a biographical sketch, a summary of the teacher standards, and an outline of the portfolio contents. A business card with the same theme could accompany the brochure. This strategy for marketing one's qualifications for teaching was illustrated in figure 2.1 (page 66).

If the portfolio system is linked to "checkpoint" courses, instructors may need to convert ratings to letter grades. For example, a course or teaching seminar (e.g., Gateway to the Profession) may be offered as a companion to student teaching. The weighted rubric in the Web-Based Employment Portfolio Assessment on page 94. could be used to make an overall judgment about the employment portfolio. In this example, note that the employment portfolio is Web based for easy access and review. A form such as the Employment Portfolio Rating Form on page 95 is another tool that can be used to assess employment portfolios.

Summary

Have you achieved the expected outcomes (see page 50) for this chapter? You should have acquired the knowledge and skills needed for developing professional portfolios for teacher candidates in physical education. The professional portfolio is an authentic way for physical education teacher candidates to document their competence. Developing and implementing a portfolio system includes the following steps:

1. Determine the primary and secondary purposes of the teacher candidate portfolio.

2. Select the types of teacher candidate portfolios that will be included in the system.

3. Identify the standards around which the teacher candidate portfolio will be organized.

4. Choose an implementation strategy that matches the advising philosophy and commitment of the PETE program.

5. Determine how various processes of involvement will be included in the teacher candidate portfolio system.

6. Identify options for organizing, maintaining, and storing the teacher candidate portfolio.

7. Decide *what, how, who,* and *when* relative to the selection of required and optional artifacts for the teacher candidate portfolio.

8. Develop checkpoints and feedback procedures that will provide a formative review of the teacher candidate portfolio.

9. Establish the approaches to be used for conducting a summative review of the teacher candidate portfolio.

Through introductory, presentation, and employment types of portfolios, teacher candidates can verify the wide range of knowledge, skills, and dispositions acquired in a physical education teacher education (PETE) program. Standards for beginning physical education teachers are recommended as the basis for organizing these portfolios. Alternative strategies can be used separately or in combination to implement portfolios (i.e., adviser directed, course affiliated, committee oversight, or program phases), each of which is characterized by different processes of involvement (i.e., training, reflection, self-assessment, presentations, and conferences).

Several assembly and structural options are available for managing and storing the different types of portfolios. Electronic-based and Web-based protocols are essential to the development and implementation of a high-quality portfolio system. The selection of artifacts is dependent on the basic processes of reflection and self-assessment. The distinction between required and optional artifacts must consider the teacher standards and the type of portfolio.

Formal and informal feedback and assessment procedures should accompany any teacher candidate portfolio system. Formative assessment can include peer review and reflection and candidate-led conferences. Ongoing performance assessment is fundamental to the process including the use of standards-based scoring rubrics. Summative assessment serves the purpose of making final or exit judgments about teacher competence. Candidate-led conferences and job interview simulations are useful techniques along with performance assessment strategies.

Sample Professional Portfolio System

To synthesize the information presented in this chapter, a sample portfolio system is provided for use in a physical education teacher education (PETE) program. Although the setting for this system is hypothetical, most of the portfolio elements are typical of teacher education training programs. The system incorporates the concepts and principles advanced in this chapter. It is structured in the form of a practical handbook for physical education teacher candidates.

In addition, the CD-ROM accompanying the book provides a template (portfolio builder) to create an electronic-based teacher candidate professional portfolio using Microsoft PowerPoint®. Instructions are provided for navigating through the slides that include hyperlinks for access to the necessary files. When the portfolio is completed, it can be copied to a CD for distribution and review. It can also be uploaded to the Internet for access as a Web-based portfolio. The following components are used to organize the portfolio:

- Table of contents
- Introduction
- Resume
- Coursework
- Teacher candidate standards
- Lesson plan sample
- Student work samples
- Gallery (pictures, video clips)
- Letters of recommendation
- Teaching evaluations

Web-Based Employment Portfolio Assessment

Name: _____

	WEIGHTED SCORING RUBRIC				
	PORTFOLIO CONTENTS				
Elements*	**Not included 0**	**Included, but incomplete 1**	**Fully developed 2**	**Weight**	**Score**
1. Home page portfolio summary with links	❏	❏	❏	× 2	(4)
2. Biographical sketch/introductory statement	❏	❏	❏	× 2	(4)
3. Updated resume	❏	❏	❏	× 2	(4)
4. Organized list of relevant courses	❏	❏	❏	× 1	(2)
5. Strength of artifacts reflective statements	❏	❏	❏	× 12	(24)
6. Strength/scope of artifacts to support each standard	❏	❏	❏	× 12	(24)
7. Video clips showing teaching style/photo gallery	❏	❏	❏	× 3	(6)
8. Reflections on each teacher standard	❏	❏	❏	× 2	(4)
	PORTFOLIO QUALITY				
Criteria	**Low quality; below expectations 0**	**Satisfactory quality; meets expectations 1**	**High quality; above expectations 2**	**Weight**	**Score**
Layout/visual appeal	❏	❏	❏	× 2	(4)
Creativity/expressiveness	❏	❏	❏	× 2	(4)

* Does not include certification or licensure documents and letters of recommendation.

Comments: _____

Total score: _____

_____   A = 65-80   (80)

B = 50-64

_____   C = 35-49   Grade: _____

D = 20-34

_____   F = 0-19

Signed: _____ Date: _____

From *Professional and Student Portfolios for Physical Education, Second Edition,* by Vincent J. Melograno, 2006, Champaign, IL: Human Kinetics.

Employment Portfolio Rating Form

Name: _____ Date: _____

Portfolio Contents

Components of the employment portfolio should be verified according to the following indicators:

+ = Fully developed   ✓ = Included, but incomplete   0 = Not included

_____ Table of contents

_____ Cover letter

_____ Biographical sketch

_____ Resume

_____ Philosophy of education statement

_____ Certification/licensing documents

_____ Letters of recommendation

_____ List of relevant courses

_____ Student teaching evaluations

_____ Reflection artifacts on teacher standards

_____ Artifacts representing the teacher standards

_____ Assessments of the presentation portfolio

Comments: _____

_____

Portfolio Quality

The employment portfolio should evidence an acceptable level of quality. Use the following scale to rate each characteristic and artifact:

2 = High quality;
above expectations

1 = Satisfactory quality;
meets expectations

0 = Low quality;
below expectations

_____ Organization

_____ Layout/visual appeal

_____ Creativity/expressiveness

_____ Spelling, punctuation, grammar

_____ Artifact 1: _____

_____ Artifact 2: _____

_____ Artifact 3: _____

_____ Artifact 4: _____

_____ Artifact 5: _____

_____ Artifact 6: _____

_____ Artifact 7: _____

_____ Artifact 8: _____

_____ Artifact 9: _____

_____ Artifact 10: _____

_____ Artifact 11: _____

_____ Artifact 12: _____

_____ Artifact 13: _____

_____ Artifact 14: _____

_____ Artifact 15: _____

_____ Artifact 16: _____

Summary Evaluation

Portfolio contents: _____ Outstanding _____ Satisfactory _____ Unsatisfactory

Portfolio quality: _____ Outstanding _____ Satisfactory _____ Unsatisfactory

Evaluator signature: _____ Date: _____

From *Professional and Student Portfolios for Physical Education, Second Edition*, by Vincent J. Melograno, 2006, Champaign, IL: Human Kinetics.

Teacher Candidate Handbook
Physical Education Teacher Education (PETE)

Professional Portfolio

Wherever State University

College of Education
Department of Physical Education

CONTENTS

OVERVIEW

The physical education teacher education (PETE) program at Wherever State University (WSU) develops educators who facilitate student learning in a democratic, pluralistic, and technological society. The program offers comprehensive coursework in general education, professional education, and the major field including clinical activities, field experiences, and student teaching. By successfully completing the program, the physical education teacher candidate is fully competent to assume the role of *beginning physical education teacher* at the in-service level and to qualify for the *multiage teaching license.*

PROGRAM MODEL AND STANDARDS

Competent beginning physical education teachers can demonstrate certain knowledge, skills, and dispositions within the organizing theme "teacher as a reflective, inquiry-oriented practitioner who knows the physical education discipline and applies content and pedagogy that is sensitive to individual learner needs." Successful physical education teachers reflect on their teaching, on their decisions, on their problems and solutions to those problems, on their students, and on the processes of teaching and learning. To operationalize the organizing theme, a set of standards was sought that defines what a beginning physical educator should know and be able to do. Because of their widespread acceptance, NASPE's *National Standards for Beginning Physical Education Teachers* are targets for the physical educator. These standards are as follows:*

Standard 1: Content Knowledge

Understand physical education content and disciplinary concepts related to the development of a physically educated person.

Standard 2: Growth and Development

Understand how individuals learn and develop, and can provide opportunities that support physical, cognitive, social, and emotional development.

From *Professional and Student Portfolios for Physical Education, Second Edition,* by Vincent J. Melograno, 2006, Champaign, IL: Human Kinetics.

97

Standard 3: Diverse Learners

Understand how individuals differ in their approaches to learning and create appropriate instruction adapted to these differences.

Standard 4: Management and Motivation

Use and have an understanding of individual and group motivations and behavior to create a safe learning environment that encourages positive social interaction, active engagement in learning, and self-motivation.

Standard 5: Communication

Use knowledge of effective verbal, nonverbal, and media communication techniques to enhance learning and engagement in physical activity settings.

Standard 6: Planning and Instruction

Understand the importance of planning developmentally appropriate instructional units to foster the development of a physically educated person.

Standard 7: Student Assessment

Understand and use the varied types of assessment and their contribution to overall program continuity and the development of the physical, cognitive, social, and emotional domains.

Standard 8: Reflection

Understand the importance of being a reflective practitioner and its contribution to overall professional development and seek opportunities to sustain professional growth.

Standard 9: Technology

Use information technology to enhance learning and personal and professional productivity.

Standard 10: Collaboration

Understand the necessity of fostering relationships with colleagues, parents/guardians, and community agencies to support the development of a physically educated person.

*Reprinted from *National Standards for Beginning Physical Education Teachers* (2nd ed.) (2003) with permission from the National Association for Sport and Physical Education (NASPE), 1900 Association Drive, Reston, VA 20191-1599.

PURPOSES OF THE PROFESSIONAL PORTFOLIO

The WSU professional portfolio is an organized, goal-oriented documentation of your professional growth and achieved competence in the complex act of teaching physical education. It illustrates who you are as a teacher. Although the portfolio is a collection of documents, it provides tangible evidence of the wide range of knowledge, dispositions, and skills that you possess as a growing professional. The portfolio is a personal tool for synthesizing all these aspects. Given a highly competitive job market, you must be able to convey to others the knowledge and skills you have acquired in your professional teacher education program. The professional portfolio can help you do this. Therefore, the primary purpose of the professional portfolio is to verify the knowledge, skills, and dispositions acquired through coursework, clinical and field experiences, student teaching, and community involvements. Secondary purposes are to (1) help you grow professionally, (2) satisfy licensing requirements, and (3) enhance employment.

PORTFOLIO MECHANICS

The professional portfolio is a purposeful and systematic collection of work that shows individual effort, progress, and achievement at WSU. More specific information and guidelines are needed regarding the actual mechanics of portfolio development. In this section of the handbook, the following questions are answered: What types of portfolios will be used? How should the portfolio be organized? What portfolio processes will be employed? How should the portfolio be managed?

From *Professional and Student Portfolios for Physical Education, Second Edition,* by Vincent J. Melograno, 2006, Champaign, IL: Human Kinetics.

Types

There are four types of professional portfolios, all of which are unified by some common work samples and exhibits. They contribute to the primary and secondary purposes of the professional portfolio in their own unique ways. Each type of portfolio is briefly described, and the expected semester in which it is to be completed is identified.

- *Introductory portfolio.* The introductory portfolio introduces you as a person and as a future teaching professional in physical education. It serves as a catalyst for self-reflection and continual sharing of ideas and insights throughout the teacher education program. The introductory portfolio is completed and evaluated during the fall semester of the sophomore year.

- *Working repository portfolio.* The ongoing systematic collection of selected work samples is compiled from courses and evidence (exhibits) of school and community activities. The working repository is the framework for self-assessment and goal setting. It provides a basis for formative assessment throughout the teacher education program at planned intervals. The completion date is the spring semester of the junior year.

- *Presentation portfolio.* This includes samples of work that best reflect your achieved competence, individuality, and creativity as a professional physical educator. The presentation portfolio should be selective and streamlined. It is used during the teacher education program to satisfy different purposes (e.g., field course requirement, clinical experiences, posterlike session) and audiences (e.g., faculty members, cooperating teachers, peers). In addition, it provides for formative assessment, depending on how it is used and when. The completion date is the fall semester of the senior year.

- *Employment portfolio.* This portfolio provides a rich overview of the personality and abilities of the physical education teacher candidate. It focuses on selected artifacts to enhance job placement, and it may be customized to a particular school. The employment portfolio offers a basis for summative assessment during the spring student teaching semester of the senior year.

Organization

Regardless of the purpose or type, professional portfolios need clear and meaningful organizational schemes. Each of the four types of professional portfolios created in the WSU system requires a different organizational scheme. The section on portfolio contents that appears later in this handbook offers suggestions about the selection of required and optional artifacts, as well as other kinds of artifacts, for each type of portfolio. Specific organizational schemes for each portfolio type are presented in this section.

The *introductory portfolio* is meant for you to introduce yourself to the profession by revealing personal characteristics and your reasons for wanting to be a physical education teacher. These aspects serve as the basis for organizing the portfolio. Artifacts should be assembled that are keyed to the following topics: (1) relationships with family, friends, and professionals; (2) personal interests and hobbies; (3) teaching and professional experiences; and (4) reasons for wanting to be a physical education teacher.

The *working repository* and the *presentation portfolio* are organized around the 10 standards for the beginning physical education teacher listed previously. These standards provide a core set of expectations for teaching physical education that are written in terms of performance and knowledge. They have wide applicability. Artifacts selected for the presentation portfolio are derived from the ongoing, more quantitative-oriented collection of items found in the working repository.

Getting a job should serve as the primary goal around which to organize the *employment portfolio.* Although you should address the teacher standards, your portfolio might include artifacts representing more than one standard. Organize artifacts to exemplify the kind of position you are seeking (e.g., elementary, high school).

Processes

The portfolio should be a cumulative record of your professional growth and achieved competence. It is the thread running throughout the WSU teacher education program in physical education.

From *Professional and Student Portfolios for Physical Education, Second Edition,* by Vincent J. Melograno, 2006, Champaign, IL: Human Kinetics.

Therefore, a systematic process is in place to collect, select, and evaluate appropriate portfolio entries, including various checkpoints and periodic reviews. The system introduces the portfolio model and provides a means for bringing closure to the process.

The WSU system is course affiliated. The four types of professional portfolios are linked to selected key courses. Several processes for involvement are part of individual courses and are graded by the instructor as part of course requirements. Implementation of the system includes the introduction of the portfolio model, periodic reviews (formative), and assessment of the completed portfolio (summative). The type of portfolio and processes associated with each of the key courses in the system are identified in table 1.

Table 1 Portfolio Processes

Year	Semester Course Portfolio type	Processes
Sophomore	Fall semester PED 200—Introduction to the Physical Education Profession Introductory portfolio	**Training**—Teacher Candidate Handbook is distributed and discussed; illustrative artifacts are exhibited; sample portfolios are inspected; basic skills are developed in self-management, reflection, self-assessment, peer reflection, and conferences. **Presentation**—Introductory portfolio is presented to the entire class; two artifacts should be selected for each of the four topics identified in the previous section on organization.
Junior	Spring semester PED 310—Adolescent and Young Adult Physical Education Working repository	**Self-reflection**—Each artifact should be thoughtfully examined to reveal its meaning and value to the portfolio relative to the 10 beginning physical education teacher standards; use the Reflection Cover Sheet for Portfolio Artifacts in appendix A. **Self-assessment**—The collection of artifacts should be reviewed to determine how the working repository adheres to the teacher standards; look for ways to document a "missing" artifact or one that has "holes"; set goals and target dates for artifacts that are needed; use the Self-Assessment Checklist of Standards for the Portfolio form in appendix A. **Peer conference**—The final working repository is shared with other teacher candidates for feedback purposes; use the Structure for the Professional Portfolio Peer Conference form in appendix A.
Senior	Fall semester PED 450—Curriculum Design and Instructional Delivery Presentation portfolio	**Self-reflection**—To enhance the presentation portfolio, more extensive reflections are needed as you contemplate your selections; use the Bridging Questions for the Presentation Portfolio form in appendix A. **Self-assessment**—The strengths and weaknesses of the presentation portfolio should be assessed relative to the teacher standards; short-term and long-term goals should be set; use the Self-Assessment of Teacher Standards for the Presentation Portfolio form in appendix A. **Presentation**—The final portfolio is presented in a poster-like session that is attended by faculty members and peers; portfolio items should be carefully selected and streamlined. **Peer and faculty reflection**—Following the posterlike session, peer and faculty feedback will be provided; the Peer and Faculty Reflection Sheet for the Presentation Portfolio will be used for this purpose as shown in appendix A.

Year	Semester Course Portfolio type	Processes
Senior	Spring semester PED 499—Gateway to the Profession Employment portfolio	**Peer and instructor conferences**—The employment portfolio is shared with other teacher candidates and the instructor for feedback purposes; use the Structure for the Peer and Instructor Employment Portfolio Conferences form in appendix A. **Presentation**—An interview simulation will be conducted by a team playing the role of employers; portfolio items should be carefully selected to portray teaching competence in a succinct manner.

Management

Ultimately, the teacher candidate assumes responsibility for organizing, maintaining, and storing the types of portfolios throughout the process. Decisions about method of construction, how and where to store portfolios, and how often to "manage" portfolios depend on the type of portfolio. You need to develop a plan to handle the logistics of your professional portfolios. The "container" for collecting artifacts is a matter of personal preference. Possibilities include notebooks, expanding and accordion files, large file box, folders, satchels, pockets for electronic documents, large notebook divided into sections, and cabinet file drawers. It may be more practical to scan paper-based materials for storage on computer disks or computer hard drives. The type of portfolio will determine the most efficient way to store and manage portfolio items.

The *introductory portfolio* is a scaled-down version of a complete portfolio. Because the number of artifacts is relatively small, an accordion file or cardboard box may be all you need. By contrast, the *working repository* requires more space because the number of artifacts is high. Anything should be collected that relates to a standard, even if not required or eventually selected as an optional piece. You should continually look for ways to document standards, particularly those that may need improvement. The *presentation portfolio* should not be cumbersome or unwieldy. Sample pages from a large project might replace the entire project. A large notebook or accordion file may be all you need. Artifacts can represent more than one standard. Each artifact should be labeled with an abbreviated title for the standard so that someone viewing the portfolio will know what it means. Finally, the *employment portfolio* should be a succinct representation of your teaching competence. Employers do not have a great deal of time to peruse portfolios, so a limited number of carefully selected items should be included in a "professional" container, such as a portfolio satchel, that is easily accessible to employers. Because this may be the first impression an employer has of you, you should check spelling, grammar, and neatness carefully.

You may be good at collecting work samples and exhibits but need help managing the portfolio. Effective organizational tools that you may want to consider include (1) dividers (separate artifacts according to teacher standards, courses, or incomplete works), (2) color codes (code entries with colored dots, colored files, or markers), (3) artifact registry (record the date, item, and reason for either adding or removing an item), (4) work log (list activities and decisions about the portfolio with dates), (5) index (compile an alphabetical index of items), and (6) self-stick notes (attach to each artifact to identify the standard and explain why you collected it).

PORTFOLIO CONTENTS

Now that you are familiar with the standards, purposes, types, organizational schemes, processes, and management options, you can begin selecting portfolio items. As you create and select artifacts, keep in mind the fact that *confidentiality should be maintained. For journal entries, personal reflections, case studies, and so on, do not use the actual names of teachers, students, schools, or other identifying information.* The contents of your portfolio must include a combination of both required and optional items. Guidelines are provided for each artifact, followed by a suggestion for how to analyze the scope of your artifacts.

From *Professional and Student Portfolios for Physical Education, Second Edition,* by Vincent J. Melograno, 2006, Champaign, IL: Human Kinetics.

101

Required Artifacts

The introductory, working repository, presentation, and employment portfolios serve different purposes, and they are reviewed by different audiences. Therefore, they require different artifacts.

Introductory Portfolio

1. Relationships with family, friends, and professionals (e.g., photographs, cards or letters, mementos, keepsakes, meaningful gifts)
2. Personal interests or hobbies (e.g., tapes or CDs, ticket stubs, items from a collection, list of favorite books, leisure sport statistics)
3. Teaching and professional experiences (e.g., custom-made materials, coaching handbook, journal entries, note or letter from former student or parent, employer evaluations)
4. Reasons for wanting to be a physical education teacher (e.g., reflections, statement of philosophy, list of professional goals, essay on a controversial topic)

Working Repository

1. Index
2. Artifacts from selected courses representing each teacher standard (see table 2)
3. Reflection cover sheets for each artifact (see appendix A)
4. Self-assessment checklist of standards (see appendix A)
5. Artifacts analysis chart (see appendix A)

Presentation Portfolio

1. Creative cover
2. Table of contents
3. Artifacts representing each teacher standard selected from the working repository
4. Reflection cover sheets for each artifact selected from the working repository (see appendix A)
5. Self-assessment of teacher standards (see appendix A)

Employment Portfolio

1. Table of contents
2. Cover letter (i.e., introduce yourself, tell why you are a good job candidate, describe some pertinent experiences, point out areas of the portfolio that are exemplary)
3. Biographical sketch
4. Resume
5. Philosophy of education statement
6. Certification or licensing documents (e.g., copy of certificate, teacher exam scores, transcripts)
7. Letters of recommendation (e.g., adviser, faculty member, supervisors, employers)
8. List of relevant courses (i.e., title, credits, grade, teacher standards to which course relates)
9. Student teaching evaluations (i.e., supervisor, cooperating teacher)
10. Artifacts representing the teacher standards selected from the working repository and presentation portfolio
11. Reflections on each teacher standard relative to selected artifacts
12. Evaluations of working repository and presentation portfolio by instructors

Optional Items

A wide variety of optional artifacts can be collected as part of your *working repository*. Particular consideration should be given to school and community activities. Many of them may ultimately

Table 2   Required Artifacts for the Working Repository

Course	Primary standards	Name of artifacts
PED 200—Introduction to the Physical Education Profession	1, 2, 8	Contributions of Physical Activity paper
HED 200—First Aid and Emergency Care	2, 4, 8 1, 3, 4, 10	Case study analyses Emergency response plan
DAN 300—Dance for the Physical Educator	5, 8, 10 1, 5, 8, 9, 10	Self-analysis journal Videotape of movement presentation
PED 300—Early and Middle Childhood Physical Education	1, 2, 3, 6, 7 1, 8	Unit plan including six lessons Article critiques
PED 310—Adolescent and Young Adult Physical Education	2, 3, 4, 5, 6, 7	Analyses of middle school and high school teachers
PED 320—Kinesiology	1, 6, 7, 8	Self-selected teaching activity
PED 330—Physiology of Exercise	1, 6, 7, 8, 9	Self-designed exercise program with PowerPoint presentation
PED 340—Motor Learning and Development	1, 3, 6, 10 1, 3, 7, 10	Practice: Design and schedule Motor Assessment project
PED 350—Legal and Administrative Aspects of Physical Education	1, 4, 5, 8, 10 2, 3, 5, 6 2, 3, 4, 5, 8, 10	Policy and Procedure paper Risk assessment and audit Negligence case study analysis
DAN 400—Teaching Dance	1, 2, 3, 4, 5, 6, 7	Mini-lessons and unit plan
PED 410—Psychosocial Aspects of Physical Activity	2, 3, 4 1, 2, 3, 4, 7	Gender Reversal paper Problem-solving report
PED 420—Physical Education for Students With Disabilities	2, 3, 6, 7 2, 3, 5, 8 1, 2, 3, 5, 6, 7 1, 2, 3, 8	IEP development Attitude Toward Disabilities paper Clinical teaching descriptions Disability Types project
PED 430—Evaluation in Physical Education	1, 7, 8, 10 1, 7, 9	Test construction and administration Collection and analysis of fitness battery using a handheld computer
PED 450—Curriculum Design and Instructional Delivery	3, 4, 5, 6, 7 3, 4, 5, 6, 7, 9	Curriculum and Instruction project Videotape of field teaching
PED 499—Gateway to the Profession	3, 4, 5, 6, 7, 9 1, 8, 10	Video clips of student teaching lesson Standards-based analysis of teaching competence

be selected for the *presentation portfolio* and the *employment portfolio* in accordance with previous guidelines. All artifacts must relate to one of the beginning teacher standards. The following artifacts, with examples, show the range of options.

1. Anecdotal records (observation notes on students' skills)
2. Article summaries or critiques (reflect on an article read on your own)
3. Assessments (performance task card you developed)
4. Awards and certificates (volunteer recognition)
5. Bulletin board ideas (photograph)
6. Case studies (show knowledge of an *anonymous* child's development)
7. Classroom management philosophy (written summary including citations)

From *Professional and Student Portfolios for Physical Education, Second Edition*, by Vincent J. Melograno, 2006, Champaign, IL: Human Kinetics.

8. Community resource documents (copies of actual correspondence)
9. Computer programs (programs incorporated into teaching)
10. Cooperative learning strategies (copy of lesson plan)
11. Curriculum plans (thematic units)
12. Essays (writing on a complex social issue)
13. Evaluations (on-the-job performance assessments)
14. Field trip plans (copy of program or brochure)
15. Floor plans (sketch of space or equipment arranged)
16. Goal statements (outline perceived role as a teacher)
17. Individualized plans (show how lessons or units have been adapted for diverse learners)
18. Interviews with students, teachers, and parents (copy of questions and answers)
19. Journals (observations during field experiences)
20. Lesson plans (copies of all components)
21. Letters to parents (weekly newsletters)
22. Management and organization strategies (summary of system for grouping students)
23. Media competencies (examples of forms of media used in teaching)
24. Meetings and workshops log (reaction paper with program)
25. Observation reports (results of checklists)
26. Peer critiques (rating sheets from presentations)
27. Philosophy statement (brief position paper)
28. Pictures and photographs (show special projects or learning centers)
29. Portfolio by student (sample artifacts from a student's portfolio)
30. Position papers (scholarly defense of an educational issue)
31. Problem-solving logs (record of solving a professional problem)
32. Professional development plans (list of future workshops or meetings to be attended)
33. Professional organizations and committees list (list memberships and involvements)
34. Professional readings list (list readings and describe reactions)
35. Projects (how teaching materials were developed)
36. References (statements from supervisors)
37. Research papers (highlight knowledge of an academic subject)
38. Rules and procedures descriptions (written guidelines)
39. Schedules (show format for events in a day)
40. Seating arrangement diagrams (reflect on a particular management strategy)
41. Self-assessment instruments (questionnaire results)
42. Simulated experiences (describe role-play experience)
43. Student contracts (samples of agreement with students)
44. Subscriptions (list of journals with address label)
45. Teacher-made materials (games, videotapes, teaching aids)
46. Theme studies (lessons that show integrated curriculum)
47. Transcripts (copy of official transcript with personal analysis)
48. Unit plans (integrated plan covering several weeks)
49. Video scenario critiques (analyses of videotapes of actual teaching episodes)
50. Volunteer experience (list and briefly describe services provided)
51. Work experience (descriptions of work in a nontraditional setting)

Analysis of Artifacts

In addition to the management and assembly guidelines offered previously in this handbook, you will need to "manage" your documentation of the teacher standards. Each artifact selected for the working repository and the presentation or employment portfolios should be analyzed to help determine (1) standards that need work, (2) an overreliance on some kinds of artifacts, and (3) the need to diversify artifacts. The artifacts analysis chart in appendix A can be used for this purpose. Check marks or dates should be entered to record the range of artifacts in support of the 10 teacher standards.

PORTFOLIO ASSESSMENT

Periodic reviews not only are essential, but they are natural to a portfolio system and a teacher education program. Because the WSU system is course affiliated, assessment is an ongoing and cumulative process at each stage of program course requirements. Peer, faculty, and instructor feedback processes are associated with the working repository and the presentation and employment portfolios (i.e., peer and instructor conferences, peer and faculty reflections). However, more formal evaluation procedures will also be used. Criteria are referenced to the portfolio's *content* and *quality*. Guidelines for the formative and summative assessment of these professional portfolios are provided.

Formative

When information is sought to help decide how to adjust or improve performance during a learning process, assessment serves a formative purpose. The working repository and presentation portfolio are associated with formative assessment in the WSU system. Because the teacher standards serve as the basis for organization, they are central to the assessment instruments. Scoring rubrics for the working repository and presentation portfolio are in appendix B.

Summative

Assessment of a summative nature is used to decide the extent to which learners have been successful in mastering final outcomes (standards). In the WSU system, the employment portfolio is viewed as the final or exit portfolio. It is subject to summative assessment protocols. However, the assessment format recognizes the purposes of the employment portfolio—to synthesize the knowledge, skills, and dispositions of the teacher candidate and enhance job placement. A scoring rubric for the employment portfolio is in appendix B.

From *Professional and Student Portfolios for Physical Education, Second Edition*, by Vincent J. Melograno, 2006, Champaign, IL: Human Kinetics.

105

Reflection Cover Sheet for Portfolio Artifacts

Name: _____ Date: _____

Standard #: _____ Title: _____

Name of artifact: _____

Course/activity: _____

Rationale statement: _____

_____

_____

_____

_____

_____

_____

_____

_____

_____

_____

_____

_____

_____

_____

_____

_____

_____

_____

_____

Self-Assessment Checklist of Standards for the Portfolio

Standard	Good	OK	Artifacts needed
1. Content knowledge			Goal: Target date:
2. Growth and development			Goal: Target date:
3. Diverse learners			Goal: Target date:
4. Management and motivation			Goal: Target date:
5. Communication			Goal: Target date:
6. Planning and instruction			Goal: Target date:
7. Student assessment			Goal: Target date:
8. Reflection			Goal: Target date:
9. Technology			Goal: Target date:
10. Collaboration			Goal: Target date:

From *Professional and Student Portfolios for Physical Education, Second Edition*, by Vincent J. Melograno, 2006, Champaign, IL: Human Kinetics.

Structure for the Professional Portfolio Peer Conference

The following questions should serve as the basis for the conference:

1. What have you learned about yourself by putting your portfolio together?

2. What artifacts are you particularly proud of? Why?

3. If you could publish one thing in your portfolio, what would it be? Why?

4. What areas of your teaching performance need further improvement?

5. How do you feel about your role as a professional physical education teacher?

From *Professional and Student Portfolios for Physical Education, Second Edition,* by Vincent J. Melograno, 2006, Champaign, IL: Human Kinetics.

Bridging Questions for the Presentation Portfolio

As you contemplate your selections, ask yourself the following questions to help "bridge" individual items into the entire portfolio:

1. Why should I choose this piece?

2. What are its strengths and weaknesses?

3. Why is it important?

4. How does it fit into what I already have?

5. What if I took it out?

6. How will others react to it?

From *Professional and Student Portfolios for Physical Education, Second Edition,* by Vincent J. Melograno, 2006, Champaign, IL: Human Kinetics.

Self-Assessment of Teacher Standards for the Presentation Portfolio

Name: _____ Date: _____

Standard #: _____ Title: _____

My strengths	Knowledge	
	Skills	
	Dispositions	
My problem areas	Knowledge	
	Skills	
	Dispositions	

Peer and Faculty Reflection Sheet for the Presentation Portfolio

Date: _____

To: _____

From: _____

During the posterlike session, please review my professional portfolio and provide feedback by answering the following questions:

1. What teacher standard is documented the most effectively? Why?

2. What teacher standard is documented the least effectively? Why?

3. What artifacts really made an impression on you? Why?

4. What artifact do you feel needs the most work? Why?

5. What is your overall impression of the organization and presentation of artifacts?

Signed: _____ Date: _____

From *Professional and Student Portfolios for Physical Education, Second Edition*, by Vincent J. Melograno, 2006, Champaign, IL: Human Kinetics.

Structure for the Peer and Instructor Employment Portfolio Conferences

Conferences should be structured around a comparison of the teacher candidate's perceptions and the opinion of a peer or the instructor regarding the following:

1. Overall strengths as a physical education teacher

2. Artifacts that represent "holistic" abilities and dispositions toward teaching

3. How the portfolio verifies that the beginning teacher standards have been met

4. Teacher standards that the candidate will likely develop further as a practicing teacher

5. Teacher standards that need work as revealed by the portfolio

From *Professional and Student Portfolios for Physical Education, Second Edition*, by Vincent J. Melograno, 2006, Champaign, IL: Human Kinetics.

Artifacts Analysis Chart for the Working Repository and the Presentation and Employment Portfolios

Kind of artifact	Name of artifact	Teacher standard									
		1	2	3	4	5	6	7	8	9	10

From *Professional and Student Portfolios for Physical Education, Second Edition,* by Vincent J. Melograno, 2006, Champaign, IL: Human Kinetics.

Working Repository Scoring Rubric

Name: _____ Semester/year: _____

Course: _____ Instructor: _____

Elements	Fair	Satisfactory	Good	Outstanding	Weight	Score
Organization/form						
1. Follows directions	1	2	3	4	×1	_____ (4)
2. Clear layout/visual appeal	1	2	3	4	×1	_____ (4)
3. Creative cover	1	2	3	4	×1	_____ (4)
4. Writing mechanics	1	2	3	4	×1	_____ (4)
5. Expressiveness	1	2	3	4	×1	_____ (4)
Completeness						
1. Reflection cover sheets	1	2	3	4	×1	_____ (4)
2. Self-assessment checklist	1	2	3	4	×1	_____ (4)
3. Artifacts analysis chart	1	2	3	4	×1	_____ (4)
4. Gallery	1	2	3	4	×1	_____ (4)
5. Index	1	2	3	4	×1	_____ (4)
Standard 1: Content knowledge						
1. Required artifacts	1	2	3	4	×2	_____ (8)
2. Optional artifacts	1	2	3	4	×2	_____ (8)
Standard 2: Growth & development						
1. Required artifacts	1	2	3	4	×2	_____ (8)
2. Optional artifacts	1	2	3	4	×2	_____ (8)
Standard 3: Diverse learners						
1. Required artifacts	1	2	3	4	×2	_____ (8)
2. Optional artifacts	1	2	3	4	×2	_____ (8)
Standard 4: Management & motivation						
1. Required artifacts	1	2	3	4	×2	_____ (8)
2. Optional artifacts	1	2	3	4	×2	_____ (8)
Standard 5: Communication						
1. Required artifacts	1	2	3	4	×2	_____ (8)
2. Optional artifacts	1	2	3	4	×2	_____ (8)

From *Professional and Student Portfolios for Physical Education, Second Edition,* by Vincent J. Melograno, 2006, Champaign, IL: Human Kinetics.

Elements	Fair	Satisfactory	Good	Outstanding	Weight	Score
Standard 6: Planning & instruction						
1. Required artifacts	1	2	3	4	×2	_____ (8)
2. Optional artifacts	1	2	3	4	×2	_____ (8)
Standard 7: Student assessment						
1. Required artifacts	1	2	3	4	×2	_____ (8)
2. Optional artifacts	1	2	3	4	×2	_____ (8)
Standard 8: Reflection						
1. Required artifacts	1	2	3	4	×2	_____ (8)
2. Optional artifacts	1	2	3	4	×2	_____ (8)
Standard 9: Technology						
1. Required artifacts	1	2	3	4	×2	_____ (8)
2. Optional Artifacts	1	2	3	4	×2	_____ (8)
Standard 10: Collaboration						
1. Required artifacts	1	2	3	4	×2	_____ (8)
2. Optional artifacts	1	2	3	4	×2	_____ (8)

Grading scale

A = 180-200

B = 160-179

C = 140-159

D = 120-139

F = Below 120

Total score: _____

(200)

Grade: _____

Comments: _____

_____

_____

_____

_____

_____

_____

_____

_____

_____

_____

_____

_____

_____

Instructor signature: _____ Date: _____

From *Professional and Student Portfolios for Physical Education, Second Edition*, by Vincent J. Melograno, 2006, Champaign, IL: Human Kinetics.

Presentation Portfolio Scoring Rubric

Poster Session

Name: _____ Semester/year: _____

Course: _____ Instructor: _____

1. Required components contained in the presentation portfolio (creative cover, table of contents, reflection cover sheets, self-assessment of teacher standards)

   1 - - - - - - - - - - 2 - - - - - - - - - - 3 - - - - - - - - - - 4 - - - - - - - - - - 5

   Included but incomplete   Some gaps   Fully developed

   Comments: _____

   _____

   _____

2. Presentation portfolio exhibited in a dynamic, creative, and informative manner

   1 - - - - - - - - - - 2 - - - - - - - - - - 3 - - - - - - - - - - 4 - - - - - - - - - - 5

   Poor display   Marginal display   Impressive display

   Comments: _____

   _____

   _____

3. In general, artifacts clearly and convincingly represent each teacher standard

   1 - - - - - - - - - - 2 - - - - - - - - - - 3 - - - - - - - - - - 4 - - - - - - - - - - 5

   Weak evidence   Satisfactorily documented   No doubt

   Comments: _____

   _____

   _____

4. Connection between artifacts and each teacher standard according to the following rating scale: + = impressive; ✓ = acceptable; 0 = needs work

   _____ Standard 1: Content knowledge

   _____ Standard 2: Growth and development

   _____ Standard 3: Diverse learners

   _____ Standard 4: Management and motivation

   _____ Standard 5: Communication

   _____ Standard 6: Planning and instruction

   _____ Standard 7: Student assessment

   _____ Standard 8: Reflection

   _____ Standard 9: Technology

   _____ Standard 10: Collaboration

From *Professional and Student Portfolios for Physical Education, Second Edition*, by Vincent J. Melograno, 2006, Champaign, IL: Human Kinetics.

5. Overall impression of the presentation portfolio poster session display

1 - - - - - - - - - - - - 2 - - - - - - - - - - - 3 - - - - - - - - - - - 4 - - - - - - - - - - - 5

Weak quality   Acceptable quality   Exceptional quality

Comments: _____

_____

_____

_____

_____

_____

_____

_____

_____

_____

_____

_____

_____

_____

_____

_____

_____

_____

Instructor signature: _____ Date: _____

From *Professional and Student Portfolios for Physical Education, Second Edition,* by Vincent J. Melograno, 2006, Champaign, IL: Human Kinetics.

Employment Portfolio Scoring Rubric

Name: _____ Date: _____

Portfolio contents: Components of the employment portfolio are verified and rated according to the following scale:

2 = Fully developed   1 = Included but incomplete   0 = Not included

_____ 1. Table of contents

_____ 2. Cover letter

_____ 3. Biographical sketch

_____ 4. Resume

_____ 5. Philosophy of education statement

_____ 6. Certification or licensing documents

_____ 7. Letters of recommendation

_____ 8. List of relevant courses

_____ 9. Student teaching evaluations

_____ 10. Artifacts representing the teacher standards

_____ 11. Reflections on each teacher standard relative to selected artifacts

_____ 12. Evaluations of working repository and presentation portfolio by instructors

_____ **Total**

Comments: _____

_____

_____

Portfolio quality: The degree of quality is determined by rating each characteristic and artifact according to the following scale:

2 = High quality; above expectations

1 = Satisfactory quality; meets expectations

0 = Low quality; below expectations

_____ Organization	_____ Artifact 5: _____
_____ Layout/visual appeal	_____ Artifact 6: _____
_____ Creativity/expressiveness	_____ Artifact 7: _____
_____ Spelling, punctuation, grammar	_____ Artifact 8: _____
_____ Artifact 1: _____	_____ Artifact 9: _____
_____ Artifact 2: _____	_____ Artifact 10: _____
_____ Artifact 3: _____	_____ Artifact 11: _____
_____ Artifact 4: _____	_____ Artifact 12: _____

_____ **Total** _____ **Average**

From *Professional and Student Portfolios for Physical Education, Second Edition,* by Vincent J. Melograno, 2006, Champaign, IL: Human Kinetics.

Comments: _____

_____

_____

_____

_____

_____

_____

_____

_____

_____

Summary ratings

Portfolio contents

_____ Outstanding (19-24)

_____ Satisfactory (12-18)

_____ Unsatisfactory (0-11)

Portfolio quality

_____ Outstanding (average 1.6-2.0)

_____ Satisfactory (average 1.0-1.5)

_____ Unsatisfactory (average 0.0-1.9)

Instructor signature: _____ Date: _____

From *Professional and Student Portfolios for Physical Education, Second Edition,* by Vincent J. Melograno, 2006, Champaign, IL: Human Kinetics.

Student Portfolios for K-12 Learners

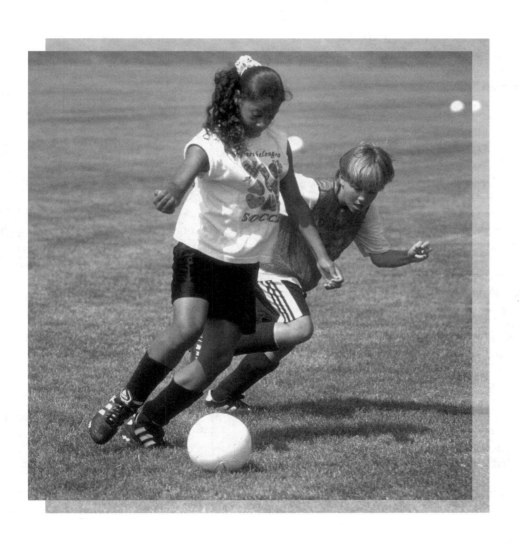

Teachers may be free to design instructional strategies and to use a variety of materials and approaches—but they are expected to get results. This means that teachers must determine the learning targets to seek, the methods for assessment, and which methods best match the intended targets. Student-involved, formative assessment—assessment *for* learning—produces significant learning gains, so assessment, learning, and teaching must be integrated. Student learning needs to be evaluated authentically in a naturalistic, performance-based manner. Skill tests, multiple-choice exams, and standardized achievement tests do not necessarily tell stakeholders what students really know and are able to do. So, how can a broader, more genuine picture of student learning be presented?

EXPECTED OUTCOMES

This chapter will help you develop student portfolios for K-12 learners in physical education. After reading this chapter, you will be able to do the following:

1. Recognize how assessment, learning, and teaching can be integrated to facilitate student-involved, classroom-level assessment *for* learning.

2. Select the types of student portfolios to be developed relative to the intended purposes.

3. Identify a framework for organizing student portfolios that considers new roles for students and teachers.

4. Determine how to construct, store, and manage student portfolios as well as how to use technology to produce student portfolios.

5. Create processes for selecting portfolio artifacts; for encouraging reflection, goal setting, and self-assessment in students; and for helping students communicate through conferences.

6. Develop assessment criteria, procedures, and tools for using scoring rubrics, grading in standards-based education, and judging student portfolios.

The search for accountability in student achievement has never been more intense than it is now. Interest in assessment has also been prompted by these accountability concerns, especially the desire to organize achievement data in ways that are credible and comprehensible to all stakeholders—students, teachers, school personnel, parents, and community members. To meet these demands, teachers must develop assessment literacy. In chapter 1, assessment literacy was defined as the ability to determine what to assess (learning targets) and how to assess (methods), and then to match the proper method of assessment with the intended target. Assessment *for* learning—student-involved, formative assessment—was also advanced because it produces significant learning gains. Clearly, this means that assessment, learning, and teaching must be integrated. Student portfolios may hold the key to successful integration by cultivating desirable student habits—reflecting on learning, developing self-direction and feedback, setting goals, creating new challenges, and communicating achievement results.

To begin the chapter, the relationships among assessment, learning, and teaching are presented and a process for integration is suggested. This foundation provides the basis for using student portfolios because portfolios play a significant role in learning. A multifaceted approach is recommended for designing student portfolio systems appropriate for K-12 school physical education programs. The process of developing portfolios includes determining the purposes and types of portfolios to use; deciding how they will be organized; dealing with production and logistics concerns; establishing a process for item selection; determining student reflection and self-assessment strategies; creating a framework for conducting conferences; and choosing assessment procedures. The chapter provides materials exemplary of established content standards in physical education. To help readers synthesize this information, sample elementary school, middle school, and high school portfolio systems are presented at the end of the chapter. In addition, the CD-ROM accompanying the book provides a template (portfolio builder) for creating an electronic-based student portfolio.

Initially, designing an integrated student portfolio system can be a complex, time-consuming task involving many decisions. The following eight-step process can help with this task (Melograno, 2000a, 2000b). The steps are also identified throughout the chapter.

1. Determine the general and specific purposes of portfolios.
2. Select the types of portfolios to be used.
3. Create a framework for organizing portfolios.
4. Plan production features and logistics (construction, storage, and management).
5. Establish a process for selecting portfolio items.
6. Decide reflection, goal-setting, and self-assessment techniques.
7. Arrange student-involved conference strategies.
8. Develop quality assessment criteria and procedures.

Assessment, Learning, and Teaching

In spite of all the efforts to reform education, many still view assessment as separate from teaching. Rather, assessment should be conducted throughout teaching and learning to help teachers diagnose student needs, adjust and plan instruction, provide feedback, and help students find success. Therefore, the purposes of this section are to (1) justify classroom-level, student-involved assessment *for* learning; (2) match learning targets with assessment methods; (3) relate various teaching models with assessment techniques; and (4) suggest a process for integrating assessment, learning, and teaching. Note that the term *classroom-level* refers to the physical education setting.

Student-Involved Formative Assessment

Accountability for student achievement is accepted among educators today because world-class standards for student achievement have been set and rigorous testing systems have been implemented. The problem is that although some students respond favorably to the intimidation and the rewards or punishments associated with testing, there are just as many students for whom this model does not work. High-stakes assessment *of* learning—offering a look at achievement status at a point in time—is simply insufficient to maximize learning for all students.

Student achievement improves through assessment *for* learning—assessment that promotes student achievement during the learning process. Such formative assessment is used to adapt teaching to meet student needs. Formative assessment is more than testing frequently. It is even more than using student information to plan next steps. Formative assessment in the context of assessment *for* learning also means that students are involved in their own assessment and goal setting, record keeping, and communication. Student-involved assessment includes anything that helps students understand learning targets, engage in self-assessment, watch themselves grow, talk about their learning growth, and plan next steps for learning. In physical education, student-involved assessment is evidenced, for example, when students do the following:

1. Engage in regular self-assessment, with movement standards held constant so that they can track their growth over time
2. Communicate with the teacher, other students, and family members about their achievement status and improvements (e.g., student-led conferences, portfolio reflections)
3. Assist in developing scoring criteria for various sport skills
4. Create assessment rubrics including criteria and descriptive indicators for each level of excellence
5. Plan their own next steps for learning based on a comprehensive skill analysis (i.e., goal setting)
6. Maintain fitness records relative to learning targets

Learning and Assessment

Quality assessments are essential to fulfill the demands of student achievement, school improvement, and educational accountability. Teachers are the key to quality assessments. Assessment-literate teachers are able to match the proper method of assessment with the intended learning targets. This section is organized around these teacher functions (Stiggins, Arter, Chappuis, & Chappuis, 2004).

Learning Targets

Teachers *and students* must have access to dependable and accurate information about learning—that is, clearly specified and appropriate achievement expectations. What students are expected to know and be able to do should be clear. Teachers who do not have a clear picture of expectations will have great difficulty developing appropriate assessment criteria and activities. The popular terms that define these expectations are *content standards, benchmarks,* and *grade-level indicators.* What are needed more precisely, however, are the specific classroom-level learning targets that underpin these overarching national, state, or local standards. They should be the focus of classroom-level, student-involved assessment. Learning targets that are clearly stated are those that everyone concerned with their attainment understands. Because content standards are normally stated at a very general level, they need to be "unpacked," or broken down into their component parts. These learning targets then become the focus for classroom-level assessment. Within the classroom (physical education context), the assessment development process begins with this precise vision of what it means to succeed. The following types of learning targets emerge:

- *Knowledge and understanding.* The mastery of subject matter content (both knowing and understanding it) is the foundation for learning. Knowledge includes both targets that are learned outright through memory (facts, concepts, relationships, principles) and those that rely on information retrieved from reference material. All subject matter has a conceptual core that combines basic knowledge to form generalizations and theories. These conceptual ideas, referred to as essential understandings, become important, developmentally appropriate learning targets for students. Examples include motor concepts such as opposition and follow-through and fitness principles such as frequency, specificity, and progressive overload.

- *Reasoning.* Students should be able to use their knowledge and understanding to reason, to figure things out, and to solve problems. For example, students might (1) analyze the relationship of body parts in performing the forehand drive in tennis, (2) compare the similarities and differences of several aerobic exercise programs, (3) infer inductively and deductively when designing a dance routine, and (4) evaluate opposing offensive and defensive strategies in soccer. If these kinds of learning targets are valuable, it is important to define precisely what is meant by reasoning and problem-solving proficiency. Students who can reason analytically are able to take things apart and see what is inside them.

- *Performance skill.* This learning target is particularly relevant to physical education. The measure of attainment is students' ability to demonstrate that they can perform or behave in a certain way. For example, at the elementary level, students are expected to exhibit fundamental movement skills. Depending on developmental levels, secondary students might be expected to demonstrate a range of aquatics, fitness, dance, recreational, individual sport, and team sport skills. General behavioral skills are also included as learning targets such as working productively as a team or cooperative group member, carrying out the steps in a learning sequence, and performing in self-directed activities.

- *Product development.* By creating tangible entities, students present evidence that they have mastered knowledge, reasoning and problem-solving proficiencies, and specific production skills. The assessment challenge is defining clearly and understandably the key attributes that the product should possess. Examples of products include work samples, reports, projects (e.g., personal fitness plan), and some of the artifacts that might be contained in a student portfolio. At the end of the chapter, several kinds of product options are included in the sample portfolio systems. The Volleyball Sportfolio for the middle school level (pages 206-215) includes a game play video, scouting report, and volleyball "box score." The Fitness for Life portfolio system for the high school level (pages 216-233) includes a fitness journal, food log, and workout schedule. The K-12 student portfolio builder on the accompanying CD-ROM includes the production of artifacts in support of established learning targets.

- *Dispositions.* There is some expectation that students will acquire positive behaviors and affect—favorable attitudes, self-confidence, or interest in something—that motivates them to act or not to act. Preferably, students will display approach, or "moving toward," behaviors rather than avoidance, or "moving away from," behaviors when it comes to a desire to acquire knowledge, move skillfully, think critically, or show respect for others. Because these attitudes, values, and interests are broad and complex, thoughtful assessment is essential. At the least, learning targets should be defined by the characteristics that represent the dichotomy of positive and negative.

Regardless of the type, learning targets should be restated in student-friendly language appropriate to students' developmental levels. This helps students understand or "see the target," and it helps teachers clarify learning expectations. For example, one of the National Association for Sport and Physical Education (NASPE, 2004) content standards, "Demonstrates competency in motor skills and movement patterns needed to perform a variety of physical activities" might be translated to "Demonstrates mature form for all basic manipulative, locomotor, and nonlocomotor skills." The standard might be further subdivided to, "Throws different kinds of objects with both accuracy and force (e.g., playground ball, Frisbee, football).

Methods of Assessment

Different types of learning targets require different methods of assessment. No single assessment method can cover the range of learning targets. Without a clear focus on the expectations to be assessed, devising effective assessment tasks and scoring procedures is impossible. That is why alternative assessment techniques have captured the attention of teachers. Although many of the so-called "new" techniques are actually familiar procedures that have been improved, they should not be used to the exclusion of traditional approaches. Multiple sources of information are desirable, characterized by (1) tasks that *directly* examine desired behaviors, (2) an emphasis on *quality* of performance, (3) *criterion-referenced* measurement, and (4) *student involvement* in developing and using assessment approaches (NASPE, 1995a).

Traditional teacher-directed techniques include (1) achievement tests to measure perceptual motor skills, motor ability, physical fitness, and sport skills; (2) observational checklists and rating scales for recording cognitive, motor, and affective behaviors; and (3) written tests to measure knowledge and higher-level abilities such as application, analysis, and synthesis. Some alternative techniques transfer partial responsibility to others. In peer assessment, one student or a group of students apply criteria established by the teacher against the ability of another student. Students develop assessment skills and a sense of responsibility by giving and receiving constructive feedback. Self-assessment allows students to make critical and valid assessments of their own abilities. Performance is compared to individual learning targets, peer standards, teacher-established criteria, or all of these.

Note that portfolios are not considered an assessment *method*. Because student portfolios are usually assembled from several assessments using multiple assessment modes, they are considered devices for collecting and communicating about student learning and teaching competence. A portfolio is an ongoing feedback system that documents student learning through actual exhibits and work samples. Although a portfolio can be assessed as a whole, its true purpose is to enrich the ability to learn, the desire to learn, and the learning itself. Students are involved in selecting and judging the quality of their own work (Melograno, 1997).

Distinguishing among what are commonly referred to as assessment options, strategies, techniques, and procedures is difficult. Regardless of the label, a sound assessment examines student achievement through a *method* that is capable of reflecting the valued target. For simplicity and analysis purposes, the various assessment methods have been placed in the following four basic categories:

1. *Selected response.* In a paper-and-pencil test format, students answer a series of questions, each of which is accompanied by a range of alternative responses. Students select (recognize) either the correct or best answer. Achievement is indexed by the number or proportion of correct answers. Common format options are multiple-choice, true–false, and matching items.

2. *Extended written response.* Students prepare (construct) an original written answer to an exercise or set of exercises. Questions might deal with content knowledge or an explanation of the solution to a complex problem. Students might also be asked to compare facts or events, interpret information, or solve open-ended problems. Typical formats are short-answer fill-in items and essay questions. The degree of achievement is determined using a point system or rubric in accordance with scoring criteria. The construction and use of rubrics is presented later in this chapter (page 178).

3. *Performance assessment.* A specified activity is actually carried out under the watchful eye of an evaluator who observes the skill or product and judges the quality of achievement. Performance assessment is based either on observations while students are demonstrating skills or on the evaluation of products. A set of scoring guides, such as rubrics, are applied against the performance task. The quality in performing motor activities is typically determined with a performance rating scale.

4. *Personal communication.* Personal communication includes questions and answers during instruction, interviews, conferences, conversations, class discussions, and oral exams. In particular, student-led conferences create a strong sense of responsibility for learning among students. Students are motivated to tell their own success stories, thus making it difficult to escape accountability. Guidelines for student-led conferences are provided later in this chapter (page 176). Student portfolios are also included as a comprehensive form of communication because they can contain many types of artifacts including, but not limited to, performance assessments and products. At the end of the chapter, several kinds of communication options are included in the sample portfolio systems. The Locomotor Skills Workbook for the elementary school level (pages 197-205) includes a partner activity, group project, and parent or guardian conference. The Fitness for Life portfolio system for the high school level (pages 216-233) includes a peer and family conference component. The K-12 student portfolio builder on the accompanying CD-ROM includes conference activities based on established learning targets.

Alignment of Learning Targets and Assessment Methods

The previous sections identified five broad types of learning targets and four general methods of assessment. Classroom-level assessment depends on a careful match of targets and methods. The task is to identify and select the most efficient and appropriate way to assess the different kinds of achievement expectations. This process of alignment yields some matches that are clearly stronger than others. For example, no doubt, the best way to assess motor proficiency is through performance assessment. But, selected response or personal communication can help the teacher determine whether students have mastered the knowledge and reasoning that underpin effective skill. Following is a discussion of the various matches of learning targets and methods of assessment.

- *Knowledge and understanding targets.* Selected response options are good for assessing discrete elements of knowledge (facts), and extended written response options are useful for assessing understanding of relationships among elements of knowledge. Personal communication through question and answer is useful, but it is a time-consuming and inefficient if there is a large amount of information and many students.

- *Reasoning targets.* Use of selected response is limited to comparative and inference patterns of reasoning. Extended written descriptions of complex solutions are good for assessing reasoning proficiency. With performance assessment, students can be observed solving some problem, but an inference must be made from what is observed. Personal communication is good for assessing reasoning by asking students to think out loud and probing more deeply with follow-up questions. Challenges include the amount time required and the need for record keeping.

- *Performance skill targets.* Performance assessment is really the only method that adequately covers performance skill targets. Teachers can observe the skills as students perform them and judge the level of achievement. The other methods can be used to determine whether students have mastered the knowledge prerequisites to skillful performance.

- *Product targets.* Through performance assessment, teachers can assess proficiency in carrying out steps in product development and attributes of the product itself. Knowledge of the prerequisites to create quality products can be assessed with the other methods.

- *Disposition targets.* Selected response items can tap student feelings, and open-ended items can probe dispositions. Teachers can also infer dispositions from performance behavior and products and by talking with students about their feelings.

Teaching and Assessment

Paradigms for teaching physical education have at least one common feature. Whether teaching is described as models, strategies, styles, reflective approaches, methods, or developmentally appropriate instruction, it should evoke the desired responses (learning targets) in students—knowledge acquisition, reasoning proficiency, problem solving, motor abilities, fitness development, normative social behaviors, self-confidence, or values clarification. In the same manner that the proper method of assessment was matched with the intended learning target, assessment-literate teachers are able to build assessment techniques into their teaching repertoires. Although it may seem simple to conceptualize assessment as an integral part of teaching, the actual integration is a difficult task.

If physical educators are to be responsive to the new vision of assessment for learning, changes in teaching behavior are needed. Traditional instructional systems in which teachers inform, direct, and predetermine priorities will not work. Although some elements of current practices can integrate alternative assessment into teaching, other changes are necessary. For example, in the use of student portfolios, the teacher facilitates, guides, and offers choices while partnerships are established among teachers, students, and parents.

The ultimate challenge for teachers is to select assessment techniques that fit their preferred teaching approaches. This section offers an analysis of patterns of teaching and a description of assessment using several teaching models. Emphasis is placed on student-involved, classroom-level assessment techniques that are used for making decisions of a formative nature. The section concludes with a discussion of the relationships among various assessment techniques and teaching models.

Teaching Patterns

Historically, the cohort pattern has been one of the most popular for teaching physical education. The teacher teaches the same thing to all students at the same time. This group focus means that students practice in the same way and at the same pace and are subject to the same kinds of standards and assessment criteria. In physical education, command and practice approaches are commonly used that are cohort in nature. Opportunities for student-involved assessment are minimal at best. Two other broad patterns of teaching physical education—individualization and interaction—offer more authentic opportunities toward the vision of achievement-based assessment *for* learning (Kelly & Melograno, 2004).

- *Individualization.* In this pattern, means and ends are interwoven through the roles of the teacher and student in an attempt to accommodate the physical, psychological, and sociological differences among students. Numerous approaches are available that can be matched with each student's interests, abilities, achievement level, and preferred learning style. Commonly used approaches are exploration, self-directed tasks, guided discovery, problem solving, contracting, programmed tasks, learning packages, tutorial programs, independent study, and computer-assisted tasks. With individualization, an assessment component is built into many of these approaches. For example, problem solving could be teacher-directed or self-directed, and could include many of the portfolio assessment techniques such as artifact reflective cover sheets, artifact analysis relative to standards or learning targets, and goal setting. At the end of the chapter, several approaches to individualization are included in the sample portfolio systems. The Volleyball Sportfolio for the middle school level (pages 206-215) includes a self-analysis of skills and goal setting based on strengths and problem areas. The Fitness for Life portfolio system for the high school level (pages 216-233) includes short-term and long-term goal setting based on fitness pretests. The K-12 student portfolio builder on the accompanying CD-ROM includes goal setting based on established learning targets, personal reflection activities, a self-assessment journal, and a gallery for photos and video clips.

- *Interaction.* The purpose of this pattern is the *process* itself, not the typical forms of communication between the teacher and students. Students seek to improve achievement while working together as partners or in small groups to discuss, question, report, and provide feedback. The chance to learn social attitudes and values is maximized. Social outcomes are sought through the use of physical education content. Commonly used approaches are reciprocal learning, role playing and simulation, and cooperative learning. Inherent to interaction approaches is giving and receiving assessment feedback with a peer or group of peers. For example, all approaches could use task cards, rating scales, and checklists designed for peer assessment. The artifacts produced from selected observations (e.g., checklists, rating scales, anecdotal recordings) and performance sampling techniques (e.g., reflections, video clips) could be integrated into these interaction approaches and then stored in a student portfolio. At the end of the chapter, several forms of interaction are included in the sample portfolio systems. The Locomotor Skills Workbook for the elementary school level (pages 197-205) includes a partner activity and group project. The Fitness for Life portfolio system for the high school level (pages 216-233) includes a peer and family conference component. The K-12 student portfolio builder on the accompanying CD-ROM includes conference activities based on established learning targets.

Teaching Models

The integration of assessment and teaching can be described using a "models" approach (Metzler, 2000). Instructional models help teachers make and carry out decisions that lead to student achievement. An instructional model is defined as a comprehensive and coherent plan for teaching that includes needs assessment, intended learning targets, teachers' content knowledge expertise, developmentally sequenced activities, and measures of learning outcomes. The components and dimensions of the seven instructional models described in this section allow for the relationship between teaching and assessment to be verified. Assessing with each model is described relative to the potential for explicit student involvement.

1. *Direct.* Teacher-centered decisions and teacher-directed engagement patterns for students characterize this model. The purpose of direct teaching is to make the most efficient use of class time and to promote very high rates of student engagement in practice activities. Students are given many supervised practice attempts so that the teacher can observe and deliver high rates of constructive feedback. They practice a task until they achieve the criterion success rate set by the teacher. Typically, assessment occurs through the teacher's informal observation of students' performance. Student success rates can be monitored informally by having students practice in blocks of task trials. For example, a block of five trials and a criterion success rate of 80 percent (four out of five) may be appropriate. Through informal self-checks, students can determine and then report when they have reached the criterion success rate. Some practical formal assessment techniques can be used. Students can be given cards on which to record successful skill attempts, or student peer observers can use a checklist of key performance cues. Opportunities for student-involved assessment are somewhat restricted in the direct teaching model.

2. *Personalized.* The theme for personalized teaching is that students progress as fast as they can or as slowly as they need to through a sequence of prescribed learning tasks. A task analysis for each of the skills and knowledge areas is carried out. Performance criteria are provided for every learning task module. As students complete a learning task to its stated performance criterion,

they move on to the next task, without dependence on the teacher for permission or instruction. Student-involved assessment is built into the personalized teaching system through self-checks and peer checks. Individual students can be expected to maintain a personal progress chart to show successful practice trials, completed learning tasks according to the specified performance criteria, and learning pace. When students experience difficulty, they can "loop back" to repeat previous tasks or complete enrichment subtasks that lead to the next task in the sequence. Student-led conferences could focus on personal achievement data. Opportunities for student-involved assessment are considered good in the personalized teaching model.

3. *Cooperative learning.* Team rewards, individual accountability, and equal opportunity for success for all students are inherent features of cooperative learning. These attributes differentiate cooperative learning from collaborative or small-group processes. Cooperative learning is both achievement based and process based. Student interaction facilitates student achievement. Students must cooperate to learn, not necessarily learn to cooperate. The nature of assessment depends on the assigned learning task or standard being sought. If the task is to develop basic skills and content knowledge, traditional kinds of assessment can be used. When the cooperative strategy is more complex, more authentic, student-involved assessment is consistent with the meaning of cooperative learning. For example, performance assessments are typically carried out using a scoring rubric. The cooperative team could assume responsibility for creating and implementing the rubric. Following are some other techniques:

- Team portfolio, with individual achievements verified
- Critical incident reporting
- Checklists of "approach" (positive) and "avoidance" (negative) social interaction behaviors to monitor frequency
- Team work logs listing who did what
- Reflective journals

Opportunities for student-involved assessment are good in the cooperative learning teaching model.

4. *Sport education.* The structure of sport education (Siedentop, Hastie, & van der Mars, 2004) is adapted from real-world, organized sport. It includes roles that need to be carried out (e.g., players, coaches, officials, score keepers, administrators), support staff (e.g., managers, public relations personnel, reporters), and other aspects (practice time, schedule of games, league rules, equipment). All students are players, but they also learn one or more other roles. They learn the skills, decisions, customs, and responsibilities that go with these roles. The goals of sport education are to develop competent, literate, and enthusiastic sport persons. The six key features of sport education are seasons, affiliation, formal competition, culminating event, record keeping, and festivity. Assessment should focus on outcomes for two key roles—as players and in duty jobs. In the role of player, basic skills can be assessed by student coaches and teammates using criteria checklists designed by team "officials" (i.e., other role students). Likewise, a team membership checklist of behaviors can be devised, with team members filling it out on themselves and each other periodically. A similar checklist for good sporting behavior could be administered by students before, during, and after the "season." Students in the other job roles can assess themselves using authentic assessment checklists. Opportunities for student-involved assessment are considered good in the sport education teaching model.

5. *Peer.* Peer teaching is a variation of direct teaching. Instructional interactions during and after students' learning trials are delegated to student peers, called tutors, who have been trained to observe and analyze other students' practice attempts. Even though practice time is cut in half because students must carry out the role of tutor, peer teaching reduces the problem of too little teacher observation of practice attempts and limited feedback. In the learning role (practicing), each student has a private tutor for each practice attempt. In the tutor role, the student is cognitively engaged, which can increase comprehension and contribute later to improved practice. Socially, students develop a reciprocal relationship based on shared responsibility. Criteria checklists

and frequency index scales, rather than rating scales, are common assessment tools. The tutor is trained on what to watch and how to determine whether a movement or outcome is correctly executed. The number and complexity of checklist items depend on the tutor's ability to discern them in motion. The student benefits from specific feedback on each performance component, while tutors are reminded of the key performance cues when it is their time to practice. In addition, peer conferencing is a natural assessment technique. Opportunities for student-involved assessment are considered average in the peer teaching model. At the end of the chapter, peer involvement is included in the sample portfolio systems. The Locomotor Skills Workbook for the elementary school level (pages 197-205) includes a partner activity and group project. The Fitness for Life portfolio system for the high school level (pages 216-233) includes a peer conference component.

6. *Inquiry.* This model is actually a combination of strategies that is often referred to as exploration, guided discovery, or problem solving. Basically, questions are used to guide learning, particularly in the cognitive domain. However, cognitive engagement can serve as a prerequisite or stimulus for answers or solutions experienced through movement. The development of students' intellectual abilities—knowledge, reasoning, problem solving, and making judgments—help students become expressive, creative, and skillful in the motor domain. Assessment can be carried out in several ways including student–peer observation with a checklist, peer critiques of students' answers, student self-assessment with a checklist, student journals explaining how answers or solutions were derived, and student-designed movement and media presentations. Opportunities for student-involved assessment are considered good in the inquiry teaching model.

7. *Tactical games.* In this model, developmentally appropriate games and gamelike activities that focus on tactical problems for students to solve are sequenced. The most essential tactics needed to play the game are learned first and then applied through the execution of skilled motor performance. Students progress from simple to more complicated simulations of game situations. Assessment should focus on the ability to make and execute tactical decisions while playing a full game, a modified game, or a game form that represents the game situation. In this respect, the assessment is authentic because of its real-life context. One way to do this is to record objective game statistics (e.g., shots on goal, shot location, time of possession, turnovers, errors) followed by self-reflection and goal setting. Another way is to evaluate tactical decision making and skill execution using a criteria checklist. Typically, the teacher observes and records instances of tactical knowledge and performance on selected components (e.g., soccer restarts). Student self-assessment of tactical game performance could follow. Opportunities for student-involved assessment are somewhat limited in the tactical games teaching model.

Alignment of Teaching Models and Assessment Techniques

The importance of target–method match was previously established to maximize student-involved, classroom-level assessment. Of equal importance is the nature of student-involved assessment and the degree to which it is accomplished within the context of teaching. As outlined in this section, opportunities vary across the range of teaching patterns and models. But, many assessment techniques are natural to the meaning and purpose of the varied teaching constructs. The relationships among student-involved assessment techniques and teaching models are identified in table 3.1. Intersections are coded (strong, moderate, limited) to indicate these relationships. Note that teacher-directed assessment techniques (e.g., achievement tests, written tests, observational inventories) are not included in this analysis. The focus is on techniques that involve students at the classroom level, specific to physical education.

Process for Integration

Assessment literacy has been defined as the ability to properly match the method of assessment with the intended learning target and to relate assessment techniques with teaching models. These alignments—learning targets with assessment methods (e.g., selected response, constructed response, performance assessment) and teaching models with assessment techniques (e.g., rating

Table 3.1 Alignment of Teaching Models and Assessment Techniques

	ASSESSMENT TECHNIQUES (RELATIONSHIP CODE: ••• = STRONG; •• = MODERATE; • = LIMITED)						
Teaching models (Metzler, 2000)	Self-check criteria and rating sheets	Peer task cards, rating scales, and checklists	Logs and journals	Self-ratings and personal reflections	Self-reports	Rubric design and implementation	Student-led conferences
Direct	••	••	•	•	•	•	•
Personalized	•••	•••	•••	•••	•••	•••	•••
Cooperative learning	•••	•••	•••	•••	•••	•••	•••
Sport education	•••	••	•••	•••	•••	•	•
Peer	•	•••	•	•	•	•	•••
Inquiry	•••	•••	•••	•••	•••	•	•••
Tactical games	••	•	••	•	••	•	•

131

scales, checklists, logs, peer task cards, self-reports, rubrics)—have been described in the context of student-involved, classroom-level assessment. Ultimately, teachers need to integrate learning targets, teaching patterns and models, and assessment methods and techniques. No doubt, the synthesis of these three variables is a complex and challenging task. The following five-step integration process will help:

1. *Determine the contexts for assessment.* What are your achievement expectations or learning targets? What are your preferred teaching approaches or models? What are your students' learning styles and assessment preferences and needs? What is the nature of the selected content to which assessment is applied?

2. *Rethink the assessment function.* Seek a balance between assessment *of* learning and assessment *for* learning. The need for summative assessment exists for practical and educational reasons (i.e., documenting achievement status, verifying mastery of standards, certifying competence to the public, grading, advancement). However, effective teachers use a recurring process: assess–plan–teach–assess–modify plans–teach–assess (Glatthorn, 1993). This process describes formative assessment, in which information is sought for deciding how to adjust or improve the instructional system while corrections are still possible. It permits changes in the learning process while changes can still affect final performance and provides feedback concerning the teaching–learning process. Thus, the current overemphasis on summary judgments should be balanced with formative assessment, including classroom-level student involvement using self-assessment, goal setting, record keeping, and communication.

3. *Begin with the end in mind.* The traditional approach to assessment is sequenced as follows: (1) Design the curriculum, (2) plan instructional strategies, (3) implement instruction and learning experiences, (4) design the assessment, and (5) conduct student assessment. In a standards-based approach, however, teachers should begin with the intended content standards and corresponding learning targets (see figure 1.1, page 11). They should identify the desired results, determine acceptable evidence, and then plan learning experiences and instruction. This "backward" design is a purposeful task analysis that answers the question, How do I get there? The approach, which is logically forward, but backward in terms of conventional habits, is sequenced as follows: (1) Select or write content standards, (2) design the assessment, (3) establish performance levels, (4) design the curriculum, (5) plan instructional strategies, (6) implement instruction and learning experiences, (7) conduct student assessment, and (8) evaluate and refine the sequence. This concept can also be conceived as planning down and implementing up (Kelly & Melograno, 2004). The information about alignment of learning targets and assessment methods can facilitate this step (page 126).

4. *Use alternative teaching behaviors as needed.* Teachers are responsible for integrating assessment into teaching. To enhance this integration, they need to (1) deliberately plan for student involvement (strategies are needed to ensure student input; it cannot be left to chance); (2) provide time for tasks that encourage decision making and reflection (they should not become overanxious because tasks look passive); (3) demonstrate expected behaviors (i.e., model expectations); actually show students what is being sought; (4) help students manage their peer or self-assessment (i.e., provide assistance just as they would guide students through a difficult motor task); (5) develop positive interactive behaviors (students need to know where they stand; feedback and encouragement are needed because of the emphasis on self-management); and (6) actually use interactions to guide teaching; information derived from assessment could result in a decision to change what is taught. Table 3.1 can be used to facilitate this step.

5. *Convert assessment data to grades, as necessary.* An expanded assessment repertoire means that the quantity and quality of evaluation information is also expanded. With more authentic student-involved assessment, conventional grades may be replaced with anecdotal records, progress reports, performance samples, and student profiles. Despite new attempts to restructure report cards that emphasize performance, social skills, problem-solving abilities, and other meaningful outcomes, traditional grades still dominate. It may be more practical to supplement report cards with descriptive progress reports to communicate students' accomplishments, their strengths and difficulties, and their development. In the case of portfolios, for example, scoring rubrics can be used to assess individual artifacts, selected key items, or the entire portfolio.

The view of some physical education teachers regarding assessment is that they have too many students and not enough time. The reality is that many teachers manage students first and deliver some kind of instruction second. Assessment, particularly student-involved assessment, may be a distant third. Most of the new techniques, however, demand greater student responsibility (e.g., self-management, self-assessment, reflection, goal setting, record keeping, student-led conferences). Once a *system* of assessment *for* learning is understood and applied, time restrictions and sheer numbers are minimized. Use of self-directed assessment tasks, partners, and small groups can reduce the effects of high student–teacher ratios. Obviously, the system of student-involved assessment needs to be well planned and organized.

The justification and means for integrating assessment, learning, and teaching have been clearly established. What is needed is a practical technique to carry out this integration. Portfolios offer the way to involve students deeply in the overall process of classroom-level assessment *for* learning. The rest of the chapter is devoted to the development of student portfolio systems for physical education.

Purposes and Types of Student Portfolios

Like other teachers, physical educators think about why they use a particular drill or lead-up game or why they guide a class in a certain direction through skill practice. They also want a clear sense of what they are trying to accomplish when they assess students. Teachers need reasons for doing what they do. Before deciding on student portfolios, physical educators need only to look at a comparison between what seems to be traditional testing practice and the characteristics of portfolios as a collecting and communicating tool (Tierney, Carter, & Desai, 1991).

Testing practices usually

1. cover a limited content area and may not truly represent what students have learned;
2. rely on teacher-scored or mechanically-scored results with little student involvement;
3. examine all students on the same dimensions;
4. minimize teacher–student and student–student collaboration;
5. address summative achievement only; and
6. separate assessment, learning, and teaching.

In physical education, testing practices have resulted in end-of-unit skills tests with little relationship to what students may have actually learned. Performance results are determined in artificial or contrived settings (e.g., skill tests) rather than in more naturalistic, real situations (e.g., game play). Testing of this nature is not considered authentic.

Portfolios, on the other hand,

1. represent a wide range of student work in a given content area;
2. engage students in goal setting, reflection, self-assessment, record keeping, and communication;
3. allow for student differences;
4. foster collaborative assessment;
5. focus on improvement, effort, and achievement; and
6. link assessment and teaching to learning.

In physical education, these elements have always existed as part of any broad-based assessment process that uses achievement data derived from drills, practice, and game settings. Portfolios offer a way to organize, manage, and communicate these performance results. The assessment artifacts that are contained in portfolios are considered authentic in nature.

Although portfolios seem to offer dynamic visual presentations of students' true abilities, strengths, and areas in need of improvement, teachers should look at the "big picture" to determine the primary and secondary uses of portfolios. They need to answer some hard questions.

Why involve students in the process of gathering artifacts? In the end, will it make a difference? What are the potential overuses and abuses of portfolios for assessment purposes and beyond? Once they have answered these critical questions, teachers can initiate with students a system of portfolio assessment, assuming that the purposes are clear to all. Therefore, the initial phase in developing a student portfolio system involves determining the purposes (step 1 of the portfolio-designing process) and the types of portfolios (step 2 of the portfolio-designing process) that can best achieve these purposes.

Purposes

The reason for creating student portfolios is twofold—to serve student needs and to serve teacher needs. These two broad reasons may seem obvious, but often they are not. Students are served by being empowered and motivated to learn and encouraged to engage in goal setting, reflection, self-assessment, and communication. Teachers are served by being given opportunities to examine instructional methodologies and assess teaching performance. As the first step in building a portfolio system, purposes for both students and teachers should be considered. How could artifacts be selected without first deciding for what and for whom the portfolio is intended?

Portfolio purposes can be derived from three primary sources. First, purposes should reflect the content that is important for students to learn (i.e., physical education subject matter). Second, purposes should reflect the processes of learning that promote motor abilities, cognitive development, and attitude formation among learners (e.g., skill practice, higher-order thinking, problem solving, acquiring interests, formulating attitudes). And third, purposes should accommodate the diversity that exists among students (e.g., learning styles, multiple intelligences, physical abilities, multicultural differences).

Another question that arises is, How many purposes should a portfolio have? Even though the number of possible purposes of portfolios is unlimited, it makes sense to be practical. Teachers are better off setting a manageable number, particularly in the beginning. This is an important decision because the purposes will govern what goes into the portfolio. Given the needs of students and teachers and the many purposes of portfolios, it is useful to think of portfolios as serving both general and specific purposes.

General Purposes

General purposes of portfolios, gathered from various places, are applicable across subject areas and grade levels. They are global in nature and serve any kind of student portfolio system. Following are some general purposes (Murphy & Smith, 1992):

- Keeping track of students' progress and growth toward learning targets
- Providing students with an opportunity to assess their own accomplishments
- Assisting the teacher in instructional planning
- Determining the extent to which established learning targets have been achieved
- Helping parents understand their children's effort and progress
- Serving as a basis for program evaluation
- Determining student placement within and outside of class

Specific Purposes

Specific purposes of portfolios relate directly to physical education as a teaching discipline. They focus on subject matter, learning processes, and accommodations represented by the student portfolio system in physical education. Following are some specific purposes:

- Helping students practice healthy lifestyles
- Communicating student's strengths and weakness in gross and fine motor skills

- Determining the degree of personal and social development in an adventure education program
- Developing the student outcomes associated with the definition of the physically educated person
- Documenting the status of physical education content standards and corresponding benchmarks and grade-level indicators

Types of Portfolios

The lists of widely varying general and specific purposes suggest that portfolios can go in several directions. A portfolio that emphasizes personal fitness, for example, would look much different from one that documents content standards and benchmarks. Once the purposes for implementing a portfolio system are clear, the second step is to determine the type of portfolio that can best achieve these purposes. The following list of portfolio types is not meant to be exhaustive. The types can be used alone, in combination, or with other ideas to satisfy established purposes.

Personal Portfolios

To introduce themselves to their peers and teachers or to share their interests, students may include in their portfolios items from outside school that show hobbies, community activities, musical or artistic talents, sports, family, pets, or travel. To form a more holistic view of students, the portfolio could contain pictures, awards, videos, or other memorabilia. For example, a student might prepare an introductory portfolio that presents herself as a "sports enthusiast." Another possibility is the autobiography portfolio that traces life events and reflects on the future in terms of school or career goals. The personal portfolio can serve as a catalyst for self-reflection and continual sharing of ideas and insights throughout the K-12 experience.

Record-Keeping Portfolios

This maintenance type of portfolio can be kept by the teacher and the student either separately or in combination. For teachers, it contains necessary assessment and evaluation samples and records that may be required by the school district (e.g., written exams, standardized tests, proficiency tests) and not chosen by the student. To enhance student-involved assessment, the record-keeping portfolio that is managed by students could include observational information (e.g., anecdotal notes, frequency index scales, narrative descriptors, behavior checklists) as well as progress reports to supplement traditional report cards. Students could also track their growth toward their own learning targets.

Thematic Portfolios

A thematic portfolio would relate to a unit of study with a particular focus. The unit would normally last from two to six weeks. For example, with teamwork as the theme, entries could reflect an understanding of offensive and defensive strategies (cognitive), sports skills that facilitate team patterns of play (motor), and behavior processes that show working toward a common goal (affective). Other themes in physical education might be socialization through sports, aerobics for real, spatial awareness, or self-expression. For example, at the end of the chapter, the Fitness for Life portfolio system for the high school level (pages 216-233) is considered a thematic portfolio.

Integrated Portfolios

To provide a picture of the "whole" student, portfolios could include works from all the disciplines showing connections between or among subjects. Selected items, either required or optional, could be drawn from several or all subjects. Students could reflect on the most and least favorite aspects of each subject or discuss what concepts and skills transfer across several subjects and outside the school setting. Subjects that could be easily integrated with physical education include health (e.g., fitness, stress), science (e.g., laws of motion, stability), language arts (e.g., nonverbal communication), art (e.g., expression, manipulation), and music (e.g., rhythm, creating).

Showcase or Celebration Portfolios

In the showcase or celebration portfolio, a limited number of items are selected to exhibit achievement growth over time and to serve a particular purpose. This portfolio usually houses only the student's best work. Students must decide what accomplishments and achievements they are most proud of. Because it is streamlined and customized, it can be presented to others in different ways, such as in small groups, large groups, posterlike sessions, or exhibitions. The showcase or celebration portfolio, for example, could be focused on growth in a sport, fitness gains, or development of a gymnastics routine. At the end of the chapter, the Locomotor Skills Workbook for the elementary school level (pages 197-205) and the Volleyball Sportfolio for the middle school level (pages 206-215) are considered showcase or celebration portfolios.

Employment Portfolios

Students are often required to collect evidence of their employment skills. This portfolio is found mostly at the secondary level, particularly among graduating seniors. Students need to show artifacts that demonstrate the ability to communicate, work cooperatively, and work responsibly. The extent to which work samples and exhibits from physical education might contribute to the employment portfolio depends on the nature of the artifact and the nature of the prospective job. A student will also benefit from compiling a sample portfolio in preparation for a mock job interview.

Scholarship Portfolios

In the scholarship portfolio, information is compiled to show student eligibility for academic or athletic college scholarships. Although transcripts, attendance records, standardized test scores, and recommendations are normally included, other items from physical education might be selected (e.g., physical fitness status, videos, projects). The scholarship portfolio is normally managed by the student and facilitated by a school counselor.

Other Portfolios

Other kinds of portfolios build off the individual types of portfolios described thus far. Some of these represent true portfolios that would be subject to typical portfolio formats and expectations. Others are not really portfolios but represent ways to organize and manage portfolios. Some misconceptions about these types of portfolios need to be clarified.

- *Multiyear portfolio.* In this type of portfolio, stored at the school, students collect items from a cluster of grade levels over two, three, or four years. For example, student reflections on changes in fitness status could occur periodically over a three-year period during middle school.

- *Group portfolio.* In the group portfolio, members of a cooperative learning group contribute items that show individual strengths. These are included along with group items (e.g., samples, pictures, community project) to demonstrate the effectiveness of the entire group. The characteristics of cooperative learning are retained—namely, interdependence, individual accountability, heterogeneity (i.e., skill level, gender, race, or cultural background), cooperative behaviors, and a group "score" that is a collection of individual scores. For example, the sport education teaching model discussed earlier lends itself to the group portfolio.

- *Working portfolio.* The so-called working portfolio is not really a portfolio. It is a working repository or holding folder for the ongoing, systematic collection of student work samples and exhibits. This collection of daily, weekly, monthly, or unit work products forms the framework for self-assessment and goal setting, and it provides all possible artifacts from which to make

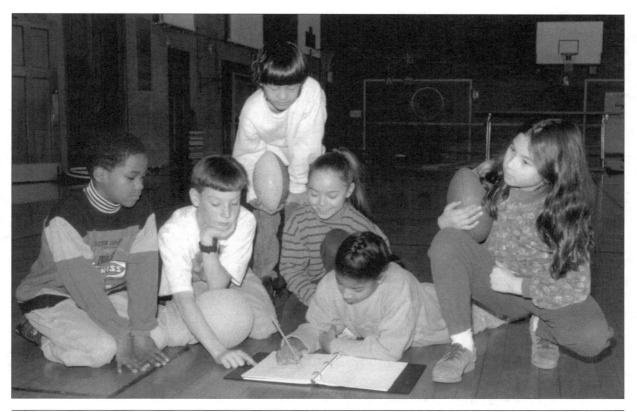

Cooperative learning can be facilitated by a group portfolio.

selections for other types of portfolios (e.g., thematic, integrated, showcase/celebration). The working portfolio is managed and kept by the student. The term *working repository* is used in this book to reflect its true meaning.

- *Electronic portfolio.* Another misconception is represented by the terms *electronic portfolio* or *e-portfolio*. All of the identified types of portfolios can be constructed, stored, and managed electronically, including on the Internet. For this reason, "electronic portfolios" are not included as a type of portfolio. Technological advances have made electronic management, storage, and portfolio-related processes a reality. However, if portfolios are simply software databases—storage for pictures, sound, or words—they are really no different from hanging files or milk crates. The content of portfolios and the process of creating them are the most important concerns. Multimedia writing tools, scanners, digital cameras, and recordable CD-ROM drives have all helped in creating true portfolios. For example, the accompanying CD-ROM contains a universal portfolio template that can be used to build student portfolios at all educational levels. Self-reflection, data sharing, and evaluation can be built in. Teachers could identify individual student needs, determine class performance, communicate with parents about student achievement, and document program effectiveness. Electronic and Web-based information and guidelines for constructing, storing, and managing portfolios are covered later in this chapter (pages 150-155).

Organizing Scheme

Developing a student portfolio system requires decisions of a practical nature. The mechanics of portfolios must be decided, and they serve as a guide for the remaining components. Given the complexities of portfolios, these decisions are critical because they affect the ongoing process of assessment and the daily lives of teachers and students.

Regardless of the purpose or type of portfolio, a clear and meaningful organizing scheme is needed (step 3 of the portfolio-designing process). Student portfolios can be organized around any number of goals, competencies, concepts, outcomes, and other constructs. The following section discusses some of these alternative organizers. Ultimately, established K-12 physical education content standards and corresponding grade-level expectations are recommended as the basis for organizing "academic" types of portfolios. A successful portfolio system is also dependent on the role of both teacher and student. Because these roles are likely to be new, expectations should be clear. Therefore, these roles are outlined and discussed.

To a large extent, the purpose and type of student portfolio will direct its organizational scheme. For example, perhaps the purpose is to monitor the progress of students' development of locomotor skills, and a showcase portfolio is to be used. The portfolio would likely be organized around the concepts and skills associated with the walk, run, jump, hop, gallop, slide, skip, and leap. Students might be expected to select their best work for each movement (e.g., task sheet, drawing of exercise, matching worksheet) and to demonstrate the movements to a small group of peers who provide feedback using a criteria checklist. The Locomotor Skills Workbook for the elementary school level that appears at the end of the chapter (pages 197-205) is designed for this purpose. To further illustrate, suppose that the purpose is to determine achievement of health-related fitness learning targets and a record-keeping portfolio is selected. The predetermined individual targets for cardiorespiratory endurance, muscular strength and endurance, flexibility, and body composition could be the basis for organizing the portfolio. These targets would need to be validated with artifacts (e.g., logs, journals, pretest and posttest comparisons, attitude inventory, fitness project). The Fitness for Life portfolio for the high school level that appears at the end of the chapter (pages 216-233) is designed for this purpose.

Alternative Organizers

Although purposes are the primary means for organizing the portfolio, there are other useful possibilities. For example, existing school district goals or outcomes can be translated into criteria and indicators of performance specific to physical education. The result would be portfolios that reflect levels of achievement referenced to the performance indicators. Similarly, state-mandated standards are excellent sources for determining the organizational basis for the portfolio. The following additional frameworks for organizing portfolios apply to the "academic" types of portfolios identified previously in this chapter (i.e., record-keeping, thematic, integrated, showcase/celebration, group, and multiyear portfolios). They would not be relevant for the other, more private types of portfolios (i.e., personal, employment, and scholarship portfolios).

Mission Statement

Oftentimes, the school district has a stated mission, which in turn is translated into program mission statements. Elements of such a statement could serve as the focus for organizing portfolios. For example, teachers and students could collect, rationalize, and organize artifacts around the following mission: "Through physical education, students will develop into healthy, physically active, socially adjusted, emotionally stable, and intellectually stimulated persons by attaining the knowledge, skills, and attitudes and values appropriate to these outcomes."

Physically Educated Person

Clearly developed, publicly stated outcomes can provide the basis for organizing portfolios. The original focus areas that defined the physically educated person could serve as useful organizing elements. According to NASPE (1992), the physically educated person

- has learned skills necessary to perform a variety of physical activities,
- is physically fit,
- participates regularly in physical activity,

- knows the implications of and the benefits from involvement in physical activities, and
- values physical activity and its contributions to a healthful lifestyle.

Learning Dimensions

Students need to grow and mature physically, intellectually, emotionally, socially, and spiritually. Because these developmental needs can be satisfied explicitly through participation in physical activities, they are valuable organizing constructs for the portfolio. Artifacts could be planned for each of the dimensions as represented by the following educational domains:

- *Cognitive:* Knowledge and intellectual abilities and skills ranging from simple recall tasks to synthesizing and evaluating information.
- *Affective:* Likes and dislikes, attitudes, values, and beliefs ranging from the willingness to receive information and respond to stimuli to the development of an established value system; encompasses the process of socialization.
- *Psychomotor:* All observable voluntary human motion ranging from reflex movements to the ability to modify and create aesthetic movement patterns.

Multiple Intelligences

Although some common learning outcomes should be sought by all students, physical educators must respect the learning diversity among students. Not all students can achieve outcomes in the same manner. The theory of multiple intelligences (Gardner, 1999) suggests that people possess several capacities for learning and creating products. Artifacts from physical education could be selected for each intelligence depending on content and individual student preferences. The portfolio could be organized around these eight domains of learning:

- *Verbal/linguistic:* Relates to written and spoken language (e.g., reactions to videos, written fitness program)
- *Logical/mathematical:* Deals with deductive thinking, reasoning, and recognition of abstract patterns (e.g., calculating energy expenditure, biomechanical analysis of sports skills)
- *Kinesthetic:* Involves using the body to solve problems, create products, and convey ideas and emotions (e.g., adventure education challenges, designing free-exercise routines)
- *Visual/spatial:* Relies on the sense of sight and the ability to visualize an object and create mental images (e.g., charting plays, sketching out routines)
- *Musical:* Includes recognition of environmental sounds and sensitivity to rhythm and beats (e.g., creating a dance step, moving to a drum beat)
- *Interpersonal:* Reflects the ability to understand and work effectively with others (e.g., planning a cooperative game, role-playing sportsmanship)
- *Intrapersonal:* Refers to knowledge about and awareness of one's own emotions and self (e.g., reflective fitness journal, describing feeling of being a pro golfer)
- *Naturalist:* Refers to the ability to recognize, categorize, and draw on features in the environment or natural world (e.g., outdoor pursuits, wilderness camping)

Organizing Centers

The physical education curriculum often lacks a focus, some frame of reference around which the curriculum is designed. The "organizing center" helps to identify elements that can serve as focal points (Melograno, 1996). Organizing centers combine concepts, skills, attitudes, and values that underlie physical education goals content. They are global in nature. The resulting program is a series of organizing centers sequentially arranged over various time periods (e.g., single lesson, series of lessons, unit, semester, academic year, four-year high school program, comprehensive K-12 curriculum). In the same manner that organizing centers provide a curriculum focus, they also provide the basis for organizing portfolios. Organizing centers range from comprehensive themes such as Education for a Global Community, Worthy Citizenship, or Meeting the Challenge of a Changing Society to specific emphases such as Body Awareness, Teamwork, or Solving a Problem. Intermediate ideas can also be used, such as Growth and Development, Success, or Decision Making. Regardless of their complexity, organizing centers offer a rationale for the selection of artifacts.

Content Standards

Given the variety of the organizing options already presented, it should be clear that a universal construct for organizing portfolios does not exist. However, there is general agreement about what students should know and be able to do as a result of their physical education program (NASPE, 2004). These physical education content standards and general descriptions were detailed in table 1.1 (pages 13-14). The six content standards, as common themes across the curriculum, offer a vertical (sequential, progressive) and integrated structure of the physical education subject matter. Because of their widespread acceptance, they are recommended as the basis for organizing student portfolios. For each content standard, the student expectations for the four grade levels (grades K-2, 3-5, 6-8, and 9-12) are presented in table 3.2. They will also be used in subsequent sections of this chapter that deal with the other phases of portfolio development.

Changing Roles

Implementing portfolio practices requires a profound shift in the responsibilities and roles of teachers and students. The reality of too many students, not enough time, and the need to provide

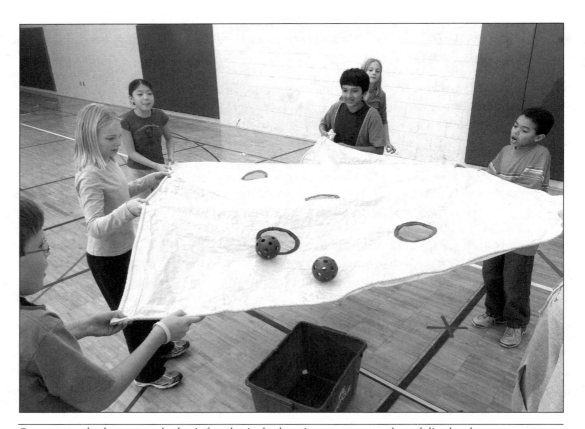

Content standards serve as the basis for physical education programs and portfolio development.

Table 3.2   Grade-Level Student Expectations for Physical Education Content Standards

Grades K-2	Grades 3-5	Grades 6-8	Grades 9-12
STANDARD 1			
DEMONSTRATES COMPETENCY IN MOTOR SKILLS AND MOVEMENT PATTERNS NEEDED TO PERFORM A VARIETY OF PHYSICAL ACTIVITIES			
At the end of grade 2, students are expected to achieve mature forms in the locomotor skills, demonstrate smooth transitions, show progress toward more complex manipulative skills, and demonstrate control in traveling, weight-bearing, and balance activities.	At the end of grade 5, students are expected to develop versatility in fundamental motor skills, achieve mature forms in nonlocomotor and manipulative skills, use skills in dynamic and complex environments and in combination, and acquire some specialized skills basic to a movement form.	At the end of grade 8, students are expected to participate with skill in a variety of modified activities, achieve mature forms in the basic skills of more specialized activities, use the skills successfully in modified activities, and demonstrate use of tactics within sport activities.	At the end of grade 12, students are expected to possess motor skills and movement patterns, demonstrate basic/advanced skills and tactics in at least one activity, and demonstrate basic skills and tactics in at least five additional activities.
STANDARD 2			
DEMONSTRATES UNDERSTANDING OF MOVEMENT CONCEPTS, PRINCIPLES, STRATEGIES, AND TACTICS AS THEY APPLY TO THE LEARNING AND PERFORMANCE OF PHYSICAL ACTIVITIES			
At the end of grade 2, students are expected to apply concepts, identify and perform concepts of effort and relationships, identify and use elements of correct form, and use feedback to improve motor performance.	At the end of grade 5, students are expected to comprehend and apply more complex concepts and principles, use performance feedback, use critical elements or motor principles to provide feedback to others, and transfer concepts.	At the end of grade 8, students are expected to exhibit discipline-specific knowledge; identify principles of practice and conditioning; understand and apply movement concepts and principles, game strategies, and characteristics of highly skilled performance; know when, why, and how to use strategies and tactics; and use information from a variety of sources.	At the end of grade 12, students are expected to develop scientifically based activity plans; use complex movement concepts and principles to refine and learn new skills; integrate advanced activity to develop the ability to learn, self-assess, and improve movement skills independently; and recognize elite-level performance.
STANDARD 3			
PARTICIPATES REGULARLY IN PHYSICAL ACTIVITY			
At the end of grade 2, students are expected to engage primarily in nonstructured physical activities outside of class, participate in wide variety of gross motor activities, participate in activities during leisure time that are moderate to vigorous, recognize that activity has temporary and lasting effects, and utilize acquired skills and knowledge during leisure time activity.	At the end of grade 5, students are expected to be aware of participation in physical activity as a conscious personal decision, voluntarily participate in moderate to vigorous physical activity outside class, make use of opportunities for regular participation in physical activity, use critical elements and movement concepts, and use information from various sources to regulate activity participation.	At the end of grade 8, students are expected to independently set activity goals; participate in individualized programs based on goals, interests, and fitness assessments; use practice procedures and training principles; be aware of opportunities for participation; and participate regularly in moderate to vigorous physical activities in school and nonschool settings.	At the end of grade 12, students are expected to desire physical activity to maintain healthy lifestyle, willingly participate in physical activities on a regular basis, assume a mature role in managing participation, possess movement capabilities and behavioral skills, independently apply appropriate training principles, and understand adult patterns of physical activity participation changes throughout life.

(continued)

Table 3.2 (continued)

Grades K-2	Grades 3-5	Grades 6-8	Grades 9-12
STANDARD 4			
ACHIEVES AND MAINTAINS A HEALTH-ENHANCING LEVEL OF PHYSICAL FITNESS			
At the end of grade 2, students are expected to enjoy physical activities, accumulate a relatively high volume of total activity, recognize physiological signs associated with moderate to vigorous physical activity, and possess basic knowledge of the components of health-related fitness.	At the end of grade 5, students are expected to participate in physical activity for improving fitness, participate in moderate to vigorous activity without tiring, engage in activities related to components of fitness, monitor physiological indicators, complete standardized fitness testing and achieve desired levels, and interpret information provided by formal measures of fitness.	At the end of grade 8, students are expected to participate in moderate to vigorous activity without undue fatigue; engage in activities that address components of health-related fitness; know components of fitness and relation to overall fitness status; monitor own heart rate, breathing rate, perceived exertion, and recovery rate; assess and use personal fitness status; and know principles of training and their use.	At the end of grade 12, students are expected to assume greater self-responsibility in own lives, demonstrate responsibility for own health-related fitness status, engage in activities to maintain health-related fitness, assess independently own personal fitness status, and interpret information from fitness tests to plan and design own programs.
STANDARD 5			
EXHIBITS RESPONSIBLE PERSONAL AND SOCIAL BEHAVIOR THAT RESPECTS SELF AND OTHERS IN PHYSICAL ACTIVITY SETTINGS			
At the end of grade 2, students are expected to discover joy of playing with friends; apply safe practices and physical education class rules; use acceptable behaviors for physical activity settings; work independently and productively; work independently and with improved motor skills; and gain appreciation for working in cooperative movement, sharing, solving a problem, and/or tackling a challenge.	At the end of grade 5, students are expected to work independently and with small groups; identify purposes for and follow activity-specific safe practices, rules, procedures, and etiquette; develop cooperation and communication skills; work independently and productively; and develop cultural/ethnic self-awareness, appreciate own heritage, and appreciate differences in others.	At the end of grade 8, students are expected to understand physical activity as a microcosm of culture and society, recognize role of activity in understanding diversity, reflect upon role in activity settings and benefits of activity, have well-developed cooperation skills, seek greater independence from adults, make appropriate decisions to resolve conflicts, and practice appropriate problem-solving techniques to resolve conflicts.	At the end of grade 12, students are expected to initiate responsible personal and social behavior, function independently, positively influence the behavior of others, demonstrate leadership, respond to potentially explosive interactions by settling conflicts, evaluate knowledge regarding the role of activity in a diverse society, make enlightened personal choices, and develop a personal philosophy of participation reflecting inclusion.
STANDARD 6			
VALUES PHYSICAL ACTIVITY FOR HEALTH, ENJOYMENT, CHALLENGE, SELF-EXPRESSION, AND/OR SOCIAL INTERACTION			
At the end of grade 2, students are expected to be physically active because they enjoy merely participating, like the challenge of experiencing new movements and learning new skills, feel joy as they gain competence, and begin to function as members of a group; work cooperatively for brief periods of time.	At the end of grade 5, students are expected to identify activities they consider to be fun, be challenged by learning a new skill or activity, attribute success and improvement to effort and practice, choose an appropriate level of challenge in an activity so as to experience success, and engage in activity with students of different and similar skill levels.	At the end of grade 8, students are expected to seek activity experiences for group membership and positive social interaction, appreciate skills performance, use activities as a positive outlet for competition and to gain recognition, increase self-confidence and self-esteem, develop confidence toward independence, be challenged by high levels of competition and in learning different activities, and experience greater awareness of feelings through self-expression.	At the end of grade 12, students are expected to be more comfortable with new interests and physiques; enjoy challenge of working hard; feel satisfaction when successful; enjoy regular participation in selected activities, either alone or with friends; and explain why participation in activities is enjoyable and desirable.

Reprinted from *Moving Into the Future: National Standards for Physical Education*, 2nd edition (2004) with permission from the National Association for Sport and Physical Education (NASPE), 1900 Association Drive, Reston, VA 20191-1599.

some kind of instruction often means that teachers believe that using portfolios for assessment purposes is unmanageable. However, portfolios demand a high level of student responsibility in terms of reflection, self-management, self-assessment, record keeping, communicating results, peer reflection, conferences, and evaluation. The number of students in a class can seem smaller when they are working as partners, in small groups, and at self-directed tasks. Students should learn to use portfolio systems incrementally, which will ultimately minimize the restriction of time and the effect of large numbers of students. Comprehensive planning, careful management, and gradual implementation are necessary. Before going any further with this system, let's look at the teacher's and students' roles more closely.

Role of the Teacher

Although elements of current instructional delivery systems could foster student-involved, classroom-level formative assessment, changes are needed to implement portfolios in physical education. Traditional teaching roles, in which teachers inform, direct, and predetermine priorities, will not work. In the portfolio model, the teacher facilitates, guides, and offers choices. Teachers become reflective practitioners. Instead of judging students' work against their own or other mandated standards, teachers become accomplished facilitators in the process of student self-assessment. Partnerships are established among teacher, students, and parents or guardians. More specifically, in the portfolio system, teachers need to do the following:

1. *Deliberately plan for student involvement.* Strategies are needed to ensure student input; involvement cannot be left to chance. Learning should be made available, not imposed.

2. *Provide time for tasks that encourage decision making and reflection.* Teachers should not become overanxious because certain tasks appear passive. Instead they can become intermediaries between students and the environment.

3. *Demonstrate expected behaviors (e.g., self-management, self-assessment).* By actually modeling for students what they are expecting, teachers can train them in decision making.

4. *Help students manage portfolios.* Teachers should provide assistance similar to guiding students through a difficult motor skill.

5. *Develop positive interactive behaviors.* Students need to know where they stand. Feedback and encouragement are needed because of the emphasis on self-management.

6. *Actually use interactions to guide instruction.* Information derived from portfolios as they are developed could influence what is taught. These kinds of adjustments are formative in nature.

7. *Rethink the environment.* Designating space so that students can become more actively involved in compiling their portfolios (e.g., portfolio storage, project work area, conference area, videotaping station) can be helpful. However, a successful portfolio system can still be implemented without any of these considerations.

Role of the Student

Because portfolios emphasize process as well as product, students must become independent. Acquiring these skills does not come easily to all students, nor does it happen overnight. Students need to observe, practice, and refine the behaviors associated with decision making, self-management, self-directed learning, and communication. Traditional student roles may not work. Students need to become active rather than passive. Instead of asking the teacher what they need to do or learning only what the teacher wants, students begin to ask themselves what is needed and to learn for themselves. Thus, students develop an increasing capacity to take responsibility for their own learning. More specifically, in the portfolio system, students need to do the following:

1. Reflect on the value of their own work; engage in metacognition (i.e., manage and assess their own learning strategies)

2. Make critical choices about what work samples and exhibits best represent learning

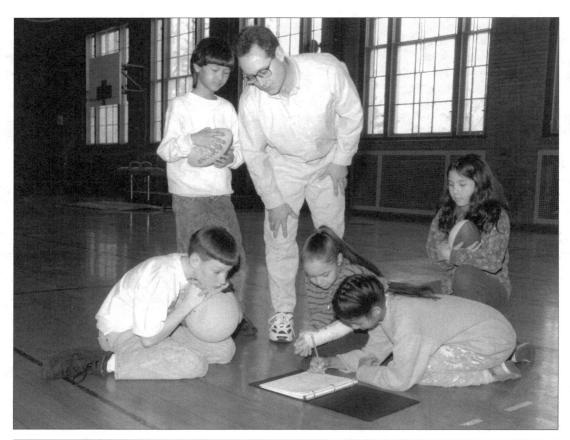

Physical education teachers need to help students manage their portfolios.

3. Trace the development of their own learning and make connections between prior knowledge and skills and new learning (i.e., transfer)

4. Make decisions and assume responsibility for future learning and set short-term and long-term learning goals

5. Engage in self-monitoring, self-management, and self-assessment

6. Collaborate within the physical education class setting (e.g., sharing best works, peer tutoring, peer reflection, student-led and peer conferences)

Production and Logistics

Planning a way to handle the production and logistics of a student portfolio system is a major expectation for teachers (step 4 of the portfolio-designing process). Decisions are needed about the method of construction, how and where to store portfolios, and how and when to manage portfolios. This section presents various options for constructing and storing portfolios that might help in developing the plan. Then, some management tools are offered for assembling and maintaining portfolios. Finally, information and guidelines are provided for using technology to facilitate the construction, storage, and management of student portfolios. Recall that a distinction was made between the working repository (holding folder), consisting primarily of hard-copy artifacts, and the various types of portfolios. The suggestions that follow apply to both the working repository and the actual portfolio depending on volume and purpose.

Construction and Storage

Perhaps the initial concern with production and logistics is how to collect and maintain all the possible items that could comprise the portfolio. At least two planning decisions must be made: the method of portfolio construction and how and where to store portfolios. Several options are depicted in figure 3.1.

Managing portfolios in physical education is different from managing them in a contained classroom. The physical education setting is not like a single room, nor is it usually the "home base" for students, so it is more difficult to centralize the portfolio system. Also, the physical education teacher must accommodate the portfolios of all students across many different classes, whereas an elementary classroom teacher, for example, may need to manage only 20 to 30 portfolios. Therefore, the physical education teacher may need to establish a common method of construction. It may not be feasible to allow the "container" for collecting artifacts to be a matter of personal preference. Possibilities include file folders, notebooks, hanging files, albums, large envelopes, accordion files, pocket folders with spiral bindings, and boxes. Every item should be dated, and a cumulative list of items should be maintained in the front of the portfolio.

Portfolios should be stored in locations that are accessible to students. Obviously, if students are responsible for storing their own portfolios, then the method of storage is a matter of personal preference. However, consideration must be given to access of the portfolio for teacher, peer, or parent review. If portfolios are stored in the physical education setting, the primary consideration is space. Depending on space, possibilities include file cabinets, file drawers, milk crates, shelves, large cardboard boxes, cereal boxes cut like magazine holders, pizza boxes, and large notebooks with jacket folders.

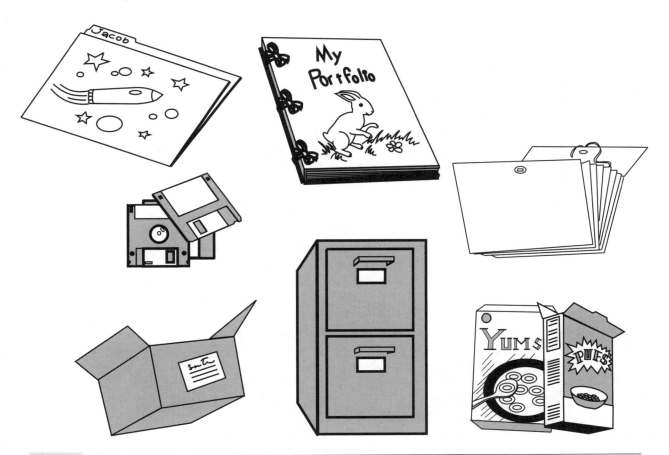

Figure 3.1   Selected construction and storage options for student portfolios.

Another storage option is a computer disk, regardless of whether the student or teacher assumes responsibility for storage. Written work, logs, scoring rubrics, journals, computer simulations, and digitized video can be kept on computer disks depending on available technology (e.g., personal computers, scanners, camcorders, digital cameras, recordable CD-ROM drives, software). Use of technology is fully covered later in this section. Lastly, portfolios can be stored in a central location (e.g., media center) for easy access and review. However, this storage option requires a great deal of coordination and cooperation among students and school personnel.

Ultimately, construction and storage decisions depend on the types of portfolios. For example, the working repository requires sufficient container space because the overall number of artifacts is high (e.g., a large notebook divided by sections, expanding and accordion files). By contrast, more selective types of portfolios (e.g., personal, thematic, integrated, showcase/celebration) may contain a relatively small number of artifacts because they are drawn from the working collection. Therefore, file folders or a small notebook may be all that is needed. The construction and storage of other specialized types of portfolios (e.g., record-keeping, group, multiyear, employment, scholarship) will vary according to purpose, number of artifacts, nature of artifacts, and who is going to review the portfolio.

A final aspect of storing portfolios relates to access. Although students' access to their own portfolios should be as hassle-free as possible, how and whether to allow access by others must be decided (e.g., peers, parents, other teachers, other school personnel). *Student confidentiality and privacy must be protected.* Certain portfolio sections or items may be designated as public, whereas others are private. Color codes, labels, stickers, or some other means of designation can be used. In any case, accessibility and confidentiality guidelines should be established from the beginning and strictly enforced thereafter by teachers and students.

Management Tools

Students vary in their ability to manage all the loose ends associated with assembling and maintaining a portfolio. Some students, regardless of grade level, are natural "organizers." Others struggle trying to keep things in order. Portfolio management skills should be taught in the same way that a motor skill is taught. Teachers need to demonstrate and model management behaviors, have students practice the behaviors, and reinforce the behaviors repeatedly. In addition, portfolios should be managed regularly by both teachers and students to avoid the overaccumulation of items at the end of a given collection period. Certain management tools are effective in handling the logistics of portfolios. They can be used separately or in combination.

Dividers

Whatever kind of container is used, divided notebook folders or divider pages can be used to separate artifacts according to the content standards or any other category that makes sense (e.g., themes, sport, unit, goal, works in progress, reflections, finished works). A filing system should be created so that the standards or categories are easily identified. Each section could be labeled with a shortened version of the standard.

Color Codes

To facilitate management, colored dots or colored files could be used to code entries in the portfolio. Artifacts could also be coded using different color markers. A code for the colors needs to be included (e.g., red for "not yet" work, blue for reflection, orange for group work, yellow for self-assessment, green for finished work).

Table of Contents

It is generally a good idea to include a list of all of the entries and page numbers in the front of the portfolio. Whether required or optional, items other than student work samples should also be listed in the table of contents (e.g., reflection sheets, peer reflections, self-assessment instruments, goal-setting page, teacher's scoring rubrics). For example, the K-12 student portfolio builder on the accompanying CD-ROM includes a table of contents.

Artifact Registry

A sheet could be maintained on which students record the date, item, and reason for either adding or removing an item. Because the registry is supposed to chronicle when and why items are removed or replaced, students engage in a dynamic form of reflection. See the artifact registry form on page 148.

Work Log

For a long-term project such as a portfolio, a biography of work could show the evolution of the portfolio. This would help in making necessary changes or shifting directions. The log could be as simple as a dated entry that traces all activities and decisions associated with the portfolio. A work log form is also shown on page 148.

Index

An alphabetical index of items and related topics could be compiled at the end of the portfolio. Such an organizational tool would help in the cross-referencing of artifacts that show evidence of the following organizing elements (discussed earlier): content standards and grade-level expectations, organizing centers, multiple intelligences, learning dimensions, mission statement, or NASPE's description of the physically educated person. An index, because of its complexity, would likely be found at the secondary level only.

Self-Stick Notes

Artifacts need to be cataloged so ideas are not lost over time. A self-stick note or index card could be attached to each artifact that identifies the content standard, benchmark, or other appropriate category to which the artifact relates. A brief statement explaining why the artifact was collected could be included on the card as well. Specific descriptors may help later in connecting the artifact to the standard, performance outcome, or category. Also, using a self-stick note or index card protects original works.

Stickers

Stickers are similar to self-stick notes except that they are preprinted. For example, stickers could be made representing each content standard. Students could identify the corresponding grade-level expectation, explain why they collected the artifact, or both. The standards could be indicated on the stickers with the following phrases: (1) basic/advanced movement form, (2) movement concept/principle, (3) benefits/costs of physical activity, (4) monitor/maintain health-enhancing fitness, and (5) social/personal responsibility. Other standard stickers could be produced with the following phrases:

I want this in my portfolio because . . .

This was difficult for me because . . .

This item shows that . . .

I think this is one of my best works because . . .

Stamps

To save time and to help students reflect on work samples, rubber stamps are a useful tool, particularly at the elementary level. A collection of stamps can facilitate the process of categorizing or labeling pieces. The following is a list of some sample stamp phrases:

This was fun!

Awesome!

This was easy for me.

Great!

Artifact Registry Form

Name: _____ Topic: _____

ADDITIONS		
Date	**Item**	**Reasons**

DELETIONS		
Date	**Item**	**Reasons**

Portfolio Work Log

Name: _____ Topic: _____

Date	Entry

Comments:

Best yet!

Bravo!

This was hard for me.

First try!

I could do better.

I need to be neater.

I should take more time.

I worked on _____.

I learned how to _____.

I need to work on _____.

Personalizing

The artwork, design, and layout of the portfolio allow students to interject their personalities. By personalizing the portfolio using color, graphics, and shapes, students distinguish their portfolios from others'. This can help in managing portfolios because individual students and their works will be identifiable. Original creative covers (using collage, photos, patterned and textured designs), such as the ones shown in figure 3.2, demonstrate personality. Also, children enjoy decorating things such as cereal boxes, file folders, or pizza boxes that serve as portfolio containers as illustrated earlier in figure 3.1 (page 145). Finally, students' personalities can be displayed by the tone of their portfolios. For example, depending on purpose, the appropriate tone could be humorous (e.g., cartoons, jokes, riddles, funny sketches), aesthetic (e.g., artwork, pictures, poems), or serious (e.g., no extras, straightforward design, efficient use of space).

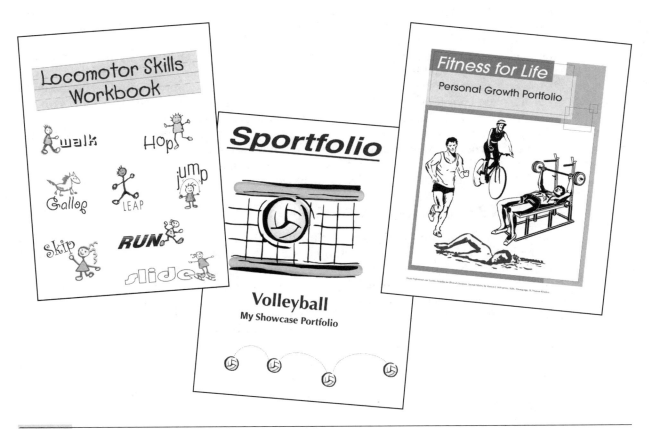

Figure 3.2 Personalized cover designs for student portfolios.

Use of Technology

The section in chapter 1 titled Technology Use in Portfolio Development should be referenced (pages 31-47). The information about hardware, storage, and software has general applicability to developing electronic-based student portfolios for K-12 physical education. Because electronic-based portfolios are an extension of paper-based portfolios, the information in this chapter on production and logistics is also applicable (pages 144-149). However, some additional information is important in regard to student portfolios for physical education programs.

Technology Standards

The national educational technology standards for students (NETS-S) developed by the International Society for Technology in Education (ISTE) are divided into six broad categories (ISTE, 2000). The standards within each category should be introduced to, reinforced with, and mastered by students. The foundation standards and corresponding grade-level (PreK-2, 3-5, 6-8, 9-12) performance indicators are identified in table 3.3. Physical education teachers can use these standards and indicators as guidelines for planning technology-related activities such as electronic-based or Web-based portfolios. The student learning, communication, and life skills reflected in the standards and the use of technology in developing portfolios can be addressed simultaneously.

Portfolio Management

Physical education classes can range from 20 to 80 or more students per class. Physical educators who wish to use electronic-based portfolios are often faced with time constraints and limited access to computers. For individualized portfolios to be practical and successful in the physical education setting, a physical educator should have access to *at least* one computer for 10 percent of the class. Operationally, students form 10 groups and rotate through a circuit of 10 stations. The circuit's computer station would then contain a computer for each student. Students could enter data or manage their personal electronic-based portfolios. Obviously, a smaller student–computer ratio is desirable.

Access to a computer lab or personal computers would facilitate moving from paper-based to electronic-based portfolios. Some physical educators require students to work on their electronic-based portfolios during time outside physical education, during school breaks, after school in the media center, or at home if they have access to a computer. When time and access to computers is limited, teachers can create task cards (step-by-step instructions) to ensure that students use their computer time efficiently. Many of the construction and management tools suggested earlier (page 145-149) can be applied to electronic-based portfolios.

Predesigned Electronic-Based Portfolios

The framework suggested in this chapter for developing student portfolios is teacher made. Although the move from paper-based to electronic-based student portfolios requires careful planning and implementation, the transition can occur in stages. Another option is to have only selected elements of a comprehensive portfolio system be electronic-based. In addition, physical education teachers can take advantage of some commercial, predesigned electronic-based portfolio systems. Although these portfolio systems use different organizational approaches, each allows students to store artifacts in an electronic format. The portfolio sections were created using FileMaker Pro, which allows the teacher to open one file and see all of the student's work on one activity or the entire student portfolio with the click of a button. While looking at an artifact, the teacher can grade it and then have the grade automatically recorded using software such as the Record Book (Bonnie's Fitware). Some popular predesigned systems are briefly described.

Table 3.3 Technology Foundation Standards and Performance Indicators for Students

TECHNOLOGY FOUNDATION STANDARDS FOR STUDENTS

1. Basic operations and concepts
   - Students demonstrate a sound understanding of the nature and operation of technology systems.
   - Students are proficient in the use of technology.
2. Social, ethical, and human issues
   - Students understand the ethical, cultural, and societal issues related to technology.
   - Students practice responsible use of technology systems, information, and software.
   - Students develop positive attitudes toward technology uses that support lifelong learning, collaboration, personal pursuits, and productivity.
3. Technology productivity tools
   - Students use technology tools to enhance learning, increase productivity, and promote creativity.
   - Students use productivity tools to collaborate in constructing technology-enhanced models, prepare publications, and produce other creative works.
4. Technology communication tools
   - Students use telecommunications to collaborate, publish, and interact with peers, experts, and other audiences.
   - Students use a variety of media and formats to communicate information and ideas effectively to multiple audiences.
5. Technology research tools
   - Students use technology to locate, evaluate, and collect information from a variety of sources.
   - Students use technology tools to process data and report results.
   - Students evaluate and select new information resources and technological innovations based on the appropriateness for specific tasks.
6. Technology problem solving and decision making tools
   - Students use technology resources for solving problems and making informed decisions.
   - Students employ technology in the development of strategies for solving problems in the real world.

PERFORMANCE INDICATORS

Grades PreK-2	Grades 3-5	Grades 6-8	Grades 9-12
All students should have opportunities to demonstrate the following performances. Prior to completion of grade 2, students will:	All students should have opportunities to demonstrate the following performances. Prior to completion of grade 5, students will:	All students should have opportunities to demonstrate the following performances. Prior to completion of grade 8, students will:	All students should have opportunities to demonstrate the following performances. Prior to completion of grade 12, students will:
1. Use input devices (e.g., mouse, keyboard, remote control) and output devices (e.g., monitor, printer) to successfully operate computers, VCRs, audiotapes, and other technologies. (1)	1. Use keyboards and other common input and output devices (including adaptive devices when necessary) efficiently and effectively. (1)	1. Apply strategies for identifying and solving routine hardware and software problems that occur during everyday use. (1)	1. Identify capabilities and limitations of contemporary and emerging technology resources and assess the potential of these systems and services to address personal, lifelong learning, and workplace needs. (2)
2. Use a variety of media and technology resources for directed and independent learning activities. (1, 3)	2. Discuss common uses of technology in daily life and the advantages and disadvantages those uses provide. (1, 2)	2. Demonstrate knowledge of current changes in information technologies and the effect those changes have on the workplace and society. (2)	2. Make informed choices among technology systems, resources, and services. (1, 2)
3. Communicate about technology using developmentally appropriate and accurate terminology. (1)	3. Discuss basic issues related to responsible use of technology and information and describe personal consequences of inappropriate use. (2)	3. Exhibit legal and ethical behaviors when using information and technology, and discuss consequences of misuse. (2)	3. Analyze advantages and disadvantages of widespread use and reliance on technology in the workplace and in society as a whole. (2)
4. Use developmentally appropriate multimedia resources (e.g., interactive books, educational software, elementary multimedia encyclopedias) to support learning. (1)	4. Use general purpose productivity tools and peripherals to support personal productivity, remediate skill deficits, and facilitate learning throughout the curriculum. (3)	4. Use content-specific tools, software, and simulations (e.g., environmental probes, graphing calculators, exploratory environments, Web tools) to support learning and research. (3, 5)	4. Demonstrate and advocate for legal and ethical behaviors among peers, family, and community regarding the use of technology and information. (2)
5. Work cooperatively and collaboratively with peers, family members, and others when using technology in the classroom. (2)	5. Use technology tools (e.g., multimedia authoring, presentation, Web tools, digital cameras, scanners) for individual and collaborative writing, communication, and publishing activities to create knowledge products for audiences inside and outside the classroom. (3, 4)	5. Apply productivity/multimedia tools and peripherals to support personal productivity, group collaboration, and learning throughout the curriculum. (3, 6)	5. Use technology tools and resources for managing and communicating personal/professional information (e.g., finances, schedules, addresses, purchases, correspondence). (3, 4)
6. Demonstrate positive social and ethical behaviors when using technology. (2)			6. Evaluate technology-based options, including distance and distributed education, for lifelong learning. (5)

(continued)

Table 3.3 *(continued)*

<table>
<tr><th colspan="4">PERFORMANCE INDICATORS</th></tr>
<tr><th>Grades PreK-2</th><th>Grades 3-5</th><th>Grades 6-8</th><th>Grades 9-12</th></tr>
<tr>
<td>7. Practice responsible use of technology systems and software. (2)
8. Create developmentally appropriate multimedia products with support from teachers, family members, or student partners. (3)
9. Use technology resources (e.g., puzzles, logical thinking programs, writing tools, digital cameras, drawing tools) for problem solving, communication, and illustration of thoughts, ideas, and stories. (3, 4, 5, 6)
10. Gather information and communicate with others using telecommunications with support from teachers, family members, or student partners. (4)</td>
<td>6. Use telecommunications efficiently and effectively to access remote information, communicate with others in support of direct and independent learning, and pursue personal interests. (4)
7. Use telecommunications and online resources (e.g., e-mail, online discussions, Web environments) to participate in collaborative problem solving activities for the purpose of developing solutions or products for audiences inside and outside the classroom. (4, 5)
8. Use technology resources (e.g., calculators, data collection probes, videos, educational software) for problem solving, self-directed learning, and extended learning activities. (5, 6)
9. Determine when technology is useful and select the appropriate tool(s) and technology resources to address a variety of tasks and problems. (5, 6)
10. Evaluate the accuracy, relevance, appropriateness, comprehensiveness, and bias of electronic information sources. (6)</td>
<td>6. Design, develop, publish, and present products (e.g., Web pages, videotapes) using technology resources that demonstrate and communicate curriculum concepts to audiences inside and outside the classroom. (4, 5, 6)
7. Collaborate with peers, experts, and others using telecommunication and collaborative tools to investigate curriculum-related problems, issues, and information, and to develop solutions or products for audiences inside and outside the classroom. (4, 5)
8. Select and use appropriate tools and technology resources to accomplish a variety of tasks and solve problems. (5, 6)
9. Demonstrate an understanding of concepts underlying hardware, software, and connectivity, and of practical applications to learning and problem solving. (1, 6)
10. Research and evaluate the accuracy, relevance, appropriateness, comprehensiveness, and bias of electronic information sources concerning real-world problems. (2, 5, 6)</td>
<td>7. Routinely and efficiently use online information resources to meet needs for collaboration, research, publication, communication, and productivity. (4, 5, 6)
8. Select and apply technology tools for research, information analysis, problem solving, and decision making in content learning. (4, 5)
9. Investigate and apply expert systems, intelligent agents, and simulations in real-world situations. (3, 5, 6)
10. Collaborate with peers, experts, and others to contribute to a content-related knowledge base by using technology to compile, synthesize, produce, and disseminate information, models, and other creative works. (4, 5, 6)</td>
</tr>
</table>

Reprinted with permission from *National Educational Technology Standards for Students: Connecting Curriculum and Technology*, copyright © 2000, ISTE (International Society for Technology in Education), iste@iste.org, www.iste.org. All rights reserved.

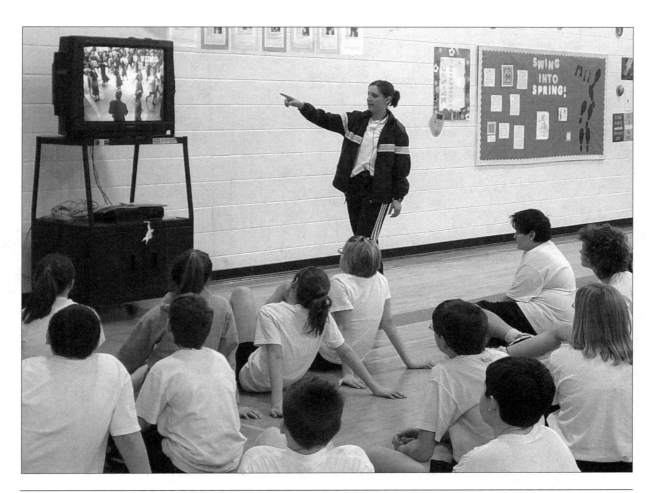

Students can analyze movement skills through various media.

- The *Health Related Fitness Tutorial/Portfolio* (Bonnie's Fitware) is a two-part commercial software program. The first part is a tutorial on health-related fitness that incorporates hypermedia so students can locate specific areas of interest. It includes cognitive concepts related to principles of fitness, safe-versus-dangerous exercises, training protocols, taking one's pulse, and warm-up and cool-down procedures, along with a variety of exercises for each fitness area. The second part is an electronic-based portfolio in which students enter fitness scores, select exercises, calculate caloric input and output, produce drawings or video clips, write journal entries, and design fitness plans. The program is set up to record fitness scores for pull-ups, push-ups, modified pull-ups, flexed-arm hang, curl-ups, back-saver sit-and-reach, shoulder stretch, trunk lift, mile run, pacer, body mass index, and skinfolds. For example, the exercise plan format is shown in figure 3.3.

- *Volleyball Complete* (Bonnie's Fitware) relates each of the eight subdisciplines of physical education (exercise physiology, motor learning, biomechanics, psychology, motor development, aesthetics, sociology, and historical perspectives) to the teaching of volleyball. This is a two-part commercial software application, similar to the Health Related Fitness Tutorial/Portfolio. One part is a tutorial, and the second part is a portfolio. Using the tutorial, students can access and interact with information on volleyball skills, techniques, strategies, training, and teamwork. Then, using the portfolio part, students enter journal writings, interactive activities, rubrics for volleyball skills, and video clips. For example, the volleying rubric is shown in figure 3.4.

Exercise Plan

Score

Week: [   ]

[Copy]

Monday	Tuesday	Wednesday	Thursday	Friday	Saturday	Sunday

(Assess) (Principles) (Concepts) (Cardiores) (Flexibility) (Endurance) (Strength) (Body Comp)

Figure 3.3   Exercise plan for electronic-based, health-related fitness portfolio.

Courtesy of Bonnie S. Mohnsen, Bonnie's Fitware Inc., Cerritos, CA; www.pesoftware.com.

Page 39

Volleying

Score [4]

Level 6 - correct technique in games
Level 5 - correct technique using qualities of movement
Level 4 - correct technique
   moves under the ball
   contacts ball with both hands
   uses finger pads
   keeps wrists stiff
   straightens arms on follow through
   extends wrists on follow through
Level 3 - intermediate
   moves under ball
   slaps at ball
   uses hands and arms
   uses little follow through
Level 2 - beginner
   slaps at ball
   contacts ball with hand then the other
Level 1 - inaccurate technique
   misses ball

[Menu] [Quit]

Figure 3.4   Analyses of volleyball skills can be accessed from electronic-based portfolios.

Courtesy of Bonnie S. Mohnsen, Bonnie's Fitware Inc., Cerritos, CA; www.pesoftware.com.

- *Physical Education Portfolio* (Bonnie's Fitware) is a commercial software package that is formatted around the six national content standards for physical education (NASPE, 2004). Students can enter fitness scores, journal entries, and video clips. It also contains rubrics for basic movement (e.g., run, hop, skip) and motor skills (e.g., throw, catch, kick). For example, the overhand throwing rubric is shown in figure 3.5. There are elementary, middle, and high school versions.

Also, a predesigned electronic-based portfolio builder for K-12 students is provided on the accompanying CD-ROM. Existing digital files, photos, video clips, spreadsheets, charts, and presentations can be used easily with this template. The components of the template are standards, learning targets, goal setting, reflections, journal (self-assessment), gallery (photos, video clips), conferences, and assessment. Instructions on how to use the CD-ROM are located at the front of the book on page xi.

Item Selection

Once the purposes, type of portfolio, and organizing scheme are determined and the production and logistics are planned, it is necessary to establish a process for selecting portfolio items (step 5 of the portfolio-designing process). This step is related closely to the type of portfolio and the elements around which it is organized. For example, an integrated portfolio organized around the learning dimensions would contain evidence of a student's development of cognitive abilities (e.g., problem solving), affective behaviors (e.g., preferences), and motor abilities (e.g., manipulative skills) across several subjects including physical education. Artifacts selected in physical education might include a problem task sheet, self-report inventory, and rating scale,

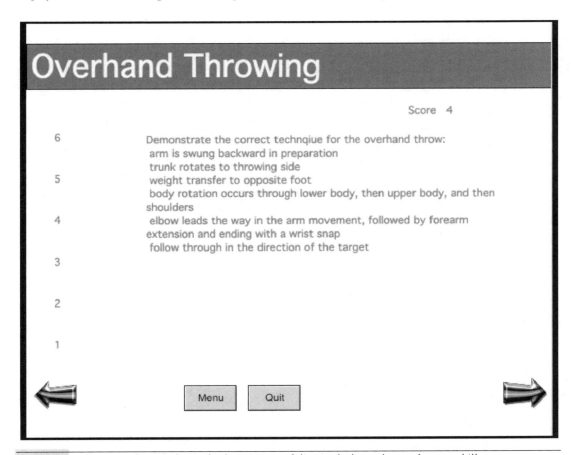

Figure 3.5 Electronic-based physical education portfolios include analyses of motor skills.

Courtesy of Bonnie S. Mohnsen, Bonnie's Fitware Inc., Cerritos, CA; www.pesoftware.com.

respectively. Each type of portfolio previously described (pages 135-137) suggests particular kinds of items that would specify what students should know and be able to do. For example, each of the three sample portfolio systems for K-12 students at the end of the chapter contains required and optional kinds of artifacts. Also, the portfolio builder for students on the accompanying CD-ROM includes artifact possibilities related to the suggested learning targets.

It is important to attend to sampling issues. The challenge is to ensure that the items chosen, for example, really do represent best or typical performance in the case of a record-keeping or growth portfolio. The number of items collected is also a sampling factor. Certain learning targets may require several items to verify achievement, whereas other targets may need only one. The challenge for teachers is to determine in advance the number and nature of items needed to support the achievement of each learning target addressed.

The process of making selections includes decisions about *what, how, who,* and *when.* What items to include depends on established criteria and standards. How to select items revolves around performance indicators and work quality. Who selects items involves decisions about which stakeholders will participate in the selection of portfolio items. When to decide on items will vary significantly depending on portfolio purposes, type, and logistics. These aspects, which are treated separately in the following sections, are not decided in any particular sequence. In fact, they are usually dealt with in conjunction with each other.

What to Select

Frequently, students' first portfolio items are "baseline" samples. A record-keeping type of portfolio managed by the teacher may be the most practical way to maintain these kinds of artifacts because of their nature and use. Information collected for entry appraisal should be included. For example, behavior sampling through informal techniques (i.e., observations, self-reports) and formal techniques (i.e., criterion-referenced measures) would yield important baseline information to ultimately show student change (learning). Likewise, other sources of entry information such as cumulative record data (e.g., previous test scores, diagnostic reviews, anecdotal records) and performance on a task sequence would also be invaluable.

When addressing the issue of what portfolios should include, educators should keep two compelling factors in mind—the students' desires and the purpose for collecting each item. Portfolios should be student centered. When students make decisions about the selection and quality of their work, they begin to establish standards by which to evaluate their own work. However, students must realize that teachers will also decide on portfolio items and that some items may be mandated by school officials. Although portfolios should not be a collection of anything and everything, the range of potential "exhibits of learning" contained in an individual portfolio is unlimited. Following is a list of the kinds of artifacts portfolios may include:

- Preassessment inventories
- Task sheets
- Self-assessment checklists
- Frequency index scales
- Rating scales
- Performance checklists
- Peer reviews
- Attitude surveys
- Self-reports
- Workbook pages
- Logs
- Journals
- Reflections

- Projects
- Independent contracts
- Videotapes and video clips
- Anecdotal statements
- Parent observations or comments
- Skill tests
- Quizzes
- Written tests
- Commercial instruments

What is ultimately selected for the portfolio depends on its organizing scheme. The focus could be on physical education subject matter, different learning processes, a special project or unit, or the previously identified organizing elements (i.e., NASPE's description of the physically educated person, mission statement, learning dimensions, spectrum of multiple intelligences, organizing centers, content standards). The various kinds of artifacts are grouped into three categories: observations, performance samples, and tests and testlike procedures. Illustrative artifacts for these three categories in physical education are identified in table 3.4 (see pages 159-164). Some of the artifacts are partial in nature because they are offered for illustrative purposes only.

1. *Observations.* These kinds of behavior cues are seen in everyday class activities. Behaviors that show movement abilities, interests, social conduct, and thinking can be recorded through observational formats (e.g., rating forms, checklists, anecdotes).

2. *Performance samples.* These tangible products or artifacts represent students' accomplishments. These kinds of formats are not as readily available in physical education settings because learning is usually centered on movement forms rather than "documents." However, many samples of performance should be considered (e.g., projects, videotapes).

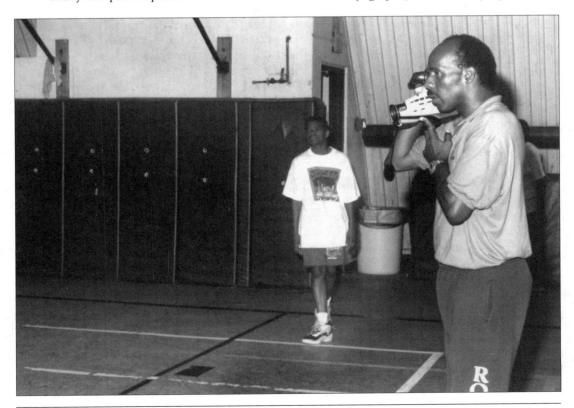

Video clips of skill performance can be included as portfolio artifacts.

3. *Tests and testlike procedures.* These include the full range of instruments (e.g., teacher-designed, commercial). The term *test* does not necessarily imply a formal, teacher-directed procedure. Informal inventories and end-of-unit tasks are valuable in documenting student learning.

How to Select

In connection with what artifacts can be included in portfolios, some decisions are needed as to how items are selected. The criteria established for evaluation, developed later in this chapter, could be used for this purpose. Other criteria, however, should be considered. For example, an item might be selected that represents "something that was hard for you to do," "something that makes you feel really good," or "something that you would like to work on again." Some additional suggestions for selecting items are a "best" or "most representative" skill (e.g., gymnastic stunt), work in progress with written plans for revision (e.g., dance routine), and samples organized chronologically according to a theme (e.g., personalized physical fitness program such as the Fitness for Life sample portfolio at the end of the chapter on pages 216-233).

Teachers and students can also create their own criteria for selection. Doing so can ensure that the portfolio contains representative work while also offering students some choice. Some selection categories include media such as cassettes, slides, videos, photos, and computer programs; group work items such as projects, performances, and group feedback; individual work items such as worksheets, logs, journals, task cards, and tests; processes such as work biography, rough and final drafts, and beginning and final attempts; and reflections such as self-assessments, short-term goals, and artifact registry (Burke, Fogarty, & Belgrad, 2001). The three sample portfolio systems for K-12 student learners at the end of the chapter include a variety of these kinds of artifacts.

Finally, when deciding how to select items, teachers and students should consider whether they demonstrate established standards. The recommended physical education content standards and student expectations for four levels (grades K-2, 3-5, 6-8, and 9-12) detailed in table 3.2 (pages 141-142) should be analyzed relative to artifact selection. The artifact selection planning matrix on page 165 can be used to "manage" the documentation of the content standards and corresponding grade-level student expectations. The matrix should facilitate diversity by ensuring that standards and expectations are adequately covered and that the portfolio does not rely too heavily on certain kinds of artifacts. On the artifact selection planning matrix, the name of the artifact is entered to show its support of the expectation. The number of artifacts for each expectation is a matter of priority. Also, some kinds of artifacts are ongoing and may, therefore, appear across all expectations (e.g., log, journal).

Who Will Select

Deciding who selects portfolio artifacts is dictated by the purposes and type of portfolio. If the purpose is to provide students with an opportunity to assess their own accomplishments through a showcase/celebration portfolio, then students should have a major voice in selection. The teacher's role may be to establish selection categories and criteria and to assist students in making selections. If the purpose is to determine students' status relative to district standards, the teacher should select artifacts according to local mandates.

Physical educators need only look at the "players" in the portfolio system to know who may select artifacts. For the most part, consideration needs to be given to the following stakeholders: students, peers, parents or guardians, or significant others, teachers, and local or state mandates. The responsibility should not fall primarily on the teacher. A powerful learning opportunity is minimized when the subject of the portfolio—the student—is not also responsible for its creation. When students ultimately assume responsibility for collecting, analyzing, and sharing their portfolios, their ability to learn, their desire to learn, and the learning itself deepens (Stiggins, Arter, Chappuis, & Chappuis, 2004). When teachers and students recognize that the role of others is a matter of degree, they can make selections separately or in combination.

Table 3.4 Portfolio Artifacts Possibilities

Category	Kind of artifact	Illustrative artifact (partial)
Observations	Rating scale	*Tennis forehand*

Tennis forehand

	Not yet (1)	(2)	(3)	(4)	(5) Awesome
• Contacts ball when even with front foot	☐	☐	☐	☐	☐
• Keeps wrist firm; swings with whole arm from shoulder	☐	☐	☐	☐	☐
• Rotates trunk so hips and shoulders face net on follow-through	☐		☐	☐	☐

Frequency index scale

Behavior trends	FIRST OBSERVATION					SECOND OBSERVATION					Rating average
	Never	Seldom	Fairly often	Frequently	Regularly	Never	Seldom	Fairly often	Frequently	Regularly	
1. Limits interactions to friends	5	4	3	2	1	5	4	3	2	1	
2. Shares equipment	1	2	3	4	5	1	2	3	4	5	
3. Takes turn at circuit stations	1	2	3	4	5	1	2	3	4	5	

Performance checklist

Forward roll

	Trial 1	Trial 2	Trial 3
• Tucks head with chin to chest	☐	☐	☐
• Shifts body weight forward until off balance	☐	☐	☐
• Accepts body weight with arms	☐	☐	☐

(continued)

159

Table 3.4 (continued)

Category	Kind of artifact	Illustrative artifact (partial)			

Rubric

BALL SKILLS

LEVELS OF EXCELLENCE

Criteria	Novice	Emerging	Proficient	Exemplary
Dribbling	Ball consistently leaves self space; slapping the ball; dribbles off own foot	Ball occasionally leaves self space; palm often used; ball bounce varies	Stationary most of time; a little palm is used; ball bounce varies sometimes	Stationary in self space; uses fingers; ball bounces below hip, above knee
Throwing	Steps with same foot; no hip and shoulder points; misses partner completely	Steps with opposite foot; no hip and shoulder point; hits partner "head to toe"	Points shoulder; steps with opposite foot; hits partner "head to waist"	Points opposite shoulder and hip; steps with opposite foot; hits partner's hands
Catching	Catches with belly button	Cradles ball with arms into body	Uses two hands; accepts ball into body	Uses two hands only; ball does not touch body

Peer review

Partner checks performance according to the criteria.

Cartwheel Criteria

	Perfect	Acceptable	Needs improvement
• Faces mat with preferred foot forward; same-side arm vertical	☐	☐	☐
• Throws weight on preferred foot; leans forward, placing same-side hand on mat	☐	☐	☐
• Throws opposite leg up at the same time, placing same-side hand on mat	☐	☐	☐

Log

Fitness calendar showing aerobic training workout schedule:

Day	Time	Program	Level	Training description
Monday	7:30 a.m.	Jogging	3	220 yards; 110 yard relief; 4 repeats
Wednesday	6:00 p.m.	Swimming	5	50 yards; 90 second relief; 8 repeats
Friday	7:30 a.m.	Jogging	4	330 yards; 110 yard walk relief; 3 repeats

Anecdotal statement

Notes about a student's abilities during movement exploration activities.

"In games of tag and dodging, Craig has difficulty moving his entire body rapidly in different directions and in response to unexpected situations; needs to improve his ability to change direction and make sudden stops and starts. He also had problems putting a hula hoop at different levels in relation to his body."

Performance samples **Task sheet**

Draw a line from the locomotor movement in the picture to the word (Hopple, 1995).

Jump Walk Hop Run

(continued)

Illustration reprinted, by permission, from C.J. Hopple, 2005, *Teaching for Outcomes in Elementary Physical Education* (Champaign, IL: Human Kinetics), 84.

Table 3.4 (continued)

Category	Kind of artifact	Illustrative artifact (partial)

Self-assessment checklist

Evaluate your own ability according to the criteria.

Golf Grip (bottom hand)

	I have acheived	Working to achieve
• Place on club first, fingers as close together as possible	❑	❑
• Thumb close to hand at the first joint	❑	❑
• Wrist is directly above shaft	❑	❑
• Thumb forms V; forefinger points over opposite shoulder	❑	❑

Journal

DOUBLE-ENTRY JOURNAL

Starting my tennis program	One month after my tennis program
1. My goals are:	1.
2. My fears are:	2.
3. I feel good about:	3.

Reflection

For secondary students:

Circle the words that describe how you feel (mostly) about gymnastics:

Interesting   Too easy   Useless   Dull   Helpful   Worthless   Fun   Important   Boring   Too hard

Super   Others: _____   _____

For elementary students:

Check (✔) the face you wear when you look at this picture:

❑ ☺   ❑ 😐   ❑ ☹

Project	**Personalized fitness program** • Plot a personal physical fitness profile based on ratings for cardiorespiratory endurance, muscular strength and endurance, flexibility, and body composition. • Generate fitness goals based on ratings for health-related components. • Select exercise or leisure activities in terms of contribution to fitness goals. • Design a program based on goals, activity selection, and activity schedule.
Independent contract	**Badminton contract** • Improve performance in six of eight skills by at least one ability rating. • Use mechanical principles, points of contact, and possible uses as criteria to compare and contrast: (1) overhead clear vs. forehand drive, (2) smash vs. overhead drop, and (3) long serve vs. short serve. • Write a brief report (four to five pages) on the history of badminton. • Create a test on badminton terms, rules, and strategies; test and grade three classmates.
Videotape	Free exercise routine; swimming stroke; game play

Tests and testlike procedures	**Preassessment inventory**	On the diagram, draw diagonal lines to show the area that is used during a singles game in tennis. Place an X where the server stands to begin a game, and an O where the server stands when the score is 30 to 15.

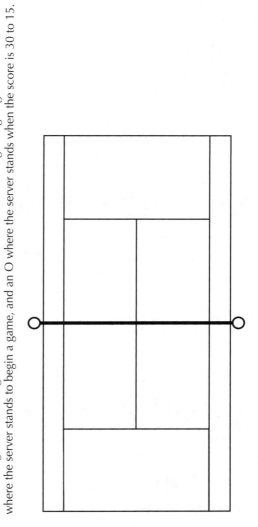

(continued)

Table 3.4 *(continued)*

Category	Kind of artifact	Illustrative artifact (partial)

Self-report

Check the space that shows how you feel most of the time. Coed volleyball is:

Exciting						Dull
Boring						Fun
Worth the time						Waste of time
Stupid						Great
Interesting						Uninteresting

Scoring: Exciting — 5 4 3 2 1 — Dull   Boring — 1 2 3 4 5 — Fun

Skill test

Balance

	Pre	Post	% change
1. Stand on line; one foot; eyes open; hands on hips	___ sec.	___ sec.	___
2. Stand on line; one foot; eyes closed; hands on hips	___ sec.	___ sec.	___
3. Repeat #1; jump and turn 180°; land on line; hold momentarily	___ sec.	___ sec.	___

Quiz

For each pair of descriptions, indicate the associated component

	Strength	Endurance
1. (a) One maximal contraction	☐	☐
(b) Sustained contraction	☐	☐
2. (a) Light weights, many reps	☐	☐
(b) Heavy weights, few reps	☐	☐
3. (a) Greater hypertrophy	☐	☐
(b) Greater capillarization	☐	☐

Commercial instrument

- Bruininks-Oseretsky Test of Motor Proficiency (Bruininks, 1978); sports skills tests (Strand & Wilson, 1993)
- Ohio State University SIGMA test of gross motor development (Loovis & Ersing, 1979)
- Test of Gross Motor Development (Ulrich, 2000)
- Sports skills tests (Strand & Wilson, 1993)
- Brockport Physical Fitness Test (Winnick & Short, 1999)
- Assessment strategies for elementary physical education (Schiemer, 2000)
- Performance-based assessment for middle and high school physical education (Lund & Kirk, 2002)
- *FITNESSGRAM* test of health-related fitness and skill- or sport-related fitness (Cooper Institute for Aerobics Research, 2004)

Artifact Selection Planning Matrix

Content standard: Demonstrates competency in motor skills and movement patterns needed to perform a variety of physical activities

Level: Middle school/junior high (grade 8)

Kind of portfolio artifact	STUDENT EXPECTATIONS			
	Can participate with skill in a variety of modified sport, dance, gymnastics, and outdoor activities	Achieve mature forms in the basic skills of the more specialized sport, dance, and gymnastics activities	Use the basic skills successfully in modified games or activities of increasing complexity and in combination with other basic skills	Demonstrate use of tactics within sport activities
Preassessment inventory				
Task sheet				
Self-assessment checklist				
Frequency index scale				
Rating scale				
Performance checklist				
Peer review				
Attitude survey				
Self-report				
Workbook page				
Log				
Journal				
Reflection				
Project				
Independent contract				
Videotape				
Anecdotal statement				
Parent or guardian comments				
Skill test				
Quiz				
Written test				
Commercial instrument				
Other:				
Other:				
Other:				

From *Professional and Student Portfolios for Physical Education, Second Edition,* by Vincent J. Melograno, 2006, Champaign, IL: Human Kinetics.

Students

The degree to which students can select artifacts for their portfolios can range from all the entries in the portfolio to a few. If students are to be truly responsible for their own learning, then they should be involved in selecting "best works," "works in progress," and "work that needs work." However, students and teacher can combine efforts. For example, the student could select two of five exhibits and the teacher could select one of the remaining three. Or, the teacher could provide the selection category (e.g., peer review of swimming strokes), and the student could select two criteria checklists.

Peers

Students should be able to review other students' work, provide helpful feedback, and offer an opinion about what artifacts should be selected for the portfolio. After all, other students are part of the same portfolio system and should, therefore, be able to provide an objective assessment in accordance with established criteria and indicators. Techniques such as peer reflection and peer conferences are discussed later in this chapter. Involving peers in the selection process also promotes cooperation, team building, and a learning community atmosphere.

Parents and Significant Others

One way to include parents and significant others (e.g., brother, grandparent, counselor, babysitter) is to ask them to select items. Doing so has the benefit of bringing them into the learning process. Teachers can help guide the selections by providing guidelines and criteria. Techniques such as reflection and conferences by parents or significant others are also discussed later in this chapter.

Teachers

Because of the need to satisfy subject matter and learning process goals, the teacher is critical in selecting artifacts. Even when students are given a great deal of liberty in selection, teachers may reserve some selections for progress reports, teacher-made tests, and evaluation rubrics. Teachers can provide the overall framework through selection categories such as reflections, projects, performance checklists, and journals.

Local or State Mandates

To monitor student achievement, some school districts and state education departments require certain kinds of work samples or exhibits. For example, the documentation of health-related fitness status is often mandated. Artifacts may then be placed in multiyear portfolios. Other mandates might relate to agreed-on state-level content standards and benchmarks appropriate to K-12 grade levels. Physical education teachers would also have an obligation to produce certain kinds of artifacts for portfolios that combine subject areas.

When to Select

The collection of artifacts can be an ongoing, cumulative process usually resulting in a working repository. Selection for the final portfolio is a different matter. Unless the artifacts to be contained in the final portfolio are predetermined, selection decisions are needed at some point during the assessment process. Assuming that aspects of *what, how,* and *who* are known, the remaining decision revolves around *when* to make the selections. Once again, the purposes and type of portfolio may suggest the checkpoints or occasions for final selections. Although the actual timing can vary widely, there are some natural times when artifact selections may occur.

- *Weekly or monthly.* Making regular selections may be a good way to manage portfolios. Also, entries in logs, journals, and registries can help monitor selections.

- *End of unit.* Selection can coincide with the completion of a sport unit, learning sequence, or thematic topic.

- *Scheduled conference or exhibition.* In preparation for teacher and parent conferences or displays (e.g., portfolio poster session, Portfolio Night), key selections are necessary to show learning progress.

- *End of grading period.* Presenting portfolios along with traditional reporting procedures offers more concrete information about student achievements than report card grades alone.

- *End of year.* Selections at the end of a school year should represent key learning targets, outcomes, or standards. These selections could be made from a series of portfolios maintained throughout the year.

- *K-12 intervals.* If cumulative, multiyear portfolios are maintained, then selections are needed as the interval is completed (e.g., every three years, at the end of elementary school).

Reflection and Self-Assessment

Inherent to portfolios *and* student-involved, classroom-level assessment is the chance for students to think about why certain items are included and to gain personal insights throughout the entire process. In other words, students can reflect on individual pieces and their value to the whole portfolio, and they can reflect on how they learn and why they fail to learn. Students can also engage in a self-assessment of their portfolio relative to growth in targeted areas, strengths and weaknesses, and short-term and long-term goals. Decisions about these essential processes are critical to the portfolio system. Teachers can choose from several reflection strategies and self-assessment techniques (step 6 of the portfolio-designing process).

Reflection Strategies

Students should thoughtfully examine each item involved in the portfolio, whether required or optional, teacher selected, peer selected, or self selected. By carefully reflecting on its meaning and value, students discover that each item is a "mirror" of self. Reflection can occur at various stages of the portfolio process. For example, before the start of a sport unit, students might think ahead about portfolio content and design relative to the strategies and skills of the sport. During the process, students need to monitor their portfolios as they take shape. At another stage students critically evaluate their work in terms of quality. Several reflection strategies can be used across these stages.

Visualization

A powerful strategy in developing sports skills is to visualize the successful performance of the skill. In the same manner, students can visualize how the portfolio will take shape and what it will look like. They can also envision a particular task sheet or project in its final form and the final portfolio itself.

Tag, Label, or Stamp

An easy way to reflect on portfolio items is to tag, label, or stamp each piece. Premade tag lines, self-stick notes, printed stickers, or rubber stamps can include a key phrase or comment. They may explain the value of the item or why the item has significance. They also provide an initial inventory of what is included and why it is valued. Some examples of tags, labels, or stamps are shown in figure 3.6.

Reflective Stems

To help students get started in reflection, some phrases can be used to stimulate their "inner voice." These phrases are referred to as reflective stems, examples of which are listed in figure 3.6. Although some of these stems could be used by elementary students, others may need to be reworded more simply.

Bridging Questions

Key questions can help students clarify their purposes and selections. Most of these questions should solicit *how* and *why* responses. Examples are identified in figure 3.6. Many of these questions can be reworded more simply for younger students.

Tags, Labels, or Stamps

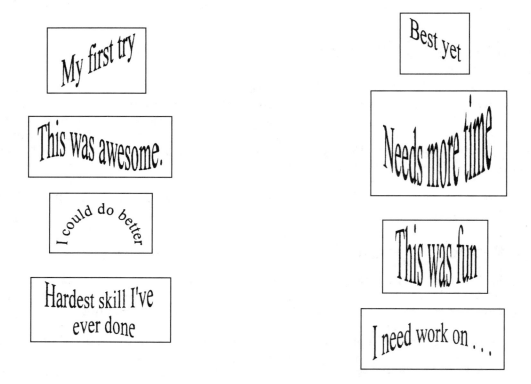

Reflective Stems

I chose this because . . .
This is important to me because . . .
I think this is my best work because . . .
This was hard for me because . . .
This was easy for me because . . .
If I could do this over again, I would . . .
This was my greatest challenge because . . .
I really like the way I . . .
When I look at this, I feel ☺ ☺ ☹
I'll remember this next year because . . .
This was my favorite piece because . . .
This will surprise many people because . . .

Bridging Questions

What have I learned from doing this?
How do I think others will react to this?
Why am I including this?
What if I took it out of my portfolio?
On a scale of 1 to 10, I would give
 this a _____. Why?
What are its strengths? Weaknesses?
Why have I chosen this?
Why is it important?
How could it have been better?
What was the hardest thing for me?
What would I like to do next?

Figure 3.6 Examples of different reflection strategies.

Benchmarking

Because portfolio development is usually a long process, students could reflect on any established benchmarks along the way that support the end result (i.e., content standards). The recommended content standards and student expectations (benchmarks) for four levels in physical education (grades K-2, 3-5, 6-8, and 9-12), detailed in table 3.2 (pages 141-142), could be used for this purpose. Each artifact could be labeled to reveal its meaning and value to the entire portfolio relative to the student expectations (benchmarks). Students get to know why an artifact was chosen for a particular benchmark in support of the corresponding content standard. Students can ask themselves, Why is the artifact filed under this benchmark? What does it say about my growing knowledge and skills? A reflection cover sheet that includes name, date, benchmark, name of artifact, and rationale, similar in format to the one presented on page 61, could be required for each artifact.

Artifact Registry

If used properly, the artifact registry is a form of reflection. Students are required to state a reason when they add or delete items. These statements comprise a useful, reflective record of portfolio management over time. The artifact registry form presented on page 148 can be used for this purpose.

Self-Assessment Techniques

Reflection is directed toward individual portfolio items. In self-assessment, a broadened view is taken by looking at the overall direction of the portfolio. In this informal self-evaluation process, students themselves are the center of the learning process. As active participants, they become more autonomous, independent, and self-monitoring. Students assume responsibility for inspecting their own performance. "They should not depend on a teacher to follow them around throughout life giving them stickers, happy faces, or A's and B's. Too many students become dependent upon authority figures with red pens to provide feedback on how they are doing" (Burke, Fogarty, & Belgrad, 2001, p. 71).

Physical education teachers can choose from a large array of self-assessment techniques that allow students to monitor their own behavior and set goals. Teachers need to accept certain realities: They are not the only ones who can carry out evaluation, and they need to empower students to become self-regulating. Several self-assessment techniques foster student ownership and responsibility.

Checklists

Probably the most fundamental way to carry out self-assessment is through behavioral checklists. Task checklists are commonly used in physical education to analyze the component parts of movement skills and social behaviors. Because observing one's own performance is difficult, except through videotape or digitized video, checklists are often used in a peer-assessment arrangement. Examples of self-assessment and peer-assessment checklists appear in table 3.4 for the golf grip and cartwheel, respectively. An example of a self-assessment checklist for a social skill is shown on page 170.

Learning Logs

To keep track of learning targets and outcomes, students can maintain daily records of activities and performance. Short, objective entries about in-class tasks and out-of-class experiences help students monitor their own progress. Logs can be used to record key ideas, make predictions, identify questions, connect ideas to other subjects, brainstorm ideas, and identify problems (Burke, 2000). Table 3.4 shows an example of a log. Entries can also be made using a variety of stem statements such as the following:

Something new I learned today was . . .

I hate it when . . .

Self-Assessment Checklist

Name: _____ Date: _____

Social behavior	Frequently	Sometimes	Seldom
Interpersonal relations in a fitness group			
1. I help others in my group.	❏	❏	❏
2. I isolate myself from my group.	❏	❏	❏
3. I interact consistently with both males and females in my group.	❏	❏	❏
4. I criticize others in my group.	❏	❏	❏
5. I show favoritism to those who are more physically fit in my group.	❏	❏	❏
6. I accept feedback from others in my group.	❏	❏	❏

One thing I'm excited about is . . .

I'm having trouble with . . .

My skill is getting better in . . .

I was surprised today at . . .

Journals

Students can use journals to monitor and reflect on goals. Unlike logs, journals are used to record more subjective feelings about learning experiences. Over time, students can trace how their feelings change as a result of new learning experiences. Table 3.4 shows an example of a double-entry journal in which students reveal some initial impressions about some topic and then wait until they have learned more about the topic to reflect a second time. Students can see their change in feelings. Journal stem statements, such as the following, can also be used to facilitate self-reflections:

The best part of this movement is . . .

I wonder why . . .

I predict that . . .

One of the interesting things about this is . . .

How could I . . .

Strengths and Weaknesses Charts

Every now and then, students can take a look at their strengths and problem areas, or "not yet" areas. It is useful for students to analyze their behaviors and abilities in all learning domains (i.e., cognitive, affective, and motor). Two formats are shown in on page 172 for conducting this kind of self-assessment (Burke, Fogarty, & Belgrad, 2001).

Goal-Setting Sheets

Following reflection and other forms of self-assessment (e.g., checklists, logs, journals), students should be ready to establish short-term and long-term goals that cover all learning domains. Sometimes students will not engage in goal setting until after a portfolio conference has been held (step 7 of the portfolio-designing process) or after the final portfolio has been judged (step 8 of the portfolio-designing process). However, this technique can also be used by students before the final portfolio evaluation by applying the same criteria used by the teacher, possibly in the form of a scoring rubric. This aspect is covered later in the chapter section on evaluation. A sample physical education goal-setting sheet is shown on page 173. In addition, at the end of the chapter, several approaches to goal setting are included in the sample portfolio systems. The Volleyball Sportfolio for the middle school level (pages 206-215) includes goal setting based on strengths and problem areas. The Fitness for Life portfolio system for the high school level (pages 216-233) includes short-term and long-term goal setting based on fitness pretests. The K-12 student portfolio builder on the accompanying CD-ROM includes goal setting based on established learning targets.

Conferences

Portfolio-related conferences are important to the portfolio process (step 7 of the portfolio-designing process). In some cases, student conferences involving the physical education teacher, parents or guardians, or other students are held at the end of a portfolio cycle after the final portfolio is evaluated. The conferences are treated as a culminating event because they are summative in nature. They are used to communicate about learning that has already occurred—assessment *of* learning. Summative conferences certainly make sense, and the idea should not be abandoned if it is practical.

My Strengths and Problem Areas: Physical Education

Name: _____ Grade: _____

My strengths	Performing sports skills	
	Understanding game strategies	
	Showing teamwork and cooperation	
My problem areas	Performing sports skills	
	Understanding game strategies	
	Showing teamwork and cooperation	

Signed: _____ Date: _____

Analysis of My Strengths and Problem Areas: Physical Education

Old me
(weaknesses)

_____
_____
_____
_____
_____

New me
(strengths)

_____
_____
_____
_____
_____

I still need improvement in:

_____
_____
_____
_____
_____

Signed: _____ Date: _____

From *Professional and Student Portfolios for Physical Education, Second Edition,* by Vincent J. Melograno, 2006, Champaign, IL: Human Kinetics.

Physical Education Goal Setting

Name: _____ Date: _____

Topic: _____ Time period: _____

Short-term goals	Target date
1.	
2.	
3.	

Long-term goals	Target date
1.	
2.	
3.	

From *Professional and Student Portfolios for Physical Education, Second Edition,* by Vincent J. Melograno, 2006, Champaign, IL: Human Kinetics.

Portfolio-related conferences are also recommended during the artifact collection, selection, reflection, and self-assessment phases. Such conferences are formative in nature because they can be used to give or receive feedback, help students formulate goals, or create an intervention—assessment *for* learning. Conferences can range from simple, informal dialogues between student and teacher—or peers, parents, or guardians—to more involved, formal meetings among the same parties. Because conferences are viewed as an ongoing process of portfolio development, they are presented before the evaluation phase. Conducting portfolio conferences after portfolio evaluation may still be desirable, however.

Regardless of decisions about participants or timing, conferences should be consciously planned and implemented. Although some "conferences" may occur spontaneously and last only a few minutes (i.e., miniconferences), more substantive ones require careful decision making regarding purposes and procedures. The following framework for conducting portfolio conferences describes the purposes and types of conferences, the varied conference participants, and the strategies for carrying out conferences in the physical education setting.

Purposes and Types

Conferences offer another kind of self-reflection and a chance for students to demonstrate their autonomy as learners. In portfolio development, the most common mode of communication is through paper and electronic artifacts (e.g., logs, checklists, written reflections, task cards, projects, tests, inventories). Dialogue adds another dimension to the quest for student-involved, authentic assessment, particularly in cognitive and affective learning. The opportunity to verbally express one's accomplishments enhances self-responsibility. The contents of individual portfolios can be shared at a deeper level of inspection. Because of the emphasis on teacher and school accountability, multiple measures of learning are desirable. The conference provides another vehicle for matching student products with content standards and grade-level expectations. The general purposes of conferences—be they informal or formal, simple or complex—can be placed in these five categories (Stiggins, Arter, Chappuis, & Chappuis, 2004):

- *Offering feedback.* Students receive information that provides an "outside" opinion about the strengths and weaknesses of their work. The information offers insight so that students can continue to improve on their learning targets.

- *Fostering goal setting.* During conferences, students confer with others to set short-term or long-term goals for learning. They should be guided toward the target content standards, however, not just their own goals. Personal goals serve as a basis for artifact selection, and they are an important aspect of reflection and self-assessment. It follows that, through conferences, progress toward goals is reinforced. Students could structure goals in response to the following reflective stems: *I need to learn . . ., My 'before' picture looks like . . ., My plan is to . . ., I need help from/with . . ., I will be ready to show my learning on . . .,* and *My 'after' picture will look like . . . .*

- *Planning an intervention.* Students having difficulty with behavior, work habits, or achievement will need a plan for improvement. A conference may be held when a student's performance is significantly above or below expectations to adjust instruction or to recommend a particular placement within the regular class setting. Accurate data are central to the effectiveness of these conferences.

- *Demonstrating growth.* The focus of some conferences may be on improvement on a single learning target or growth over time spanning a number of learning targets within physical education. Students who have engaged in self-assessment and goal setting will have worked on one or more learning targets. Sharing their improvements will help them notice and take pride in their learning. Students could prepare by making lists under the following headings: My Learning Targets, Evidence of Where I Started, Evidence of Where I Am Now, What I Did to Improve, What I Can Do Now That I Could Not Do Before, and What to Notice About My Work.

- *Communicating achievement.* During a conference, information can be shared about a student's current status. The topic of discussion is the student's level of achievement, competence with respect to learning targets, or evidence of having met goals. To create and sustain student motivation, students should be involved in achievement conferences.

Given these general purposes, the specific focus of the conference should also be decided. Several directions can be taken, as described in the following list of conference types (Burke, Fogarty, & Belgrad, 2001). These types of conferences, which can be used separately or in combination, can help orient students as they further narrow their artifact selections for the conference.

- *Achievement.* Significant achievements are given primary attention as revealed, for example, by learning logs, performance video clips, projects, or improvement in skill tests.
- *Goals.* The status of goals is presented based on portfolio items that show how students have met or surpassed their goals. For example, health-related fitness goals could be documented through selected artifacts.
- *Learning process.* Artifacts would be selected and discussed around a particular process. In physical education, the focus might be on solving movement problems, becoming an effective dancer, or being a team player.
- *Personal satisfaction.* Students select items for the conference that have the greatest meaning to them. Preferably, the items represent achievements that students feel best about.
- *Group accomplishment.* Students as a group present their cooperative efforts and successes as a community of learners. The results of adventure or risk activities, cooperative games, or sport education would be applicable to physical education.
- *Total portfolio.* This holistic conference should survey students' strengths and successes versus weaknesses and failures. Overall performances are assessed and discussed.

Participants

Depending on the purpose and type of conference, decisions are needed about who will participate in conferences. These decisions can be made by the student alone, by the teacher alone, or by the student and teacher together. The student whose portfolio is under review could be involved at different conference levels. The range is from one-on-one dialogues with the teacher, a parent or guardian, or a peer to a presentation and discussion at a portfolio display with numerous people.

Teacher

Naturally, the teacher is primarily involved either alone or with others (e.g., parents or guardians, other students). Teachers can have a role to play in all of the conference options, but their participation is particularly critical if the purpose of the conference is to plan an intervention. If the conference is led by the teacher, questions can be prepared in advance to help guide the student. For example, if the conference focuses on goals, some questions might be, How do you want to grow as a tennis player? What do you need to do to improve? What are your goals for the rest of the year?

Parents or Guardians

Although parent–teacher conferences are still common, the nature of such conferences can be changed. Because the portfolio offers a full view of student learning not represented by grades and report cards, portfolio conferences can give parents or guardians the opportunity to celebrate their child's accomplishments, thus providing a more personally satisfying experience than a traditional parent–teacher conference might provide. Child–parent portfolio conferences can also promote family involvement. The physical education teacher could provide parents or guardians with a portfolio conference guide that suggests questions to ask, such as, What have you found out about yourself by completing the wellness portfolio? What parts of your wellness portfolio do you like the most? What are you going to do now that you have completed the wellness portfolio? Parents and guardians play a significant role in the conference when achievement is the focus and when placement in a specialized program is the recommended intervention.

Peers

Several options exist for student–student conferences. Conferences with a peer can be helpful because peers are involved in their own portfolio development. Therefore, they are qualified to review others' work and give feedback or help with goal setting. The conference can center on answers to questions such as, What items are you proud of and why? If you could publish one thing in your portfolio, what would it be? What areas of fitness need improvement? What items should be taken out of your portfolio and why?

Conferences could also be held among a group of peers to solicit more dialogue and diverse opinions. Group-based conferences are particularly relevant if the physical education setting promotes cooperative learning or the concept of a community of learners. Another form of peer conference is a "conference" held with a pen pal via electronic mail. Obviously, artifacts would need to be exchanged in advance in written form, as e-mail attachments, or on computer disks. Finally, students can hold conferences with students of various ages who have experience in the portfolio process.

Significant Others

For individual students, conferences with other family members (e.g., grandparents, brother, sister) and other people in their lives (e.g., baby-sitter, coach) may be particularly meaningful. Also, an exhibition of portfolios (e.g., Portfolio Night) would afford another chance for conversation about the portfolio with a potentially varied audience.

Strategies

Unlike classrooms, the physical education setting is unique for conducting portfolio conferences during the regular instructional routine. Devoting time for conferences may also be more difficult than in classrooms because the conference activity itself is not as easily integrated into typical physical education learning experiences. Obviously, out-of-class conferences could be held in an office or a classroom. Because of these limitations, some ideas for conducting portfolio conferences in physical education are miniconferences, conference stations, and student-led conferences.

Miniconferences

Teachers can create conference time within the organizational flow of the physical education teaching–learning process. For example, while students are engaged in self-directed tasks, practice activities, or game play, individual students can be taken aside for miniconferences. The teacher could even post a conference schedule so that students can prepare in advance. Selected aspects of the portfolio could then be available for the conference, as necessary. Peer conferences could also be organized in this format.

Conference Stations

Learning stations are commonly used in physical education. Circuit training and rotated self-directed tasks are examples of stations arranged in a gymnasium or outdoor facility to foster variety and independent learning. On selected occasions, one of these stations could be devoted to portfolio conferences in which students could engage in group-based discussions or one-on-one dialogues with peers or with the teacher.

Student-Led Conferences

Students can benefit greatly from planning and leading portfolio conferences with the teacher, peers, parents or guardians, and others. Autonomy and ownership are reinforced when students are responsible for handling the date and time, as well as the conference protocol. Other benefits are increased communication and increased commitment to learning through responsible and self-directed behavior. Students are capable of establishing their own conference goals. For example, the elementary school student might want to tell how he learned to be a gymnast, the middle

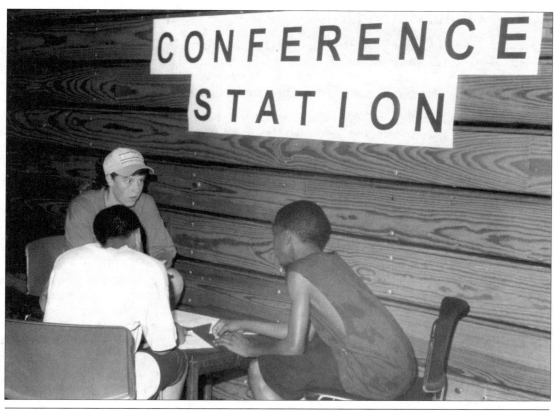

A station can be established for conducting in-class teacher and peer miniconferences.

school student might want to show how she improved her volleyball skills, and the high school student might want to present an analysis of the effects of a personal weight training program.

Typical formats are two-way (student and parent or guardian), three-way (student, parent or guardian, teacher), and showcase (student, others, teacher). In preparation for leading conferences, students need to collect evidence; reflect on selected items; assess their strengths, needs, and goals; set the conference agenda; rehearse the conference (e.g., role play); and invite other participants. Parents and guardians need to review and comment on work samples that may have been taken home; speculate on strengths, needs, and goals; and plan to attend the conference. Teachers need to help students prepare; determine the student's strengths, needs, and goals; help organize the logistics (time, place, materials, equipment); and validate student roles and responsibilities.

Assessment

The emphasis on assessment in today's world of educational accountability has been clearly established. In chapter 1, quality assessment was identified as a major educational trend (page 8) and the principles of assessment literacy, including assessment *for* learning and authentic assessment, were explored (pages 19-26). Earlier in this chapter, the integration of assessment, learning, and teaching was substantiated along with the need to match assessment methods with learning targets and to implement student-involved, formative assessment (pages 123-133).

All teachers must be able to collect, organize, and report achievement data in credible and comprehensive ways. However, the process of assessment (step 8 of the portfolio-designing process) is only as effective as its product—student achievement results. This section covers many important aspects of assessment by answering several questions: What are the standards for quality assessments? What role do rubrics play in performance assessment, and how are rubrics developed? How should teachers grade in standards-based education? Should teachers make judgments about student portfolios?

Quality Standards

Sound and productive classroom-level assessments can be measured against a set of quality control standards. Basically, teachers need to assess accurately and use assessment to benefit students, not merely to grade and sort students. Quality assessments are built around the following five key dimensions (Stiggins, Arter, Chappuis, & Chappuis, 2004):

1. *Clear purpose.* Quality assessments serve clearly articulated and appropriate purposes. Why is the assessment being conducted? Is there a clear picture of who will use the results and how they will be used? Is the distinction between assessment *for* and *of* learning clear? How do the purposes of the assessment fit into the bigger plan for assessment over time?

2. *Clear targets.* Quality assessments arise from clear and appropriate student learning targets. Achievement expectations should be defined clearly and completely. Is there a clear picture of what is being measured? Are learning targets even stated and easy to find? Would teachers agree on what they mean? Are they appropriate? Do they represent the discipline, and are they worth the instructional and assessment time devoted to them? Are they clearly connected to standards? Do they reflect a bigger plan across grade levels—previous and next learning—in a vertical curriculum?

3. *Sound assessment design.* Quality assessments are designed with learning targets and purposes in mind. The assessment uses an appropriate method, samples student achievement to make appropriate inferences, and avoids potential sources of bias that could distort results. Are the assessment methods best for the learning targets being assessed (is there a balance between most accurate and practical)? Is the scoring guide (rubric) clear, and does it cover the most important aspects of quality? Does the assessment gather enough information to generalize about student achievement of the target? Is there anything about the assessment or the way it is carried out that would not allow students to really demonstrate what they know and can do?

4. *Effective communication.* Quality assessments are planned to serve the needs of users. Can information from the assessment be managed and reported in ways that will satisfy users? Has communication been planned as part of the assessment? Is assessment information accurately recorded over time and appropriately combined for reporting? Will users of the results understand them and find them useful?

5. *Student involvement.* Quality assessments involve students in record keeping, self-assessment, and communication. If appropriate, does the assessment incorporate elements of student involvement? Were learning targets made clear to students? Was descriptive feedback provided to students? Are students engaged in self-assessment, tracking progress, and setting goals? Do students communicate about their own learning?

Use of Rubrics

Rating scales and checklists are relatively easy-to-use, efficient assessment techniques. Some examples were provided in table 3.4 (pages 159-164) and figure 3.4 (page 154). Responses to performance tasks and open-ended questions can be judged with two kinds of rating scales. Bipolar scales are used to respond to statements about students' responses or performance, such as, *The overhead smash was executed correctly.* The scale for rating it might be, Strongly disagree (–2), Disagree (–1), Not sure (0), Agree (1), or Strongly agree (2). Hierarchical scales can be used to evaluate student abilities along a continuum of levels of quality or proficiency. A commonly used scale is, Poor (1), Fair (2), Good (3), or Excellent (4). Checklists contain categories for evaluation and rating options for each category. The rating options could be Yes or No or be presented as a narrow scale such as Never, Seldom, Sometimes, Frequently, or Always. Although rating scales and checklists are simple to apply, they do not offer the detailed, explicit criteria found in scoring rubrics (McTighe & Ferrara, 1994).

A rubric is a scoring guide designed to assess the quality of a student's performance. A scoring rubric consists of a measurement scale of criteria that explains the possible levels of performance for a learning task. However, the purpose of the rubric is to define quality, not just provide a scoring device or justify a grade. Rubrics are used to inform students about intended learning targets or standards and levels of quality. For this reason, scoring rubrics have emerged as a popular assessment tool in conjunction with student portfolios.

Usually, the rubric has three to five levels. For example, a three-point scale might include criteria for the following levels: Needs improvement, Acceptable, and Exemplary. On a four-point scale, criteria could be determined for descriptive levels such as Novice, Apprentice, Proficient, and Distinguished. Performance on a task is compared to the criteria at each level. It is recommended that students be involved in developing the criteria and descriptive indicators by which their performance tasks will be assessed. In this manner, they can internalize the criteria, but they must be guided toward good criteria.

In the previous section, a distinction was made between grading portfolio artifacts and grading the portfolio itself. Similarly, scoring rubrics can be designed for and applied to specific performance tasks, and they can provide general criteria for judging the overall portfolio. For illustrative purposes, several rubrics are provided that represent the range of learning dimensions. In figure 3.7, two examples are shown for the elementary school level, the rubric in figure 3.8 could be used at the middle school level (see page 181), and figure 3.9 offers a rubric appropriate for use at the high school level (see page 182). Finally, a sample weighted scoring rubric is presented on page 183 for judging the whole portfolio. With these rubrics as models, teachers need guidelines for developing rubrics, determining the quality of rubrics, and converting rubric scores to grades, if necessary.

Developing Rubrics

As the samples show, rubrics can be structured differently. However, each shares a common definition. A rubric is a particular format for performance criteria. It is a written-down version of the criteria, with all score points described and defined. The best rubrics are worded in a way that covers the essence of what teachers and students look for when judging quality, and they reflect the best thinking in the field as to what constitutes good performance. Rubrics are frequently accompanied by examples of products (anchors) or descriptions of performance that illustrate the various score points on the scale (Arter & McTighe, 2001).

In standards-based education, an authentic or performance-based assessment tool is needed to define and communicate what constitutes excellence or quality. A rubric is a declaration of expectations (learning targets) and a means of self-assessment. Students are more likely to perform well if they know what constitutes quality. Regardless of structure, rubrics also share common elements. When designing rubrics, teachers should incorporate the following elements: (1) standards or levels of excellence, (2) specific criteria for assessment, and (3) specific indicators describing what the various levels of excellence look like for each of the criteria (Jacobs, 1997). These elements are defined and illustrated in figure 3.10 (see page 184).

Constructing rubrics can be a time-consuming, difficult activity when developing performance-based assessments. There are two types of rubrics. Generalized rubrics are universal to assess broad traits rather than criteria specific to a single task. For example, a game play rubric might consider execution, strategy, shot placement, and court movement. A task-specific rubric is used for a single performance-based assessment (e.g., golf swing). Although the types of rubrics may vary, there are seven basic steps to follow when constructing a rubric (Lund & Kirk, 2002):

1. Envision the desired student performance on the assessment.
2. Determine the criteria.
3. Pilot the assessment.
4. Write levels for the rubric.
5. Create a rubric for students.
6. Administer the assessment.
7. Revise the rubric.

Resources are available to assist in developing physical education rubrics such as *Elementary Physical Education Teaching & Assessment: A Practical Guide* (Hopple, 2005), *Creating Rubrics*

Theme: Space awareness
Task: Design, refine, and perform a movement sequence with a partner.
Learning dimensions: Physical, intellectual, social
Level: Grades 3-4
Criteria: Use at least two directions and two levels with a definite beginning and ending shape.

3. Achieved	Sequence clearly shows • two (different) directions and two levels, • a definite beginning and ending, and • excellent refinement (no visible breaks in continuity and smooth transitions between movements).
2. Needs improvement	Sequence shows • one or two different directions or levels, • a beginning and ending shape, although they may not be held long enough, and • an attempt at refining the sequence (breaks in continuity and smoothness may appear by one or both partners).
1. Working to achieve	Sequence • lacks any planned directions, levels, or a beginning and ending shape, and • no or few attempts have been made to refine the sequence (one or both partners have repeated losses of execution, smoothness, or memory).

Theme: Kicking
Task: Design and play a game with a small group (2-on-2, 3-on-3) of students of similar skill level.
Learning dimensions: Physical, intellectual, social
Level: Grades 5-6
Criteria: Use the skills of kicking and punting toward a goal area.

2. Outstanding	Student clearly and consistently demonstrates the ability to • cooperate with others and help create the rules and boundaries for the game, • work with others in a (physically and verbally) positive manner, • abide by group decisions when playing, • use the offensive strategies of keeping the body between the ball and the defender and of creating space by moving to get open, and • use the defensive strategy of keeping the body between the opponent and the goal.
1. Acceptable	Student usually shows the ability overall to • cooperate with others and help create the rules and boundaries for the game, • abide by and accept decisions of the group (any challenging is done in a nonthreatening manner), • keep the body between the ball and the defender and move to pass and receive the ball, and • keep the body between the opponent and the goal.
0. Deficient	Student • does not cooperate with others in a positive way; • contributes barely or not at all to developing the rules and boundaries for the game; • has difficulty abiding by and accepting decisions made by the group, and may interact with others in a nonpositive manner; • when on offense, is consistently unable to (or doesn't try to) use the offensive strategies of keeping the body between the ball and the opponent or of moving to open spaces; and • when on defense, is consistently unable to keep the body between the opponent and the goal.

Figure 3.7 Rubrics for performance assessment at the elementary school level.

Adapted, by permission, from C.J. Hopple, 1995, *Teaching for Outcomes in Elementary Physical Education* (Champaign, IL: Human Kinetics), 22-23.

Theme: Leisure pursuits
Sport: Tennis
Task: Execute the forehand drive in returning a real serve.
Learning dimensions: Physical, emotional
Level: Grades 7-8
Type of assessment: ❑ Teacher   ❑ Peer   ❑ Self (videotape)

Criteria/elements *(Circle letter of elements that need work.)*	Scale			
	1 All silence	2 Scattered applause	3 Round of applause	4 Standing ovation

1. Criterion: Grip
  a. Base knuckle of thumb centered on top of grip
  b. Palm is behind handle
  c. Thumb overlaps and is next to middle finger with index finger spread
  d. Fingers evenly spread
  e. Butt end just protrudes from hand
	❑
	Comments:
		❑	❑	❑

2. Criterion: Backswing
  a. Move as quickly as possible into position after opponent hits ball
  b. Turn both shoulders and pivot hips so forward shoulder points in direction of ball flight
  c. Racket drawn back approximately parallel to body between waist and knee height (below intended point of contact)
  d. Straight-back technique with racket
  e. Racket at comfortable length from body; grip hand hidden from opponent
	❑
	Comments:
		❑	❑	❑

3. Criterion: Forward swing
  a. Dictate body and racket position at impact by "going after" ball
  b. As forward foot hits the ground, front knee is bent so that eyes are closer to line of flight of ball
  c. Arm and racket move forward as a unit with racket head trailing wrist during early stage; racket head catches up with wrist before contact; racket moves forward and upward
  d. At impact, racket is laid back (hyperextended); ball struck in line with or slightly in front of lead foot
  e. Wrist kept firm, not changed from original position during forward swing; vertical racket head in line with wrist at impact
	❑
	Comments:
		❑	❑	❑

4. Criterion: Follow-through
  a. Wrist and racket stay together as a unit for short time during early follow-through
  b. Watch spot where contact was made to avoid pulling eyes off ball
  c. Head remains in precisely the same position as when ball was contacted
  d. Stroke completed with full sweep of arm close to chin with body balanced to move to next shot
	❑
	Comments:
		❑	❑	❑

Figure 3.8 Rubric for assessing the tennis forehand drive at the middle school level.

Theme: Expressive movement
Task: Choreograph and perform own dance routine.
Learning dimensions: Intellectual, physical
Level: Grades 9-12

Criteria	Elements	Scale			Score
		1	2	3	
Creativity	Shows innovative patterns	Little	Partial	Complete	
	Includes original moves	None	A few	Many	
	Contrasts speed	Same pace	Some change	Varied pace	
Fluidity	Coincides with rhythm of music	Off-beat	Off-and-on beat	Right on beat	
	Connects moves to patterns	No fit	Some fit	Fits together	
	Brings together beginning, body, and ending	Can't tell	Somewhat	Clearly evident	
				Total:	

Figure 3.9 Rubric for assessing a choreographed dance routine at the high school level.

for Physical Education (Lund, 2000), and *Performance-Based Assessment for Middle and High School Physical Education* (Lund & Kirk, 2002). In addition, general rubric builders are accessible through the following Web sites:

- The Rubric Builder: www.rubricbuilder.on.ca/
- Teach-nology: http://teachers.teach-nology.com/web_tools/rubrics/
- Rubistar: http://rubistar.4teachers.org/index.php
- Worksheets: http://makeworksheets.com/Samples/

Creating Quality Rubrics

Rubrics for physical education come from two primary sources. As indicated in the previous section, many rubrics can be found in the literature or through the World Wide Web. The other source is teachers, who customize rubrics to specific teaching settings and students. In either case, teachers need a basis for selecting ready-made rubrics or judging rubrics that they have constructed. A "metarubric" was developed that contains criteria for judging the quality of rubrics—a rubric for rubrics. Although the complete metarubric is not provided, following is a summary of the traits (criteria) (Stiggins, Arter, Chappuis, & Chappuis, 2004):

1. *Content.* This trait defines what to look for in a student's product or performance to determine its quality. Content truly is the final definition of standards because a rubric describes what will "count."

   - Can I explain why each thing included in the rubric is essential to a quality performance?
   - Can I cite references that describe the best thinking in the field on the nature of quality performance?
   - Can I describe what was left out, and why it was left out?
   - Do I ever find performances or products that are scored low (or high) that I really think are good (or bad)?
   - Is this worth the time devoted to it?

Physical Education Portfolio

Weighted Scoring Rubric

Name: _____ Date: _____

Title: _____ Teacher: _____

Criteria	1	2	3	Weight	Score
Appearance	❑ Messy No attempt to individualize	❑ Neat Some attempt to individualize	❑ Creative Individual touches added	× 1	(3)
Organization	❑ Poor layout Can't follow Many missing items	❑ Layout OK Hard to follow Some missing items	❑ Clear layout Follows all directions All items complete	× 3	(9)
Form/style	❑ No variety Weak sentences Many mechanical errors	❑ Some variety Good sentences Some mechanical errors	❑ Wide variety Variety of sentences No mechanical errors	× 3	(9)
Understanding of subject matter	❑ Inaccurate Basic information No originality	❑ Some inaccuracies Limited use of ideas Some originality	❑ Very accurate Applies new ideas Shows much originality	× 4	(12)
Quality of items	❑ No depth to reflections Lacks thoroughness Not very expressive	❑ Some vague reflections Several gaps Limited expressiveness	❑ Thoughtful reflections Very thorough Highly expressive	× 5	(15)

Comments: _____

_____

_____

_____

_____

Scale

A = 43-48

B = 38-42

C = 33-37

D = 28-32

Total: _____
(48)

Grade: _____

From *Professional and Student Portfolios for Physical Education, Second Edition*, by Vincent J. Melograno, 2006, Champaign, IL: Human Kinetics.

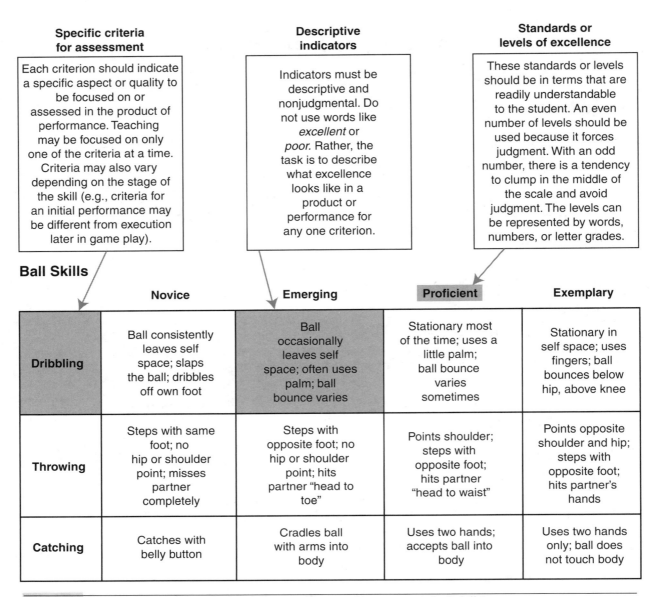

Specific criteria for assessment

Each criterion should indicate a specific aspect or quality to be focused on or assessed in the product of performance. Teaching may be focused on only one of the criteria at a time. Criteria may also vary depending on the stage of the skill (e.g., criteria for an initial performance may be different from execution later in game play).

Descriptive indicators

Indicators must be descriptive and nonjudgmental. Do not use words like *excellent* or *poor.* Rather, the task is to describe what excellence looks like in a product or performance for any one criterion.

Standards or levels of excellence

These standards or levels should be in terms that are readily understandable to the student. An even number of levels should be used because it forces judgment. With an odd number, there is a tendency to clump in the middle of the scale and avoid judgment. The levels can be represented by words, numbers, or letter grades.

Ball Skills

	Novice	Emerging	Proficient	Exemplary
Dribbling	Ball consistently leaves self space; slaps the ball; dribbles off own foot	Ball occasionally leaves self space; often uses palm; ball bounce varies	Stationary most of the time; uses a little palm; ball bounce varies sometimes	Stationary in self space; uses fingers; ball bounces below hip, above knee
Throwing	Steps with same foot; no hip or shoulder point; misses partner completely	Steps with opposite foot; no hip or shoulder point; hits partner "head to toe"	Points shoulder; steps with opposite foot; hits partner "head to waist"	Points opposite shoulder and hip; steps with opposite foot; hits partner's hands
Catching	Catches with belly button	Cradles ball with arms into body	Uses two hands; accepts ball into body	Uses two hands only; ball does not touch body

Figure 3.10 Rubric elements described and illustrated for a performance task (ball skills).

2. *Clarity.* Teachers, students, and others should interpret the statements and terms in the rubric the same way. In addition to including important content, the rubric should be stated clearly.

   - Would two teachers be likely to give the same rating on a product or performance?
   - Can I find examples of student work or performance that illustrate each level of quality?
   - Could I show someone else sample student work or performances that specifically illustrate each score point on each dimension?

3. *Practicality.* Having clear criteria that cover appropriate content means nothing if the system is too cumbersome to use. Practicality refers to ease of use.

   - Can teachers and students understand and use it easily?
   - Does it give them the information they need for instructional decision making and tracking student progress toward important learning outcomes?
   - Can the rubric be used for more than just assessing students?
   - Can it also be used to improve the achievement being assessed?

4. *Technical quality and fairness.* It is important to have "hard" evidence that the performance criteria adequately measure the target being assessed, that they can be applied consistently, and that there is reason to believe that the ratings actually do represent what students can do. Although this might be beyond the scope of what individual teachers can do, teachers still have the responsibility to ask hard questions when they adopt or develop a rubric.

- Is it reliable? Will different raters give the same score?

- Is it valid? Do the ratings actually represent what students can do?

- Is it fair? Does the language adequately describe quality for all students? Are there racial, cultural, or gender biases?

Grading in Standards-Based Education

Although this chapter section is about assessment, grading is related to assessment because it is usually derived from assessment scores. Changes in the ways students are taught and assessed are having an impact on traditional grading practices in which the focus is on sorting, selecting, and justifying grades. The development of standards, greater access to information about student achievement, and an emphasis on self-directed learning styles have resulted in authentic learning (i.e., relevant to students and the real world) and authentic assessment (i.e., an accurate picture of what students really know, can do, and believe). Dramatic changes have occurred in the underlying perspectives on grading. We need to move away from traditional grading and toward using grading to inform learning (O'Connor, 2002).

Consider what is communicated to students and parents or guardians by the factors traditionally used to evaluate performance in physical education. These factors typically include some or all of the following: attendance and punctuality, preparation for class (dressed out), attitude, effort, participation, knowledge, or performance. What do factors such as attendance, being prepared for class, attitude, or effort communicate to students and parents or guardians? How much credit do students typically receive in other content areas such as math and science for showing up to class on time with pens and papers and smiles on their faces? Although these factors are important for learning to occur, they are prerequisites, not learning targets. It is the student's responsibility to come to class, to be dressed appropriately, and to be ready to learn. Students are smart. If they can earn a passing or acceptable grade simply by showing up and not misbehaving, then that is what they are going to do. If the only way they can earn a passing grade is by demonstrating certain knowledge and performance on the learning targets defined in the curriculum, then that is where they will focus their efforts. Teachers should make sure that assessment criteria match what they want students to focus on. Note that the terms *attitude* and *effort* as used here refer to subjective judgments made by the teacher. These should not be misinterpreted as being the same as learning targets related to attitude and persistence that are defined in the curriculum (Kelly & Melograno, 2004).

Guidelines

A standards-based environment carries many grading challenges. The goal should be to provide information that communicates the current status of achievement of standards. Unfortunately, many grading systems in schools continue to use traditional letter grades that fail to provide specific information about standards-based learning targets. Following are guidelines for grading in standards-based systems to support learning and to encourage student success (O'Connor, 2002):

1. Relate grading procedures to the intended learning targets or goals (i.e., standards).

- Use learning targets or goals (standards or some clustering of standards such as strands) as the basis for grade determination.

- Use assessment methods (e.g., skill tests 20 percent, project 30 percent) as the subset, not the set.

2. Use criterion-referenced performance standards as reference points to determine grades.
   - The meaning of grades (letters or numbers) should come from clear descriptions of performance standards.
   - If students hit the target or goal, they get the grade (i.e., no bell curve).
3. Limit the valued attributes included in grades to individual achievement.
   - Grades should be based on achievement (i.e., demonstration of the knowledge and skill components of the standards). Attendance, dressing for class, effort, participation, attitude, and other behaviors should be reported separately.
   - Grades should be based on individual achievement.
4. Sample student performance—do not include all scores in grades.
   - Provide feedback on formative performance—use rubrics, rating scales, or checklists.
   - Include information only from varied summative assessments to determine grades.
5. Grade in pencil—keep records so they can be updated easily.
   - Use the most consistent level of achievement with special consideration for more recent evidence of achievement.
   - Provide several assessment opportunities (vary method and number).
6. Crunch numbers carefully—if at all.
   - Avoid using the mean; consider using the median or mode.
   - Think "body of evidence" and professional judgment—determine, don't just calculate, grades; weight components to achieve the intent of final grades.
7. Use quality assessments and properly record evidence of achievement.
   - Meet standards for quality assessment (e.g., clear targets, clear purpose, appropriate target–method match, appropriate sampling, and avoidance of bias and distortion).
   - Record and maintain evidence of achievement and behaviors (e.g., portfolios, tracking sheets, journals, productions).
8. Discuss and involve students in assessment, including grading, throughout the teaching–learning process.
   - Ensure that students (age appropriately) understand how their grades will be determined.
   - Involve students in the assessment process, in record keeping, and in communication about their achievement and progress.

In summary, these guidelines suggest that to be *truly* standards based, teachers' grading practices should (1) separate achievement from behavior, (2) exclude formative assessments, (3) emphasize recent achievement, and (4) avoid the mean and the effect of zeros. Clearly, some radical changes in grading practices are needed if grading is to be aligned with standards. Because of negative community reaction, attempts to remove grades from report cards have not been successful, even though traditional grades may be of questionable worth.

Rather than fight the battle of eliminating the symbol of grades, it would be more productive to design grading and reporting systems that emphasize clear reference points such as learning targets and standards. An accepted practice has been to supplement traditional grades with diagnostic reviews or progress reports such as the example on page 187.

A more comprehensive approach is recommended that reflects standards-based education and the guidelines identified earlier. The sample report card on pages 189-190 is based on physical education content standards and eighth-grade performance indicators (NASPE, 2004); learning and social behaviors are separate from these achievement behaviors. Because of the existing pressure to assign traditional grades, the report card accommodates this need. The performance indicators should be rewritten in student-friendly language. They could also be substituted with grade-level performance outcomes that are specific to the actual physical education content that is taught, such as the following examples:

Physical Education Progress Report

Grades 3-4

Student: _____ Date: _____

Teacher: _____

___ 1st qtr. (Nov.)   ___ 2nd qtr. (Feb.)   ___ 3rd qtr. (April)   ___ 4th qtr. (June)

	Working to achieve	Needs improvement	Achieved
Intellectual			
1. Knows rules and procedures governing movement activities and games.	❏	❏	❏
2. Recognizes the effects of space, time, force, and flow on the quality of movement.	❏	❏	❏
3. Applies basic mechanical principles that affect and control human movement.	❏	❏	❏

Comments: _____

	Working to achieve	Needs improvement	Achieved
Social			
1. Respects rights, opinions, and abilities of others.	❏	❏	❏
2. Shares, takes turns, and provides mutual assistance.	❏	❏	❏
3. Participates cooperatively in student-led activities.	❏	❏	❏

Comments: _____

	Working to achieve	Needs improvement	Achieved
Emotional			
1. Assumes responsibility for giving and following directions.	❏	❏	❏
2. Makes decisions on an individual basis.	❏	❏	❏
3. Responds freely and confidently through expressive bodily movement.	❏	❏	❏

Comments: _____

	Working to achieve	Needs improvement	Achieved
Values			
1. Carries out tasks to completion.	❏	❏	❏
2. Displays preferences for various forms of movement.	❏	❏	❏
3. Engages in movement activities voluntarily.	❏	❏	❏

Comments: _____

	Working to achieve	Needs improvement	Achieved
Physical			
1. Executes all locomotor movements in response to rhythmic accompaniments.	❏	❏	❏
2. Controls body while balancing, rolling, climbing, and hanging.	❏	❏	❏
3. Shows body control in manipulating playground ball while stationary and moving.	❏	❏	❏

Comments: _____

Standard 1 (competency in motor skills and movement patterns)
- Serves a volleyball overhand using mature form
- Places the ball cross-court during a tennis rally (forehand and backhand)
- Designs and performs a dance routine

Standard 2 (understand movement concepts, principles, strategies, and tactics)
- Designs a personal fitness program that reflects training principles
- Corrects errors in golf swing based on performance results
- Explains at least three offensive game strategies in playing soccer

Standard 3 (regular participation in physical activity)
- Sets health-related physical activity goals through selected activities outside of school
- Maintains a weekly physical activity log including progress toward goals
- Accumulates number of target miles for a month as part of a personal running program

Standard 4 (health-enhancing level of physical fitness)
- Participates in activities that apply principles of threshold, overload, and specificity
- Meets age and gender standards for health-related fitness program
- Achieves muscular endurance goals following a six-month weight training program

Standard 5 (responsible personal and social behavior)
- Accepts opponent's line calls during a competitive game of tennis
- Spots others equally in gymnastics regardless of gender, race, ethnic, or ability differences
- Contributes and remains on task during an outdoor camping activity

Standard 6 (values physical activity)
- Accepts new skills and activities as challenging
- Encourages peers to participate in unfamiliar activities, regardless of ability
- Seeks to improve skills through voluntary activities outside of class

Conversion of Rubric Scores to Grades

There is no need to convert rubric scores to letter grades if the purpose of assessment is to communicate about student achievement. The points and descriptions corresponding to the score provide clear, focused feedback. When a grade is required, a plan is needed for converting rubric ratings to grades. For illustrative purposes, refer to figure 3.11, which shows Laura's assessment record of achievement over an entire grading period focused on leisure time pursuits (see page 191). She has completed 13 elements, some of which were rated on all six criteria (scale scores), and some of which were only partially rated. Note that in this situation, the entire grade is based on rubric ratings only. The following methods of calculation can be considered (Arter & McTighe, 2001; Stiggins, Arter, Chappuis, & Chappuis, 2004):

Method 1: Overall Percentage of Points Possible
- Add up the total points Laura received from all assessment items and divide it by the total points possible from all assessment items. What grade would Laura get? (167 / 200 = 84%)
- What if Laura failed to turn in her Internet project and got zeros for Knows Facts and Basic Information and Analyzes Movement Forms? Now what grade would Laura get? (157 / 200 = 78%) Should missing one project make this much difference?

Method 2: Average Percentages of Points Possible on Each Assignment
- Calculate the percentage of points Laura earned on each assessment item (the total earned on each assessment item divided by the total possible for each assessment item). Average these percentages. What grade would Laura get? (1,157 / 13 assessment items = 89%)

Physical Education Report Card

Eighth Grade

Student name: _____ Teacher: _____ School: _____ School year: _____

RATING SCALE FOR ACHIEVEMENT STANDARDS

4	EXCEEDS expectation of grade-level indicator
3	MEETS expectation of grade-level indicator
2	PROGRESSING toward expectation of grade-level indicator
1	LIMITED PROGRESS toward expectation of grade-level indicator
—	Not assessed as this time

Standard	Performance indicators	Quarter			
		1st	2nd	3rd	4th
1. Demonstrates competency in motor skills and movement patterns needed to perform a variety of physical activities.	1-1 Can participate with skill in a variety of activities.				
	1-2 Achieves mature forms in basic skills of specialized sports, dance, and gymnastics activities.				
	1-3 Demonstrates use of tactics within sport activities.				
2. Demonstrates understanding of movement concepts, principles, strategies, and tactics as they apply to the learning and performance of physical activities.	2-1 Identifies principles of practice and conditioning that enhance movement performance.				
	2-2 Understands and applies movement concepts/principles and game strategies, elements of movement skills, and characteristics of highly skilled performance.				
	2-3 Knows when, why, and how to use strategies and tactics within a game.				
	2-4 Uses information from a variety of sources to guide and improve performance.				
3. Participates regularly in physical activity.	3-1 Independently sets physical activity goals; participates in activities based on personal goals, interests, and results of fitness assessments.				
	3-2 Selects and uses practice procedures and training principles appropriate for the activity goals.				
	3-3 Participates regularly in moderate to vigorous physical activities in school and nonschool settings.				

RATING SCALE FOR LEARNING AND SOCIAL BEHAVIORS

+	Exemplary demonstration of behaviors
✓	Demonstrates behaviors consistently
O	Needs improvement/below expectations
—	Not assessed at this time

Learning behaviors	Quarter			
	1st	2nd	3rd	4th
Works independently				
Listens attentively				
Follows directions				
Stays on task				
Is prepared (dressed)				
Completes tasks/assignments on time				
Produces quality work				
Displays effort to learn				
Accepts responsibility for actions				
Follows class rules				
Manages feelings				

Social behaviors	Quarter			
	1st	2nd	3rd	4th
Works, plays, shares cooperatively				
Demonstrates self-control				
Demonstrates respectful behavior				
Accepts others' differences				
Gives/receives feedback appropriately				

(continued)

From *Professional and Student Portfolios for Physical Education, Second Edition,* by Vincent J. Melograno, 2006, Champaign, IL: Human Kinetics.

Standard	Performance indicators	Quarter			
		1st	2nd	3rd	4th
4. Achieves and maintains a health-enhancing level of physical fitness.	4-1 Participates in moderate to vigorous physical activity on a regular basis without undue fatigue.				
	4-2 Engages in physical activities that address each component of health-related fitness.				
	4-3 Knows the components of fitness and how these relate to overall fitness status.				
	4-4 Monitors own heart rate, breathing rate, perceived exertion, and recovery rate during and following strenuous physical activity.				
	4-5 Assesses personal fitness status for each component; uses information to develop fitness goals.				
	4-6 Shows progress toward knowing various principles of training and how principles can be used.				
5. Exhibits responsible personal and social behavior that respects self and others in physical activity settings.	5-1 Understands concept of physical activity as a microcosm of modern culture and society.				
	5-2 Recognizes the role of physical activity in understanding diversity; includes and supports others, respecting group members.				
	5-3 Moves from following rules, procedures, and positive forms of social interaction to reflecting on role in physical activity settings.				
	5-4 Has well-developed cooperation skills; can accomplish group/team goals in cooperative and competitive activities.				
	5-5 Seeks greater independence from adults.				
	5-6 Makes appropriate decisions to resolve conflicts arising from powerful influence of peers.				
	5-7 Practices appropriate problem-solving techniques to resolve conflicts when necessary in competitive activities.				
6. Values physical activity for health, enjoyment, challenge, self-expression, and/or social interaction.	6-1 Seeks physical activity experiences for group membership and positive social interaction.				
	6-2 Uses physical activities as a positive outlet for competition.				
	6-3 Increases self-confidence and self-esteem through enjoyment in physical activity participation.				
	6-4 Develops confidence toward independence through physical activities.				
	6-5 Is challenged by experiencing high levels of competition and in learning new and/or different activities.				
	6-6 Experiences greater awareness of feelings through self-expression provided by physical activities.				

GRADE FOR ACHIEVEMENT STANDARDS

A	Outstanding; well exceeds achievement standards
B	Good; above achievement standards
C	Satisfactory; meets achievement standards
D	Improving; below achievement standards
F	Unsatisfactory; well below achievement standards

Subject	Quarter			
	1st	2nd	3rd	4th
Physical education				

COMMENTS

1st quarter:

2nd quarter:

3rd quarter:

4th quarter:

Standards and performance indicators from *Moving into the future: National standards for physical education*, 2nd edition (2004) with permission from the National Association for Sport and Physical Education (NASPE), 1900 Association Drive, Reston, VA 20191-1599.

STUDENT'S NAME: LAURA

Leisure time pursuits: assessment items	Displays social attitudes	Exhibits interest and values	Knows facts and basic information	Applies concepts, principles, and strategies	Analyzes movement form	Demonstrates skill proficiency
Biomechanics report	1 2 3 4 5	1 2 3 4 5	1 2 3 4 5	1 2 3 4 5	1 2 3 **4** 5	1 2 3 4 5
Motor abilities	1 2 3 4 5	1 2 3 4 5	1 2 3 4 5	1 2 3 4 5	1 2 3 4 5	1 2 3 4 **5**
Tennis essentials	1 2 3 **4** 5	1 2 **3** 4 5	1 2 3 **4** 5	1 2 3 **4** 5	1 2 3 **4** 5	1 2 **3** 4 5
Tennis footwork	1 2 3 4 5	1 2 3 4 5	1 2 3 4 5	1 2 3 4 5	1 2 3 4 **5**	1 2 3 4 5
Golf essentials	1 2 3 4 **5**	1 2 3 4 **5**	1 2 3 4 **5**	1 2 3 **4** 5	1 2 3 **4** 5	1 2 3 **4** 5
Golf swing	1 2 3 4 5	1 2 3 4 5	1 2 3 4 5	1 2 3 4 5	1 2 3 **4** 5	1 2 3 4 5
Internet project	1 2 3 4 5	1 2 3 4 5	1 2 3 4 **5**	1 2 3 4 5	1 2 3 **4** 5	1 2 3 4 5
Strength training	1 2 3 4 5	1 2 3 4 5	1 2 3 4 5	1 2 3 4 5	1 2 3 4 5	1 2 3 4 **5**
Aerobic training	1 2 3 4 5	1 2 3 4 5	1 2 3 4 5	1 2 3 **4** 5	1 2 3 4 5	1 2 3 4 **5**
Cycling	1 2 3 **4** 5	1 2 **3** 4 5	1 2 3 **4** 5	1 2 3 **4** 5	1 2 **3** 4 5	1 2 3 4 **5**
In-line skating	1 2 3 4 5	1 2 3 4 5	1 2 3 4 5	1 2 3 4 5	1 2 3 4 5	1 2 3 4 5
Contributions paper	1 2 3 4 5	1 2 3 4 5	1 2 3 4 **5**	1 2 3 4 5	1 2 3 4 5	1 2 3 4 5
Backpacking	1 2 3 **4** 5	1 2 3 **4** 5	1 2 **3** 4 5	1 2 3 **4** 5	1 2 3 **4** 5	1 2 3 **4** 5
1 = Low 5 = High →	1 2 3 4 5	1 2 3 4 5	1 2 3 4 5	1 2 3 4 5	1 2 3 4 5	1 2 3 4 5
Rating totals	4, 1	2, 2, 1	4, 3	4, 2	2, 5, 2	2, 2, 4

Figure 3.11 Rubric assessment record of achievement over an entire grading period.

- Say the biomechanics report paper got a 5 on Analyzes Movement Form instead of a 4. Now what grade would Laura get? (1,177 / 13 assessment items = 91%) How can so small a change make such a big difference?

Method 3: Weight Social Attitudes and Interest/Values Twice as Heavily as the Rest

- Divide the total number of points earned by the total number of points possible. What grade would Laura earn? (207 / 250 = 83%)

Method 4: Use Logic Decision Rules for Converting Ratings to Grades

- Logic A:

Grade	Sample rule	Interpreting Laura's record
A	90% 4s and 5s	Laura's ratings are not this high.
B	At least 25% 4s and 5s, with 90% 3s or better	Laura meets both criteria with 85% 4s and 5s and 100% 3s or above; she earns a B.
C	At least 75% 3s or better	Laura's work exceeds this level.
D	25% 3s and above	Laura's work is at a higher level.
F	10% 3s and above	Laura is way above this.

- Logic B: Convert scores directly to percentages (5 = 100%, 4 = 90%, 3 = 80%, 2 = 70%, 1 = 60%). These conversions were based on how the wording in the rubric seemed to describe A, B, and so forth. Divide the number of points earned by the number of points possible. What grade would Laura get? (3,550 / 4,000 = 89%)

Method 5: Later Assignments Count More

- Because the goal might be to report current abilities—not to average current ability with beginning ability—it might be logical to count the last several items in the grade.
- If there is a series of summative assessments, such as in Laura's situation, this method is not logical.

Using each of the methods, what grade would you give Laura? The dilemma of grading performance-based assessments is revealed by these alternative methods. Consider the following recommendations (Arter & McTighe, 2001; Stiggins, Arter, Chappuis, & Chappuis, 2004):

- *Although they might seem easiest, methods 1, 2, and 3 are not recommended.* The primary reason is that a 1 would convert to 20%. Usually, an F is defined as 60%. If 1 is seen as failing, averaging a 20% in with other percentages unfairly weights failing grades. It would take a lot of 4s and 5s to bring an average containing even a single 1 up to 60%.
- *Don't use strict percentages when translating rubric scores to letter grades.* Although a percentage model could work just fine for tests and quizzes (e.g., student answered 80% of the items on a multiple-choice test correctly), they are misleading when converted from rubric scores. The preferred method is to come up with a "logic rule" for deciding on grades. For example:

If the student gets:	Then the grade should be:
No more than 10% of scores lower than a 4, with at least 40% 5s	A
No more than 30% of scores lower than a 4, with at least 10% 5s	B
No more than 10% of scores lower than a 3, with at least 20% 4 or better	C
No more than 30% of scores lower than a 3, with at least 10% 4 or better	D
Anything lower than this	F

The next best way to convert scores to grades is to decide from the descriptions in the rubric what grade each score should earn. For example, 4 and 5 might be an A, 3 might be a B, and 2 might be a C. Therefore, all 4s and 5s would convert to whatever percentage given to As (e.g., 90%), 3s would convert to 80%, 2s would convert to 70%, and 1s would convert to 60%.

- *Separate grades that describe achievement from grades for other factors (e.g., progress, effort, work completion, behavior).* Unless teachers completely agree on the elements that should be included in a grade (e.g., achievement, motivation, ability) and factor them into grading in consistent ways, the meaning of grades will vary from class to class. When this happens, students earn the same grades for very different reasons. Whatever methods are used, teachers should make sure that everyone (teachers, students, parents and guardians, and the community) understands the scheme and supports it.
- *Use systems that permit students to be in control of their own ultimate level of success.* Teachers can consider using the systems described, but give students the opportunity to improve their work and thus their grade. Students can be permitted to revise any assessment items with ratings of 3 or below, using feedback from the teacher and their peers, for reevaluation and regrading. If they attain a new level of proficiency, that grade replaces the previous (now outdated) one. Teachers can weave these ideas into contracts with students. This will help motivate special needs students. A preassessment can be used to determine a student's starting level of proficiency, and then a student-led conference can be held to agree on a profile or subsequent ratings that represents a reachable, but demanding goal for the student. In contract terms, teacher and student should agree that attainment of that level will represent an A. Decision rules for other letter grades can be established from there.

This discussion about grading in a standards-based environment leads to the role of student portfolios in the overall grading scheme. If the primary purpose of grades is to communicate about standards-based achievement, then the processes and products that characterize student portfolios serve that purpose in a unique way. For this reason, the matter of grading or judging the worth of portfolios is covered next.

Portfolio Judging

Given the nature of student-involved, formative assessment *for* learning and the role of student portfolios, is it really necessary to assess portfolios? The answer is yes! Simply collecting items for the sake of collection serves no meaningful teaching or learning function without some measure of worth. Therefore, step 8 in the portfolio-designing process includes the development of criteria and procedures for judging portfolios. It is a challenging task. However, the portfolio's purpose should help define the nature of assessment as well as the people who will do the assessing. Physical education teachers should collaborate with students so that expectations are clearly communicated.

A set of criteria that can help determine the strength or power of a portfolio is helpful in the judging phase. Teachers, students, or both must also decide among several grading options. It should be clear that assessing portfolios is not the same as grading portfolios. For example, achievement feedback can be given to students in an informal manner about their improvement in a sport as evidenced by the portfolio. A grade may not be assigned even though the portfolio is assessed to provide information feedback. No doubt, one of the most controversial and difficult portfolio issues is whether to grade the portfolio. Some options are available for each side of this issue.

Criteria

Because the student portfolio focuses on many learning targets (i.e., knowledge, reasoning, skills, products, dispositions) and processes (i.e., reflection, self-assessment, goal setting, communication), performance criteria are useful. Without some criteria, students may rely on their own views of quality. In physical education, this could mean number of attempts, following instructions, completing all tasks, or trying hard. Use of these criteria would not result in a true picture of student learning. Three types of performance criteria are useful with portfolios (Stiggins, Arter, Chappuis, & Chappuis, 2004):

1. *Criteria for individual entries.* Portfolio artifacts that reflect the learning targets should define what various levels of quality look like. In the case of performance assessment, each entry should have one or more criteria by which to judge its quality. For example, students gathering evidence of their ability to execute a volleyball overhand serve should have a rubric that defines what a high-level serve looks like. Illustrative artifacts were identified in table 3.4 (pages 159-164). The use of rubrics was discussed earlier.

2. *Criteria for self-reflection.* Most students do not know how to self-reflect. They do not know what it is, why it is important, and what quality self-reflection looks like. Students could be shown examples of "beginning," "developing," and "sophisticated" reflections and asked to select the ones they think demonstrate the best reflection and indicate why. Reflection strategies were suggested earlier in this chapter (pages 167-169). Self-assessment is a related process that requires training and practice. Techniques for self-assessment were also identified earlier (pages 169-171).

3. *Criteria for the portfolio as a whole.* Separate from the individual work samples and exhibits within a portfolio, it is sometimes helpful to look at the portfolio as a whole. A rubric for the portfolio as a product itself might contain the traits of clear targets, adequate evidence, good self-reflections, and ease in finding information. Unless the portfolio is a graded assignment, the purpose is to help students understand the nature of quality. Other criteria to consider are change over time (demonstrated growth); diversity (variety of artifacts); evidence of problem solving (analyzed, planned strategies, and worked through to a solution); organization, format, and structure (clearly arranged and sequenced); and self-reflection (thoughtful consideration of personal strengths and needs).

Not Graded

If the basis for the portfolio is growth and development over time, the portfolio itself may not be graded, even though individual pieces in the portfolio may have been graded. In this case, the portfolio is designed to showcase the student's artifacts, including reflections and self-assessments. It is still a valuable synthesis of learning for review by the teacher and parents or guardians. The final nongraded portfolio could also be integrated to represent a student's work across a certain time period (e.g., semester, school year). Items would be selected from several subject areas to profile students' accomplishments. Without the stigmas attached to grades, students are more likely to take learning risks, be more honest about their true learning, feel less constrained, and focus on *Look what I learned* instead of *What is my grade?* Self-esteem usually improves because portfolios can accommodate a greater variety of learning styles.

Traditional grading systems and report cards are a reality within the educational establishment. Translating portfolio contents into report card grades can be difficult given the fact that grades typically rate students on a curve and portfolios place students on a developmental continuum. Also, portfolios are normally skewed because students' "best" work is presented. Therefore, a full representative sample of students' actual learning should be assured. As previously suggested, report cards can be redesigned to include narrative statements or descriptive labels, but it may be more practical to supplement report cards with anecdotal progress reports. Students' accomplishments, their strengths and difficulties, and their development can be more clearly communicated with progress reports. The example shown on page 187 is based on performance indicators rather than grades. Progress is judged as Achieved, Needs improvement, or Working to achieve. Space is provided for general comments about strengths and weakness in each component. Plans for supporting learner growth can also be included. A more comprehensive standards-based physical education report card with separate learning and social behaviors appears on pages 189-190.

Graded

If the basis for the portfolio is performance, the portfolio should be graded in some manner. The assessment should be tied to established content standards and corresponding grade-level expectations. Consideration should be given to different grading options. Physical education teachers can use the following options in combination, alternate them at various times during the year, or alternate them for various purposes and types of portfolios:

- *Whole portfolio.* One grade is given for the whole portfolio, considering the entire body of artifacts. The grade is based on criteria that have been predetermined by both students and teacher, such as organization, completeness, creativity, reflectiveness, understanding of subject matter, and quality of products.

- *Separate items.* Each piece of work in the portfolio is graded separately either prior to or after the portfolio is submitted. Grades are based on predetermined criteria for each artifact or task. The portfolio as a whole could still be graded using the criteria mentioned earlier. This option can be very time consuming for the teacher, particularly if items are not graded until after the portfolio is submitted. The advantage is that students know that each item is important because each is graded.

- *Selected key items.* A number of possibilities exist with this option. For example, the teacher may predetermine and announce the two items that will be evaluated, or the student may identify the two that he or she wants graded. Another option is not to tell students which three items will be graded. Thus, students should be motivated to seek quality on all items. Key items could also be selected from predetermined categories (e.g., learning dimensions, content standards, multiple intelligences).

- *Continual tracking.* Several items from the portfolio are graded and passed on to the next physical education teacher. Each year, some items are removed and others added that are representative of the student's performance. The portfolio can be compiled and graded at key intervals (i.e., after elementary school, middle school, and high school).

Summary

Have you achieved the expected outcomes (see page 122) for this chapter? You should have acquired the knowledge and skills needed for developing student portfolios for K-12 learners in physical education. Assessment *for* learning—student-involved, formative assessment—produces significant learning gains. Clearly, this means that assessment, learning, and teaching must be integrated. Student portfolios may hold the key to successful integration by cultivating desirable student habits—reflecting on learning, developing self-direction and feedback, setting goals, creating new challenges, and communicating achievement results. Student portfolios offer a more naturalistic, genuine technique to verify student learning. Designing portfolio systems appropriate for K-12 physical education programs requires a multifaceted approach that includes the following steps:

1. Determine the general and specific purposes of portfolios.
2. Select the types of portfolios to be used.
3. Create a framework for organizing portfolios.
4. Plan production features and logistics (construction, management, and storage).
5. Establish a process for selecting portfolio items.
6. Decide reflection, goal-setting, and self-assessment techniques.
7. Arrange student-involved conference strategies.
8. Develop quality assessment criteria and procedures.

Depending on the purpose, various types of portfolios can be used (i.e., personal, record-keeping, thematic, integrated, showcase/celebration, scholarship). Alternatives exist around which these portfolios can be organized, including the mission statement, the NASPE description of the physically educated person, learning dimensions, multiple intelligences, organizing centers, and content standards. For logistics, numerous options for construction and storage as well as various management tools should be considered. Technology protocols are essential for the production and maintenance of portfolios and to enhance learning. Also, electronic-based applications are valuable for portfolio efficiency and quality.

The process of selecting portfolio artifacts includes decisions about *what, how, who,* and *when.* The range of possible artifacts in physical education is unlimited. Once selected, reflection strategies (i.e., visualization; tag, label, or stamp; reflective stems; bridging questions; benchmarking; artifact registry) and self-assessment techniques (i.e., checklists, learning logs, journals, strengths and weaknesses charts, goal-setting sheets) encourage student involvement. In addition, portfolio conferences offer another kind of self-reflection, be they informal or formal, simple or complex. Conferences should consider various participants (i.e., teacher, parents or guardians, peers, significant others) and strategies such as miniconferences, conference stations, and student-led formats.

Finally, assessment of portfolios involves the application of quality standards for assessment (i.e., clear purpose, clear targets, sound assessment design, effective communication, student involvement) and the use of scoring rubrics. Grading in a standards-based environment is critical to student-involved, classroom-level assessment *for* learning. Decisions about grading portfolios are also needed (i.e., whole portfolio, separate items, selected key items, continuous tracking).

Sample Student Portfolio Systems

To synthesize the information presented in this chapter, sample portfolio systems are provided for use at the elementary school, middle school, and high school levels. Although the settings for these systems are hypothetical, the portfolio elements are applicable to actual K-12 physical education programs. These systems incorporate the concepts and principles advanced in this chapter.

In addition, the CD-ROM accompanying the book provides a template (portfolio builder) to create an electronic-based student portfolio using Microsoft PowerPoint®. Instructions are provided for navigating through the slides that include hyperlinks for access to the necessary files. When the portfolio is completed, it can be copied to a CD for distribution and review. It can also be uploaded to the Internet for access as a Web-based portfolio. The following components are used to organize the portfolio:

- Table of contents
- Introduction
- Standards
- Learning targets
- Goal setting
- Reflections
- Journal (self-assessment)
- Gallery (pictures, video clips)
- Conferences
- Assessment

Elementary School Portfolio System

In an attempt to develop students' responsibility and self-management skills early in the educational process, an achievement portfolio is described for the elementary school level, appropriate for grades 2 or 3. The PEP (physical education portfolio) system includes a series of units. The sample presented focuses on the development of locomotor skills. It is structured in the form of a workbook for students. Because many of the terms associated with portfolios are beyond the language levels of primary-aged students, they are not used explicitly in the workbook. Although not labeled as such, the worksheets integrate many of the portfolio concepts and principles, such as reflection, self-assessment, goal setting, and conferences.

Middle School Portfolio System

A showcase type of portfolio is described for the middle school level. The portfolio focuses on the development of knowledge, skills, and attitudes in volleyball. Volleyball is one of several sports offered across the middle school curriculum in which students maintain a continual "Sportfolio" (Marmo, 1994). It is structured in the form of instructions for the volleyball sport unit.

High School Portfolio System

The type of portfolio described for the high school level is thematic in nature. The theme is Fitness for Life. The portfolio is designed for a one-semester course in physical education. It is structured in the form of guidelines for personal growth.

Physical Education Portfolio

Locomotor Skills Workbook

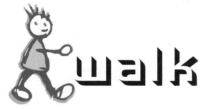 walk

Hop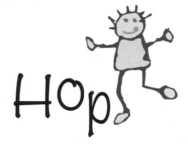

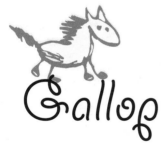 Gallop

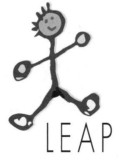 LEAP

jump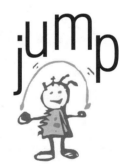

Skip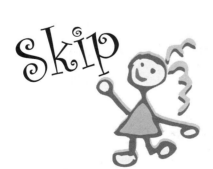

RUN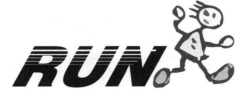

slide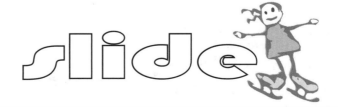

From *Professional and Student Portfolios for Physical Education, Second Edition,* by Vincent J. Melograno, 2006, Champaign, IL: Human Kinetics.

How to Make Your Container

1. Get a regular size cereal box.

2. Cut the cereal box.

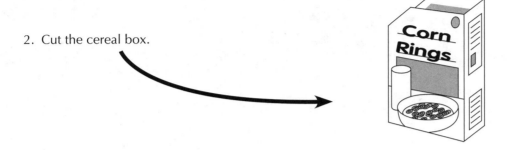

3. Cover your portfolio.

4. Put your name on the portfolio.

5. Decorate the sides of your portfolio.

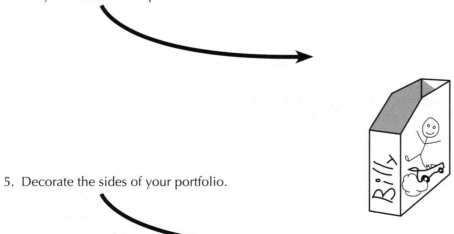

Locomotor Skills Journal

Name: _____

Instructions: During the next three weeks, write down different exercises, activities, or sports that use each locomotor skill.

Locomotor skill	Exercise, activity, or sport
Walk	1. 2. 3.
Run	1. 2. 3.
Jump	1. 2. 3.
Hop	1. 2. 3.
Leap	1. 2. 3.
Slide	1. 2. 3.
Gallop	1. 2. 3.
Skip	1. 2. 3.

From *Professional and Student Portfolios for Physical Education, Second Edition,* by Vincent J. Melograno, 2006, Champaign, IL: Human Kinetics.

199

Locomotor Skills Partner Activity

Name: _____

Partner's name: _____

Instructions: With a partner, design a *movement* sequence using four different locomotor patterns (skills). Each pattern (skill) should last for eight counts. You should repeat the sequence four times to 4/4 beat music, which will be provided. Use the chart below to design your sequence. Practice the sequence together!

Sequence	Description
First pattern or skill	
Second pattern or skill	
Third pattern or skill	
Fourth pattern or skill	

Locomotor Skills Group Project

Name: _____

Group member's name: _____

Group member's name: _____

Instructions: In a group of three, write a rhyme that you can jump to with a long jump rope. The rhyme should last at least 12 jumps. Include at least three different types of jumps (e.g., one-foot, skip-step, turns). Write out each line of your rhyme below. Show what type of jump is used for each line of the rhyme.

Rhyme	Type of jump
Line 1:	
Line 2:	
Line 3:	
Line 4:	
Line 5:	
Line 6:	

From *Professional and Student Portfolios for Physical Education, Second Edition,* by Vincent J. Melograno, 2006, Champaign, IL: Human Kinetics.

Rate Your Locomotor Skills

Name: _____

Instructions: Think about the correct way to do each locomotor skill. At the end of each week, check (✓) the face that shows how well you think you can do each locomotor skill. Record the date in the space provided for each week.

Locomotor skill	Week 1 Friday (__/__/__)			Week 2 Friday (__/__/__)			Week 3 Friday (__/__/__)		
Walk	☹ □	😐 □	🙂 □	☹ □	😐 □	🙂 □	☹ □	😐 □	🙂 □
Run	☹ □	😐 □	🙂 □	☹ □	😐 □	🙂 □	☹ □	😐 □	🙂 □
Jump	☹ □	😐 □	🙂 □	☹ □	😐 □	🙂 □	☹ □	😐 □	🙂 □
Hop	☹ □	😐 □	🙂 □	☹ □	😐 □	🙂 □	☹ □	😐 □	🙂 □
Leap	☹ □	😐 □	🙂 □	☹ □	😐 □	🙂 □	☹ □	😐 □	🙂 □
Slide	☹ □	😐 □	🙂 □	☹ □	😐 □	🙂 □	☹ □	😐 □	🙂 □
Gallop	☹ □	😐 □	🙂 □	☹ □	😐 □	🙂 □	☹ □	😐 □	🙂 □
Skip	☹ □	😐 □	🙂 □	☹ □	😐 □	🙂 □	☹ □	😐 □	🙂 □

Locomotor Skills Checklist

Name: _____

Instructions: Keep this checklist in your portfolio. It shows your progress in each of the locomotor skills. Your physical education teacher will observe you and fill it out.

Locomotor skill/criteria	1ST OBSERVATION		2ND OBSERVATION	
	Working to achieve	Have achieved	Working to achieve	Have achieved
Walk:				
• Head is up; body is erect	_____	_____	_____	_____
• Leg swings forward	_____	_____	_____	_____
• Diagonal push-off backward against ground with ball of one foot	_____	_____	_____	_____
• Arms swing in opposition to legs				
• Heel-to-toe placement of foot	_____	_____	_____	_____
• Toes point straight ahead	_____	_____	_____	_____
	_____	_____	_____	_____
Run:				
• Head is up; body leans forward	_____	_____	_____	_____
• Support foot contacts ground close to body's center of gravity	_____	_____	_____	_____
• Knee swings forward and upward	_____	_____	_____	_____
• Lower leg flexes, bringing heel close to buttocks	_____	_____	_____	_____
• Push-off sends body momentarily into air	_____	_____	_____	_____
• Arms drive in opposition to legs	_____	_____	_____	_____
• Toes point forward	_____	_____	_____	_____
Jump:				
• Crouch is taken by flexing hips, knees, and ankles	_____	_____	_____	_____
• Forceful extension of legs depending on need	_____	_____	_____	_____
• Use arms, timing them with the leg action; arms out to sides for stability	_____	_____	_____	_____
• Land softly by bending ankles, knees, and hips	_____	_____	_____	_____
Hop:				
• Body is erect	_____	_____	_____	_____
• Push off from one foot and land on same foot	_____	_____	_____	_____
• Flex hip, knee, and ankle for greater force	_____	_____	_____	_____
• Nonsupport leg is held up with knee bent, usually with foot held back	_____	_____	_____	_____
• Arms bent at elbow, slightly out from body to aid balance	_____	_____	_____	_____
• Land softly, with flexion in ankle, knee, and hip to absorb force	_____	_____	_____	_____
• Contact with ground begins with forward part of foot, shifting gradually to ball of foot, then heel	_____	_____	_____	_____

(continued)

From *Professional and Student Portfolios for Physical Education, Second Edition*, by Vincent J. Melograno, 2006, Champaign, IL: Human Kinetics.

(continued)

Locomotor skill/criteria	1ST OBSERVATION		2ND OBSERVATION	
	Working to achieve	Have achieved	Working to achieve	Have achieved
Leap:				
• Head is up; body leans forward	——	——	——	——
• Take off from one foot landing on the other foot	——	——	——	——
• Flexion in hip, knee, and ankle for thrust	——	——	——	——
• Body remains airborne to cover greater distance	——	——	——	——
• Body is more fully extended, including legs	——	——	——	——
• Arms move in opposition to legs but move upward	——	——	——	——
• Land softly by flexing hip, knee, and ankle	——	——	——	——
Slide:				
• Body is erect; head is up	——	——	——	——
• Step (leap) to side	——	——	——	——
• Transfer weight by drawing or closing step with other foot	——	——	——	——
• As weight transfers to trailing foot, lead leg reaches to side again	——	——	——	——
• Same foot leads each step	——	——	——	——
• Step is longer than draw phase of slide	——	——	——	——
Gallop:				
• Slide performed in a forward direction	——	——	——	——
• Step forward (short leap)	——	——	——	——
• Transfer weight by drawing or closing step with other foot	——	——	——	——
• As weight transfers to trailing foot, lead leg reaches forward again	——	——	——	——
• Same foot leads each step	——	——	——	——
• Step is longer than draw phase of slide	——	——	——	——
Skip:				
• Body is erect; head is up	——	——	——	——
• Initiated by taking a step forward on one foot	——	——	——	——
• Followed by a hop on the same foot; opposite foot brought forward to begin next step; lead leg lifts	——	——	——	——
• Arms move in opposition to legs; may be brought upward and forward	——	——	——	——
• Step forward performed on first beat in rhythm	——	——	——	——
• Skip is repeated with a step on the opposite foot	——	——	——	——

Locomotor Skills Letter or Conference

Name: _____

Instructions: Write a letter to your parents or guardians telling them about your locomotor skills. Use the space below. Try to answer these questions in your letter:

- What locomotor skills am I good at?
- What was fun about learning locomotor skills?
- What locomotor skills still need more work?
- What are my physical education goals?

Then, sit down and talk to your parents or guardians about your portfolio. Ask them to write their comments below and sign this sheet.

Dear _____:

_____

_____

_____

_____

_____

_____

_____

_____

_____

_____

_____

_____

_____

_____

_____

_____

Parent's or guardian's comments: _____

_____

_____

_____

_____

_____

_____

_____

_____

Signed: _____ Date: _____

From *Professional and Student Portfolios for Physical Education, Second Edition*, by Vincent J. Melograno, 2006, Champaign, IL: Human Kinetics.

Sportfolio

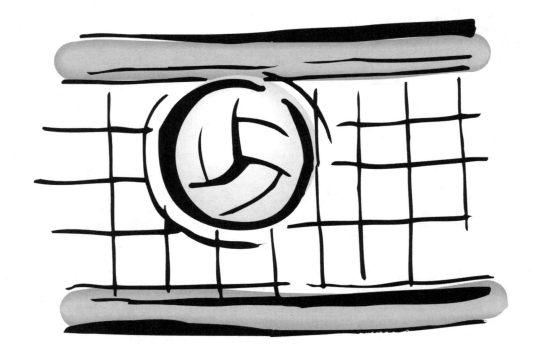

Volleyball
Directions for the Showcase Portfolio

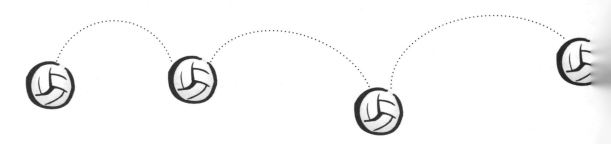

SPORTFOLIO FRAMEWORK

The Sportfolio is a series of showcase portfolios that are maintained all year throughout the physical education program. It is a way for you to continually keep track of your accomplishments in each sport.

Goal

Develop knowledge, skills, and values in a variety of individual and team sports: soccer, flag football, basketball, volleyball, team handball, softball, tennis, and golf.

Standards

A. Uses a variety of basic and advanced movement forms
B. Uses movement concepts and principles in the development of motor skills
C. Understands and practices social and personal responsibility associated with participation in physical activity

Outcomes

A1. Uses intermediate sport-specific skills for individual and team sports
B1. Understands the critical elements of advanced movement skills
B2. Uses basic offensive and defensive strategies in a modified version of a team and individual sport
B3. Understands movement forms associated with highly skilled physical activities
C1. Works in a group to accomplish a set goal in both cooperative and competitive activities
C2. Knows the difference between inclusive and exclusionary behaviors in sports
C3. Understands that sports are a vehicle for self-expression

Showcase Portfolio

Purpose: To display your *best* work in a particular individual or team sport

Description: The portfolio should be streamlined. You are *not* expected to collect and store all the day-to-day items (e.g., checklists, worksheets, task cards) that are part of the physical education program. You are expected, however, to complete certain tasks and projects for each sport that will be part of your showcase portfolio. You will be given instructions for each sport. Eventually, you will have a series of showcase portfolios that, together, make up your personal Sportfolio.

Management: You will manage your own showcase portfolio. You are responsible for collecting, organizing, storing, and maintaining any items or materials that are needed for any given showcase portfolio. Even though some items will be developed in physical education class, it is still your responsibility to manage what you need. Most items are developed outside of physical education class. *Be very careful with and protect your work samples.* A due date will be announced for each of the showcase portfolios as the different sports are covered during the school year.

TASKS

The showcase portfolio for volleyball includes several tasks that must be completed. The common set of Sportfolio categories is used to organize these tasks. Some choices are built into certain categories.

From *Professional and Student Portfolios for Physical Education, Second Edition,* by Vincent J. Melograno, 2006, Champaign, IL: Human Kinetics.

207

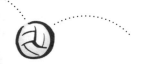

A. Tracking Growth

Description: To record your experiences, results, feelings, and perceptions, you will maintain a volleyball journal to track your growth in volleyball. Entries to the journal will be made at the end of the second, fourth, and sixth weeks. Use the form on page 210. Record the date in the space provided for each week.

Task: Maintain a journal during the volleyball sport unit.

B. Personal Skill Analysis

Description: You will be videotaped during game play. Time will be provided for you to view the videotape and to analyze each of the major skills of volleyball: overhand or underhand serve, overhead pass/front set, bump pass, spike, and block. Use the self-analysis rating sheet for these skills on page 211.

Task: Write a description of your *two best* skills, based on your self-analyses.

C. Sport Insight

Description: Through different kinds of projects, you can learn more about and gain greater insights into the game of volleyball. The following projects could be used for this purpose.

1. *Scouting report.* A class volleyball tournament will be held at the end of the unit. Once teams are selected, write a scouting report for each team, including your own team. Include an analysis of the teams' strengths and weaknesses and their offensive and defensive strategies. Predict the outcome of the tournament and the reasons for your predictions.

2. *Interview.* Conduct an interview with one of the varsity volleyball players at the high school. The interview should focus on how he or she became a volleyball player, how he or she developed skills, and what practice routines and training techniques he or she uses. Develop questions in advance. Write a script of the questions and answers.

3. *Essay.* Write an essay about the origins, history, and future of the sport of volleyball. You should also include how volleyball was introduced into the United States and the background of volleyball as an Olympic and NCAA sport.

4. *Article summaries.* Read and summarize *three* articles in sports magazines or journals about volleyball skills, practice techniques, and training and conditioning tips. Each written summary should be at least one page.

Task: Select and complete one of the Sport Insight projects.

D. Game Analysis

Description: The skills, rules, and strategies of volleyball all come together when a game is played. To show your understanding of the sport, you will have a chance to analyze a class volleyball tournament game or a high school volleyball game and to communicate your analysis in one of the following roles:

1. *Newspaper sports reporter.* Observe one of the class volleyball tournament games or a high school volleyball game. Write a newspaper article about the game. The article should include a complete analysis of individual and team performances as well as game statistics. Design a volleyball "box score" as part of the article. Include action photos if possible.

2. *Radio sports announcer.* Observe one of the class volleyball tournament games or a high school volleyball game. Record, on a tape recorder, your play-by-play commentary of the game as though you were a radio sports announcer. Select a player of the game and conduct a postgame interview on the audio tape.

3. *TV sports broadcaster.* Observe one of the class volleyball tournament games or a high school volleyball game. Record, on videotape, your play-by-play commentary of the game as though you were a TV sports broadcaster. Select a player of the game and conduct a postgame interview on the videotape.

Task: Select and complete one of the Game Analysis projects.

 From *Professional and Student Portfolios for Physical Education, Second Edition,* by Vincent J. Melograno, 2006, Champaign, IL: Human Kinetics.

E. Goal Setting

Description: You will be able to look at what you know about volleyball, what your skills are in volleyball, and how much you like volleyball. After the unit, you should be well aware of your strengths and problem areas. By looking at yourself, you should be able to establish some volleyball goals for yourself. Use the strengths and problem areas and goal-setting chart on page 213.

Task: Set goals for volleyball based on strengths and problem areas.

F. Communicating Achievement

Description: It is hoped that you will want to show others how you developed your volleyball abilities. You should be proud of your accomplishments in volleyball. Therefore, you are expected to share your showcase portfolio with your parents or guardians. Use the parent or guardian conference guide on page 214.

Task: Arrange and conduct a portfolio conference with your parents or guardians.

CONTENTS

An accordion file with dividers or a soft cover notebook with pockets would be a good portfolio container. To help you organize the portfolio, a list of required items follows.

1. *Informational cover.* Make sure your name and class are included. Your cover design is a matter of personal choice and creativity.

2. *Table of contents.* All items should be listed with page numbers. Clearly indicate your choice of projects for the Sport Insight and Game Analysis tasks.

3. *Journal.* The volleyball journal should include complete entries following the second, fourth, and sixth weeks.

4. *Description of two best skills.* Using your personal skills self-analyses, decide your two best skills and describe them in detail.

5. *Sport Insight project.* Include one of the following: (a) scouting report, (b) interview script, (c) essay, or (d) article summaries.

6. *Game Analysis project.* Include one of the following: (a) newspaper article as sports reporter, (b) audiotape as radio sports announcer, or (c) videotape as TV sports broadcaster.

7. *Goals for volleyball.* Using your identified strengths and problem areas, indicate the volleyball goals you have set for yourself.

8. *Conference results.* Include any notes from your conference with your parents or guardians and their written comments and sign-off.

ASSESSMENT

The showcase portfolio will be assessed in different ways. A simple rating scale (+, √, 0) will be used for the basic required items: informational cover, table of contents, journal, skill descriptions, goals, and parent conference. A letter grade will be assigned to the special required items: Sport Insight project and Game Analysis project. Then, the whole showcase portfolio will be assessed considering the ratings for the basic items and the grades for the special items. The criteria for the overall grade are detailed in the assessment form on page 215.

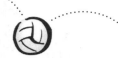

Journal

Name: _____

Questions	End of second week (__/__/__)	End of fourth week (__/__/__)	End of sixth week (__/__/__)
1. What volleyball activities were really fun?			
2. Which of my volleyball skills are pretty good or better?			
3. Which of my volleyball skills could use more work?			
4. The things I like best about volleyball are . . .			
5. The things I like least about volleyball are . . .			
6. My overall impressions of volleyball are . . .			

Self-Analysis Skills Rating Sheet

Name: _____

	Not yet	OK	Good
Overhand serve			
1. Faces net in a stride position with foot opposite striking arm forward	❏	❏	❏
2. Ball tossed two to three feet above net and in front of hitting shoulder	❏	❏	❏
3. Striking arm moves rearward at approximately shoulder height	❏	❏	❏
4. Elbow flexes, permitting forearm and hand to drop behind the head	❏	❏	❏
5. Arm rotated forward at shoulder	❏	❏	❏
6. Forearm lags behind upper arm and hand behind forearm	❏	❏	❏
7. Upper palm or heel of hand used to contact ball	❏	❏	❏
8. Ball contacted momentarily at its midpoint with little follow-through	❏	❏	❏
Underhand serve			
1. Faces net with foot opposite the striking arm in front	❏	❏	❏
2. Rests ball in nonstriking hand at about knee to waist height	❏	❏	❏
3. Striking arm moved rearward to shoulder height in a swinging action	❏	❏	❏
4. Body weight shifted rearward onto back foot at same time	❏	❏	❏
5. Hits ball off the holding hand with striking hand in an open and cupped position, a half fist for striking with heel of hand, or a fist	❏	❏	❏
6. Hitting arm swings forward and upward during hit (as in bowling a ball)	❏	❏	❏
7. Hand follows ball straight through in the direction of the flight of the ball	❏	❏	❏
Overhead pass or front set			
1. Performs "ready position" (shoulder-width stance with body weight equally distributed over both feet)	❏	❏	❏
2. Knees flexed, head tilted back to focus on ball	❏	❏	❏
3. Arms move forward and upward until upper arms are parallel with floor; elbows flexed and pointing out to sides	❏	❏	❏
4. Hands bent backward at wrist; fingers spread; hands slightly cupped	❏	❏	❏
5. Thumbs and index fingers form a triangle	❏	❏	❏
6. Extends legs and arms at same time into ball	❏	❏	❏
7. Fingers (not palms) contact ball above and in front of forehead	❏	❏	❏
8. Fingers close in a grabbing action once contact is made	❏	❏	❏
9. Follows through with continuous upward extension of body in direction of hit	❏	❏	❏
Bump pass			
1. Clasps hands together (clenched fist, curled fingers, or thumb over palm)	❏	❏	❏
2. Moves quickly to a position behind ball	❏	❏	❏
3. Knees bent, feet shoulder-width apart in forward stride position, trunk slightly forward	❏	❏	❏
4. Hands and arms extended, together and parallel with elbows locked during contact	❏	❏	❏
5. Hands point toward floor	❏	❏	❏
6. Ball contacted on the forearms above wrists	❏	❏	❏
7. Arm movement in an arc from shoulders with legs involved	❏	❏	❏

(continued)

From *Professional and Student Portfolios for Physical Education, Second Edition,* by Vincent J. Melograno, 2006, Champaign, IL: Human Kinetics.

211

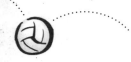

(continued)

	Not yet	OK	Good
Spike			
1. Uses step-hop, three-step, or four-step approach	❏	❏	❏
2. On last step or hop, body drives downward by flexing at ankles; knees and hips with shoulders face net	❏	❏	❏
3. Immediately, extension at knees and hips propels body upward into jump	❏	❏	❏
4. Arms held close to body in the forward and upward swinging action	❏	❏	❏
5. Striking arm moves in a straight horizontal path rearward as in the overarm throwing pattern	❏	❏	❏
6. After hips begin to rotate, striking arm starts forward at the shoulder	❏	❏	❏
7. Elbow begins extension while the wrist is bent backward	❏	❏	❏
8. Upper arm lags behind shoulder, forearm behind upper arm, and hand behind forearm	❏	❏	❏
9. Arm fully extended at contact, made in front of body above shoulder at height equal to length of fully extended arm	❏	❏	❏
10. Ball contacted slightly above its center with entire hand	❏	❏	❏
11. Trunk flexes forward with snapping of wrist as part of follow-through	❏	❏	❏
Block			
1. Ready position established after reaching position of one to two feet from net	❏	❏	❏
2. Stance is parallel with feet shoulder-width apart and knees flexed	❏	❏	❏
3. Hands held at shoulder height, elbows flexed, forearms parallel with net	❏	❏	❏
4. Jump preparation consists of flexion at ankles, knees, and hips with trunk slightly flexed forward to assume half-squat position	❏	❏	❏
5. Jump begins immediately after spiker jumps	❏	❏	❏
6. With extension of ankles, knees, and hips, arms are extended vertically over top of net on vertical jump	❏	❏	❏
7. Fingers spread and arms held firm for ball contact	❏	❏	❏
8. Reach is sustained for as long as possible	❏	❏	❏

  From *Professional and Student Portfolios for Physical Education, Second Edition*, by Vincent J. Melograno, 2006, Champaign, IL: Human Kinetics.

Setting Goals Based on Strengths and Problem Areas

Name: _____

My volleyball strengths	Performing volleyball skills	
	Understanding the rules of volleyball	
	Applying offensive strategies in volleyball	
	Applying defensive strategies in volleyball	
	Working with others on volleyball team	
My volleyball problem areas	Performing volleyball skills	
	Understanding the rules of volleyball	
	Applying offensive strategies in volleyball	
	Applying defensive strategies in volleyball	
	Working with others on volleyball team	

Volleyball goals	Target date

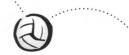

Parent or Guardian Conference Guide

Name: _____

To the Student

You are expected to direct the conference with your parent or guardian. Some of the things you could focus on are answers to the following questions:

- How did you improve your volleyball skills?
- If you could publish one portfolio item, what would it be?
- What are you most proud of?
- What aspects of volleyball need more work?
- What surprised you most about the volleyball unit?
- What do you think about the showcase portfolio? About the Sportfolio process?
- What would you change if you could?
- What was your biggest challenge?

To the Parent or Guardian

Your child would like to share his or her showcase portfolio with you. Please look it over and discuss it with your child, who will direct the conference. You may also be interested in answers to some of the questions above. After the conference, please offer your reactions below and verify the conference with your signature.

Comments:

_____
_____
_____
_____
_____
_____
_____
_____
_____
_____
_____
_____

Parent or guardian signature: _____ Date: _____

From *Professional and Student Portfolios for Physical Education, Second Edition,* by Vincent J. Melograno, 2006, Champaign, IL: Human Kinetics.

Assessment Form

Name: _____

Basic Items	0 Does not meet expectations	✓ Meets expectations	+ Exceeds expectations
Informational cover	_____	_____	_____
Table of contents	_____	_____	_____
Journal	_____	_____	_____
Descriptions of best skills	_____	_____	_____
Goals	_____	_____	_____
Conference	_____	_____	_____

Comments: _____

_____

_____

_____

Special Items	F Poor	D Fair	C Satisfactory	B Good	A Excellent
Sport Insight project	_____	_____	_____	_____	_____

❏ Scouting report ❏ Interview ❏ Essay ❏ Article summaries

	F	D	C	B	A
Game Analysis project	_____	_____	_____	_____	_____

❏ Newspaper article ❏ Radio commentary ❏ TV commentary

Comments: _____

_____

_____

_____

Overall Grade

_____ A = Portfolio is exemplary in terms of contents and quality.

_____ B = Portfolio is fully developed; there is room for improved quality.

_____ C = Portfolio includes all required items; meets all minimum expectations.

_____ D = Portfolio is not fully developed in some aspects; quality is below expectations.

_____ F = Portfolio items are incomplete or missing; quality is lacking.

Signed: _____   Date: _____

From *Professional and Student Portfolios for Physical Education, Second Edition,* by Vincent J. Melograno, 2006, Champaign, IL: Human Kinetics.

215

Fitness for Life

Guidelines for the Personal Growth Portfolio

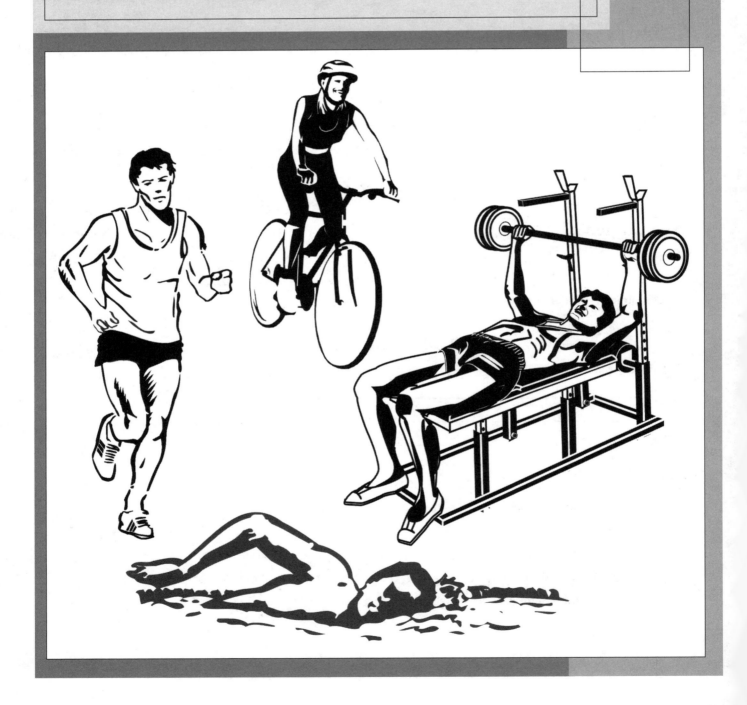

PERSONAL GROWTH PORTFOLIO

Over the next four months, you will learn why it is important to adopt a physically active lifestyle *now* and in later *adulthood*. You will discover the benefits of physical activity and physical fitness in preventing cardiovascular disease and how they improve your sleep, increase your capacity to perform daily functions, improve your mental health, and help you to maintain a desirable weight. You may also find that physical activity and physical fitness help reduce your stress, offer chances for social contacts, and even help with your academics.

You will learn about the concepts and principles of what is called "health-related fitness." This means that you will participate in learning experiences designed to improve fitness, promote health, and prevent future disease. The goal of the Fitness for Life course is to make sure you have the chance to engage in physical activity during physical education class and to encourage you to participate in physical activity outside of school and throughout your life.

Because physical fitness is a personal matter, you need a way to develop, maintain, and monitor your own program of fitness. That is what the personal growth portfolio is all about. A *portfolio* is a collection of work samples and exhibits that shows your effort, progress, and achievement. In this case, the portfolio will present a picture of your physical fitness. You probably have many questions about the portfolio process. These guidelines will help answer them.

QUESTION 1

What are the *purposes* of the personal growth portfolio?

- Help you keep track of your own fitness progress
- Encourage you to assess your own accomplishments
- Help your family members understand your effort and achievement
- Motivate you to practice a healthy lifestyle
- Help you determine your degree of personal satisfaction and social development
- Help you meet health-related fitness standards
- Show you how to monitor and adjust activity levels to meet personal fitness needs
- Help you understand how to maintain an active lifestyle throughout life
- Help you design a personal fitness program that is based on sound concepts and principles of training that include all fitness components

QUESTION 2

How should the portfolio be *organized* and *managed?*

Your personal growth portfolio should be organized in a way that is clear and meaningful. Because it is designed for the Fitness for Life course, it should be organized around aspects of fitness. The one broad *standard* that you should keep in mind as you develop the portfolio is supported by eight *benchmarks*. They define what you should know and be able to do, which indicates progress toward the standard. Your portfolio should be organized around the standard and benchmarks.

Standard

Understands how to monitor and maintain a health-enhancing level of physical fitness; achieves and maintains a health-enhancing level of physical fitness; exhibits a physically active lifestyle

Benchmarks

1. Knows personal status of cardiorespiratory endurance
2. Knows personal status of muscular strength and endurance of the arms, shoulders, abdomen, back, and legs

3. Knows personal status of flexibility of the joints of the arms, legs, and trunk

4. Knows personal status of body composition

5. Meets health-related fitness standards for appropriate level of a physical fitness test (e.g., aerobic capacity, body composition, muscle strength and endurance, flexibility)

6. Knows how to monitor and adjust activity levels to meet personal fitness needs

7. Understands how to maintain an active lifestyle throughout life (e.g., participate regularly in physical activities that reflect personal interests)

8. Designs a personal fitness program that is based on the basic principles of training and encompasses all components of fitness (e.g., cardiorespiratory efficiency, body composition, muscular strength and endurance, flexibility)

You will need to "manage" the collection of items as your portfolio is developed throughout the Fitness for Life course. This is called your *working portfolio*. It will evolve over time and serves as the repository for your work samples and exhibits. Eventually, your *final personal growth portfolio* will be made up of items selected from your working portfolio, some of which are required, others of which involve your making choices. The question of what to include in your portfolio is answered later. The following guidelines will help you assemble and maintain your portfolio.

Construction and Storage

You will have access to your own portfolio on a daily basis. You are not allowed to look into or use someone else's portfolio for any reason without permission. Likewise, your portfolio is private. Access to it is strictly forbidden without your permission. Storage options for the working and final personal growth portfolio are described next.

Working portfolio. Individual hanging files will be maintained alphabetically in milk crates on rollers. File folders will be available to help separate and organize your portfolio items by fitness topics, by the eight benchmarks, or by works in progress and finished works. Working portfolios will be stored in the physical education office until the last three weeks of the course.

Final portfolio. You are responsible for storing and maintaining the personal growth portfolio during the last three weeks of the course. Your final portfolio must be placed in a soft-cover notebook binder. Required elements are identified later.

Management Tools

You should manage your portfolio on a regular basis. The following management tools can be used separately or in combination. They should be particularly helpful with the working portfolio.

Table of contents. A list of *all* entries and file or page numbers must be maintained on a sheet placed at the front of your hanging file or attached to the inside cover of the hanging file.

Color codes. Use color stick-on dots or different color markers to organize items. Make sure a code for the colors is indicated, probably as part of the table of contents.

Registry. Record the date, item, and reason for either adding or removing an item. Use the Portfolio Item Registry form that appears at the end of these guidelines.

Self-stick notes. So that you don't forget your ideas and to protect original items, use self-stick notes (or attach index cards) to *briefly* explain why you collected each item. You may want to connect the items to one or more of the benchmarks.

Personalize. Do not hesitate to inject your personality into the portfolio through colors, graphics, and shapes.

QUESTION 3

What *items* should be included and how are they *selected?*

As you should know by now, you are really developing two portfolios. The working portfolio is the result of the regular, day-to-day collection and management of items. The final personal growth portfolio is more streamlined and includes items selected from the working portfolio. The expected contents for each are outlined.

From *Professional and Student Portfolios for Physical Education, Second Edition,* by Vincent J. Melograno, 2006, Champaign, IL: Human Kinetics.

Working Portfolio

Everything related to the Fitness for Life course should be kept in the working portfolio, including such things as handouts, class notes, journals, logs, workout sheets, project drafts, item registry, conference forms, reflections, peer assessments, and copies of articles. The items should be linked primarily to the eight benchmarks. However, certain key items are required for each of the benchmarks as shown in table 1.

Table 1   Required Items for the Working Portfolio

Benchmarks	Required items
Personal status of: 1. Cardiorespiratory endurance 2. Muscular strength and endurance 3. Flexibility of the joints 4. Body composition	Physical Fitness Profile chart 1. 1-mile walk/run (min/sec) 2. 1-RM tests (lb): bench press, standing press, curl, leg press; push-ups (#); curl-ups (#); modified pull-ups (#) 3. Shoulder lift (inches); trunk extension (inches); sit-and-reach (inches) 4. Sum of triceps and calf skinfolds (mm); food log for five days
5. Health-related fitness standards	Physical Fitness Goals sheet Compare pretest results and *FITNESSGRAM* standards for age and gender (Cooper Institute for Aerobics Research, 2004); establish short-term and long-term goals for each fitness component
6. Monitoring and adjusting activity levels to meet fitness needs	Physical Fitness Journal form Fitness Workout Schedule form
7. Maintaining active lifestyle	Physical Activity and Leisure Questionnaire Physical Activity Log for same five days as the food log
8. Personal fitness program	Project: Fitness for Life program

Final Personal Growth Portfolio

Whereas the working portfolio focuses on the eight benchmarks, the final personal growth portfolio is linked to the following broad standard established for the Fitness for Life course: *Understands how to monitor and maintain a health-enhancing level of physical fitness; achieves and maintains a health-enhancing level of physical fitness; exhibits a physically active lifestyle.*

The final personal growth portfolio is made up of several items, some of which will require you to make choices. In addition, some of the items are described later (e.g., reflections, conference records). The following items are required:

1. Creative cover

2. Table of contents

3. Reflections:
   a. Health style self-test inventory
   b. Article reviews for four different benchmarks
   c. Food and activity logs
   d. Dietary guidelines, food guide pyramid

4. Conference records:
   a. Peer
   b. Family

From *Professional and Student Portfolios for Physical Education, Second Edition,* by Vincent J. Melograno, 2006, Champaign, IL: Human Kinetics.

5. Project (select *one*):

   a. *New activities.* Identify three activities available to you that you have not experienced but think you might like; observe and participate in one of those activities; submit a report about the activity, its equipment, cost, where it is available, and so on.

   b. *Concepts scrapbook.* Describe the components of physical fitness and related principles; collect drawings, illustrations, or pictures that depict various exercises and activities to improve the components.

   c. *Interviews.* Conduct interviews of a male and female for three age groups (15-30, 31-50, 51-65 years); determine their activity patterns and evaluate them in terms of gender and age trends.

6. Fitness for Life program criteria:

   a. Plot a personal physical fitness profile based on ratings for cardiorespiratory endurance, muscular strength and endurance, flexibility, and body composition.

   b. Generate fitness goals based on ratings for health-related components.

   c. Select exercise or leisure activities based on their contributions to fitness goals.

   d. Design a program based on goals, activity selection, and activity schedule.

   e. Satisfy principles of exercise, including heart rate training zone, specificity, overload, progression, and regularity (frequency, intensity, time).

7. Fitness contract: As a result of the Fitness for Life course, it is hoped that you are interested in changing some habits so that new fitness behaviors become a normal part of your lifestyle; complete all parts of the change contract.

   a. Behaviors I want to change

   b. Reasons for wanting to change

   c. Specific outcomes

   d. Goals for four consecutive weeks

   e. Plan of action (actual activities)

   f. Plan to monitor success (diary, log, graph, or chart)

   g. Barriers and strategies to overcome barriers

   h. People who will be on my support team

   i. How I will reward myself when successful

   j. When I will start and how long I will stay with it

   k. My estimated chance of success (0 to 100 percent)

   l. Sources to refer to about my behavior change

   m. Plan for motivational strategies to enhance my success

QUESTION 4

How should *reflection* and *self-assessment* be carried out?

To gain insights throughout the portfolio process, you are expected to reflect on your work. Reflection means that you thoughtfully examine your work samples and think or write about their meaning and value. Through reflection, you will have an opportunity to think about what you have learned and how you have learned it. You should also get to know yourself better, particularly about your physical fitness status.

The Portfolio Item Registry form that you need to keep in the working portfolio is one kind of reflection. As you add or delete items, you must give a reason. In addition, you need to reflect on four items that are required for the final personal growth portfolio.

1. *Health style self-test inventory.* You will complete an inventory that covers different categories of healthy behavior. Reflect on your scores for each of the following categories: tobacco use, alcohol and other drug use, nutrition, exercise and fitness, emotional health, safety, and stress. The following questions could help your reflections: What scores surprised me? Why? What changes can I make to improve my health? How would others react to my scores?

2. *Article reviews.* Select four of the eight benchmarks and find magazine articles that relate to each benchmark. Do not simply summarize the articles. Instead, reflect on their meaning and significance in developing fitness. Questions to ask are: Why does the article relate to the benchmark? What aspects about the article could I use in my fitness program? What is the most important thing I learned from the article?

3. *Food and activity logs.* Use the results of your food and activity logs to reflect on your caloric intake versus caloric expenditure. Use these reflective stems: The thing I'll remember is . . .; I was really surprised about . . .; I really like the way I . . .; My biggest challenge now is . . . .

4. *Dietary guidelines and food guide pyramid.* Review the nine categories from "Dietary Guidelines for Americans 2005" (accessible through www.healthierus.gov/dietaryguidelines). How does your diet measure up to *each* guideline? Look at the dietary guidelines. Do you meet the daily criteria for recommended servings in each food group? Explain! What are two dietary changes you could make that would enhance your nutrition?

Although reflection is usually directed toward individual portfolio items, you should also look at the overall direction of your portfolio. That is the purpose of self-assessment. The Fitness for Life course provides many opportunities to become self-monitoring and to assume responsibility for inspecting your own performance. Self-assessment is built into several items required for the working and final personal growth portfolios, as follows:

1. Food log
2. Physical fitness goals
3. Physical fitness journal
4. Fitness workout schedule
5. Physical activity log
6. Fitness contract

QUESTION 5

What kinds of *conferences* are to be held?

Holding conferences with others is an important aspect of the portfolio process. Conferences offer another kind of self-reflection. They allow you to discuss your fitness progress, look at the status of your fitness goals, and receive feedback about your efforts and achievements. It is expected that you will engage in conferences with peers and family members, records of which are required for the final personal growth portfolio.

Peer Conferences

During the Fitness for Life course, you should hold conferences with two other students, one after the second month and the other after the third month. You should focus on the benchmarks and the items required for the working portfolio. A conference station will be available in the gymnasium for you to conduct the conference. To verify the conferences, ask the people you hold conferences with to complete the peer portfolio conference form that appears on page 231.

Family Conferences

You are expected to share your final personal growth portfolio with two family members, one of which must be a parent or guardian. This will give you a chance to show off and celebrate your achievements. The family portfolio conference guide should be given to the family member to help structure the conference. These forms should be submitted along with your final personal growth portfolio.

From *Professional and Student Portfolios for Physical Education, Second Edition,* by Vincent J. Melograno, 2006, Champaign, IL: Human Kinetics.

221

QUESTION 6

How will the portfolio be *assessed?*

Your teacher will review your working portfolio periodically and provide feedback using self-stick notes so that your original materials are protected. These reviews focus on the eight benchmarks and whether they are complete. Your final personal growth portfolio is evaluated using the portfolio scoring rubric. Criteria are used for evaluating both the *contents* and *quality* of your portfolio. The rating (score) is converted to a letter grade for the whole portfolio. Individual items do not receive separate grades. The grading scale is also shown on the rubric.

From *Professional and Student Portfolios for Physical Education, Second Edition,* by Vincent J. Melograno, 2006, Champaign, IL: Human Kinetics.

Portfolio Item Registry

ADDITIONS			DELETIONS		
Date	Item	Reason	Date	Item	Reason

From *Professional and Student Portfolios for Physical Education, Second Edition,* by Vincent J. Melograno, 2006, Champaign, IL: Human Kinetics.

223

Physical Fitness Profile

Name: _____

Component or test	Pre	Mid	Post
Cardiorespiratory endurance	_____	_____	_____
1-mile walk/run (min/sec)	_____	_____	_____
Muscular strength and endurance			
1-RM bench press (lb)	_____	_____	_____
1-RM standing press (lb)	_____	_____	_____
1-RM curl (lb)	_____	_____	_____
1-RM leg press (lb)	_____	_____	_____
Push-ups (#)	_____	_____	_____
Curl-ups (#)	_____	_____	_____
Modified pull-ups (#)	_____	_____	_____
Flexibility			
Shoulder lift (inches)	_____	_____	_____
Trunk extension (inches)	_____	_____	_____
Sit-and-reach (inches)	_____	_____	_____
Body composition			
Sum of triceps and calf skinfolds (mm)	_____	_____	_____

From *Professional and Student Portfolios for Physical Education, Second Edition*, by Vincent J. Melograno, 2006, Champaign, IL: Human Kinetics.

Food Log

Name: _____ Date: _____

(12:00 a.m. to midnight)

Time of day	Food item	Amount	Calories consumed

Physical Fitness Goals

Name: _____ Date: _____

Component	Pretest	*FITNESSGRAM* standard	REASON FOR GOAL (CHECK ONE)	
			Needs improvement	**Desire to maintain**
Cardiorespiratory endurance (1-mile walk/run)				
	Short-term goal:		Long-term goal:	
	Target date:		Target date:	
Muscular strength and endurance (curl-up)				
	Short-term goal:		Long-term goal:	
	Target date:		Target date:	
Flexibility (sit-and-reach)				
	Short-term goal:		Long-term goal:	
	Target date:		Target date:	
Body composition (sum of skinfolds; % fat)				
	Short-term goal:		Long-term goal:	
	Target date:		Target date:	

Physical Fitness Journal

Name: _____

	I wish I could . . .	I predict that . . .	I feel good about . . .	My fears are . . .
Before my fitness pretests Date: _____				
After my fitness pretests Date: _____				
One month after my fitness program Date: _____				
Two months after my fitness program Date: _____				

Fitness Workout Schedule

Day	Activity	Location	Time of day	Duration	Description of tasks
Example	Warm-up Jogging Cool-down	School track	7:30 a.m.	20 minutes	Jogging program; training level 5; 440-yard distance; 220-yard walk relief; 3 repeats; walk 220 yards
Monday					
Tuesday					
Wednesday					
Thursday					
Friday					
Saturday					
Sunday					

Physical Activity and Leisure Questionnaire

Name: _____ Date: _____

1. Which leisure activities do you engage in on a regular basis? (check all that apply)

   ❑ Playing cards   ❑ Swimming   ❑ Racket sports   ❑ Board games

   ❑ Fishing   ❑ Snow skiing   ❑ Video games   ❑ Camping

   ❑ Water skiing   ❑ Watching TV   ❑ Canoeing   ❑ Hiking

   ❑ Reading   ❑ Horse riding   ❑ Climbing   ❑ Painting

   ❑ Shooting sports   ❑ Rappelling   ❑ Sewing   ❑ Crafts

   ❑ Basketball   ❑ Volleyball   ❑ _____   ❑ _____

   ❑ _____   ❑ _____   ❑ _____   ❑ _____

2. How do you rate the amount of physical activity you perform daily?

   ❑ Very little   ❑ Slightly active   ❑ Moderately active   ❑ Very active

3. On the average (over the past year), how many hours a day have you spent performing the following activities?

   _____ Sitting   _____ Walking   _____ Moderate physical work

   _____ Standing   _____ Light physical work   _____ Heavy physical work

4. Which sports or activities do you engage in on a regular basis? (check all that apply)

   ❑ Golf   ❑ Tennis   ❑ Cycling   ❑ Bowling

   ❑ Soccer   ❑ Basketball   ❑ Archery   ❑ Skiing

   ❑ Hiking   ❑ Volleyball   ❑ Swimming   ❑ Skating

   ❑ Racquetball   ❑ Jogging   ❑ Weight training   ❑ _____

   ❑ _____   ❑ _____   ❑ _____   ❑ _____

5. How often do you exercise for fitness?

   ❑ Daily   ❑ 3-6 times weekly   ❑ Occasionally   ❑ Seldom   ❑ Never

6. How do you rate your cardiorespiratory endurance compared with others of your age and sex?

   ❑ Excellent   ❑ Good   ❑ Average   ❑ Fair   ❑ Poor

7. What can you conclude about your leisure patterns?

   _____
   _____
   _____
   _____

8. What can you conclude about your fitness or exercise patterns?

   _____
   _____
   _____
   _____

From *Professional and Student Portfolios for Physical Education, Second Edition*, by Vincent J. Melograno, 2006, Champaign, IL: Human Kinetics.

229

Physical Activity Log

Name: _____ Date: _____

(12:00 a.m. to midnight)

Time of day	Activity	Location	How long	Calories expended

From *Professional and Student Portfolios for Physical Education, Second Edition,* by Vincent J. Melograno, 2006, Champaign, IL: Human Kinetics.

Peer Portfolio Conference

Portfolio owner: _____

Conference focus: Fitness for Life benchmarks

Instructions to peer: Jot down your impressions or comments from your discussion about the following questions:

1. What aspects of fitness are you proud of? Why?

2. What areas of fitness need your attention? What are you doing about it?

3. What areas of fitness are your biggest challenges?

4. How do you feel about your portfolio?

Peer signature: _____ Date: _____

Family Portfolio Conference Guide

Dear family member:

Please review the personal growth portfolio that _____ completed for the Fitness for Life course. Ask him or her questions about his or her portfolio items and accomplishments. The following questions might help start the discussion. Thank you for your help and cooperation!

1. What did you find out about yourself by developing the Fitness for Life portfolio?

2. What part of your portfolio do you like the most?

3. What surprised you the most in putting your portfolio together?

4. What are you going to do now that you have completed the portfolio?

Please include any comments about the Fitness for Life portfolio or the conference:

_____

_____

_____

_____

_____

_____

Signed: _____   Date: _____

From *Professional and Student Portfolios for Physical Education, Second Edition,* by Vincent J. Melograno, 2006, Champaign, IL: Human Kinetics.

Portfolio Scoring Rubric

Name: _____ Date: _____

Elements	Content		Quality				Subtotal	Weight	Score
	Components of the portfolio system should be verified; required items should be present		*Organization:* Follows directions; clear layout *Form/style:* Visual appeal, writing mechanics; expressiveness *Understanding:* Shows knowledge of fitness components; application of ideas; realistic						
	1 = Included, but incomplete; 2 = Fully developed		1 = Fair 2 = Satisfactory 3 = Good 4 = Outstanding						
Creative cover; table of contents	1	2	1	2	3	4		×1	(6)
Reflection: Health style self-test inventory	1	2	1	2	3	4		×2	(12)
Reflection: Article reviews (4) for different benchmarks	1	2	1	2	3	4		×2	(12)
Reflection: Food and activity logs	1	2	1	2	3	4		×2	(12)
Reflection: Dietary guidelines and food guide pyramid	1	2	1	2	3	4		×2	(12)
Conference records: Peers (2), family members (2)	1	2	1	2	3	4		×2	(12)
Project: New activities ❏ Interviews ❏ Concepts scrapbook ❏	1	2	1	2	3	4		×5	(30)
Fitness for Life program	1	2	1	2	3	4		×6	(36)
Fitness contract	1	2	1	2	3	4		×3	(18)

Comments: _____

_____

Total: _____ (150)

Grade: _____

Scale: A = 135-150,   B = 120-134,   C = 105-119,   D = 90-104,   F = below 89

From *Professional and Student Portfolios for Physical Education, Second Edition,* by Vincent J. Melograno, 2006, Champaign, IL: Human Kinetics.

4

Professional Portfolios for Practicing Teachers

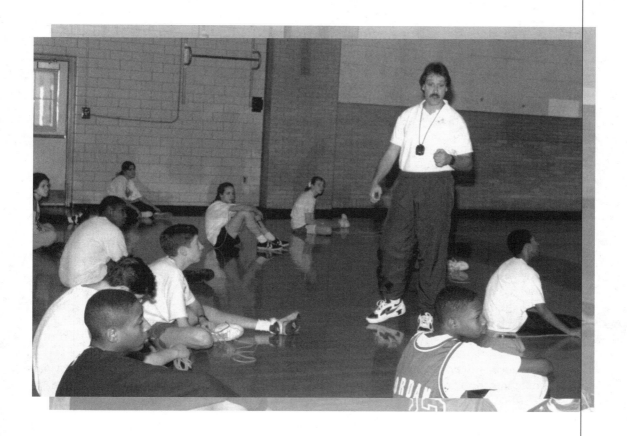

Many believe that the most important way to reform schools is to improve and strengthen the role of teaching. The opinion is that world-class schools cannot exist without world-class teachers. There exists a professional consensus on the aspects of practice that distinguish accomplished teachers. Rigorous standards for what accomplished teachers should know and be able to do have been linked to the ultimate criterion of success—student achievement. Accomplished teachers engage in professional development in pursuit of this criterion. Practicing teachers who effectively enhance student learning and demonstrate high levels of knowledge, skills, dispositions, and commitment need a "symbol" of professional competence. Their outstanding work often goes unrecognized and unrewarded. So, how can teaching excellence best be represented in the real world?

EXPECTED OUTCOMES

This chapter will help practicing teachers in physical education develop professional portfolios. After reading this chapter, you will be able to do the following:

1. Determine the purposes for documenting professional accomplishments.
2. Distinguish among different types of professional portfolios for practicing teachers.
3. Use accepted standards for teaching effectiveness as the organizing framework for professional portfolios.
4. Develop portfolio assembly, management, and storage options including the use of technology.
5. Establish guidelines for collecting and selecting artifacts for the professional portfolio.
6. Create evaluation tools and procedures for judging the worth of the professional portfolio for practicing teachers.

Pursuing teaching goals and charting one's own professional growth are worthy endeavors. Accomplished teachers continually look for ways to improve and bring distinction to their successful practices. The accountability demands that confront teachers suggest the need for a professional development plan for both personal and certification or license renewal. This chapter presents an organizational scheme—the professional portfolio for practicing teachers—that can integrate, interrelate, and communicate the knowledge, skills, and dispositions desirable for teaching effectiveness. Fortunately, there is general agreement on the advanced standards, specific to physical education, that can serve as learning and development targets for practicing teachers. The standards reflect the professional consensus about the essential aspects of accomplished practice.

In this chapter various primary and secondary purposes for documenting professional accomplishments are identified. Then, professional growth and showcase portfolios are described, followed by suggestions for organizing and managing these types of portfolios. Guidelines are also provided for collecting and selecting artifacts. Lastly, some ideas are offered for how teachers can assess their portfolios. To synthesize this information, a sample portfolio system for practicing teachers is presented at the end of the chapter. In addition, the CD-ROM accompanying the book provides a template (portfolio builder) to create an electronic-based professional portfolio for practicing teachers.

Designing an integrated, professional portfolio system for practicing teachers is a complex task involving many decisions. The following seven-step process can help with this task. The steps are also identified throughout the chapter.

1. Determine the primary and secondary purposes of the professional portfolio for practicing teachers.
2. Distinguish between the professional growth and showcase types of portfolios.
3. Use the advanced standards for accomplished teachers as the basis for organizing the professional portfolio.

4. Identify options for organizing, managing, and storing the professional portfolio for practicing teachers.

5. Select the processes of involvement that will be used in developing the professional portfolio.

6. Decide *what, how, who,* and *when* relative to the selection of artifacts for the professional portfolio.

7. Develop feedback procedures that will provide a formative and summative review of the professional portfolio for practicing teachers.

Definition and Purposes

Teacher candidates are primarily focused on satisfying physical education teacher education (PETE) program requirements and certification or licensing standards. Practicing teachers with limited experience are usually focused on adjusting to real-life teaching, meeting any provisional certification or licensing requirements, achieving tenure as soon as reasonable, and seeking graduate coursework leading to a master's degree. Experienced teachers, however, must operate under a different incentive for maintaining effectiveness—personal satisfaction, professional success, and advanced certification or licensure. Therefore, like any other professional occupation, physical education requires a systematic way to determine and recognize excellence.

Professional physical educators possess expert knowledge of the subject field, cope with unique problems, and pursue the interests of their students. These dimensions of professionalism also suggest an ethical standard—the ongoing obligation and commitment to conduct oneself as a model of an educated person. Although the knowledge, skills, dispositions, beliefs, and practices that characterize professional physical education teachers are substantial, they need to be results oriented and verified.

The professional portfolio for practicing teachers is an organized, goal-driven documentation of growth and achieved competence in the complex act of teaching. In deciding whether to engage in such a demanding demonstration of knowledge and skills, teachers face some difficult questions: Why should they involve themselves in the ongoing process of gathering information about their work? How will the portfolios be used? What is the actual intent of this developmental tool? What are the potential uses, overuses, and abuses of portfolios for assessment purposes and beyond? These questions are answered by determining the primary and secondary purposes of the professional portfolio for practicing teachers (step 1 of the portfolio-designing process).

Primary Purpose

Selecting items for a portfolio with no sense of what the portfolio represents is unimaginable. Given the real-world demands on physical education teachers, some solid reasons for spending time and energy on portfolios are needed. To help make this task easier, the professional portfolio should be an adaptable, yet incisive tool that serves multiple purposes. The primary purpose of the portfolio developed by practicing teachers is to verify the wide range of knowledge, skills, and dispositions acquired through teaching experience, professional development, advanced training, and reflection. Together, these competencies define excellence in teaching, or what is often called the "master teacher."

Secondary Purposes

The specific day-to-day purposes of portfolio engagement will vary according to personal preference, the nature of the school setting, school governance, bargaining agreement policies, or all of these. These secondary purposes will likely depend on whether a portfolio review process is voluntary or mandatory. Regardless, the following purposes could be served by a portfolio system, either separately or in combination.

Help Teachers Grow Professionally

Practicing teachers are fully capable of assessing their own progress as teachers. When they review and reflect on their accomplishments, they are involved in a process that fosters lifelong professional advancement. By examining their strengths and weaknesses, teachers can monitor their own growth. They should know from their experiences as teacher candidates and practicing teachers that this cumulative process is just as valuable as the product (e.g., student work samples, student performance scores, instructional videos).

Monitor Goals

By compiling their own professional portfolios, teachers model how to use portfolios. Completed short- and long-term goals can be validated with artifacts. For example, sport education could be a goal for the next semester. Unit plans, lesson plans, performance records, partner checklists, student notebooks, and tournament schedules could be collected to show goal achievement.

Satisfy Evaluation Procedures

Teachers may be required to engage in preconferences and postconferences with their supervisors for evaluative purposes. The professional portfolio could be structured around preestablished criteria (e.g., student achievement levels, positive learning environment, accommodating diversity) as well as those agreed on by the teacher and supervisor during the preconference.

Show Contribution to Educational Mission

It is reasonable to expect teachers to seek to fulfill their school's and program's stated mission. The extent to which a teacher has contributed to this mission can be documented through the portfolio. For example, teachers could collect and rationalize artifacts in support of the following mission: "Through physical education, students will develop into healthy, physically active, socially adjusted, emotionally stable, and intellectually stimulated people by attaining the knowledge, skills, and attitudes and values appropriate to these outcomes."

Track Action Research

Physical educators often engage in site-based "research" in an attempt to systematically and objectively evaluate the outcome of educational activities. For example, a teacher might, following pretests, teach tennis skills using method A in one class and method B in another. The combined test results would then be compared to determine whether the two instructional conditions resulted in a significant difference in student performance. The portfolio could be the vehicle used to organize, assemble, reflect on, and assess this kind of endeavor.

Guide Career Path

Many school districts have implemented "career ladders" or "individual professional development plans" to facilitate advancement within the system. A multiyear portfolio would be a natural way to organize progress along a career path at appropriate intervals.

Enhance New Job Opportunities

The prospects of increased job mobility, new career opportunities, and higher salary are attractive to most teachers. Although the professional portfolio offers no guarantees, it can go a long way in helping teachers build a case for themselves when seeking alternative job placements.

Types of Portfolios

Unlike teacher candidates and students, practicing teachers do not need a wide variety of portfolios. The two types of portfolios recommended here seem adequate—professional growth and showcase portfolios. However, the distinction between them should be clear (step 2 of the portfolio-designing process). They will be covered again in subsequent sections of this chapter that deal with organization and management, selection of artifacts, and assessment. Before the types of portfolios are described, it is necessary to clarify some misconceptions.

- *Working portfolio.* As with teacher candidate portfolios (see chapter 2), the so-called "working portfolio" is not really a portfolio. It is a working repository or holding folder. The work samples systematically collected on an ongoing basis for this working repository come from work products, student-related work samples, videos of teaching, and evidence (exhibits) of school or community activities. This process is a continual "work in progress" and serves as the repository for everything associated with the advanced standards for accomplished teachers. The collection of artifacts and work products forms the framework for reflection, self-assessment, and goal setting, and it provides all possible artifacts from which to make selections for the other types of portfolios. The *working repository*—the term that has been used throughout this book—is managed and kept by the practicing teacher. It can also provide a basis for monitoring goals, teaching evaluations, certification or licensure renewal, or advanced national certification.

- *Electronic portfolio.* Another misconception is represented by the terms *electronic portfolio* or *e-portfolio.* All types of portfolios can be constructed, managed, and stored electronically, including on the Internet. For this reason, "electronic portfolios" are not included as a type of portfolio. Technological advances have made electronic management, storage, and portfolio-related processes a reality. However, if portfolios are simply software databases—storage for pictures, sound, or words—they are really no different from hanging files or containers. The content of portfolios and the process of creating them are the most important concerns. Multimedia writing tools, scanners, digital cameras, and recordable CD-ROM drives have all helped in creating true portfolios. Self-reflection, data sharing, and assessment can be built in. Electronic and Web-based information and guidelines for constructing, managing, and storing portfolios are covered later in this chapter (pages 240-247).

Professional Growth Portfolio

The ongoing, systematic collection of teacher artifacts and related student work samples that constitutes the professional growth portfolio should occur on a weekly basis or, preferably, as part of a daily routine. The overall collection forms the framework for goal setting and reflection by exhibiting professional growth over time. It also provides a basis for review by colleagues and self-appraisal at planned intervals during a given school year or teaching career, facilitating assessment of a formative nature. The professional growth portfolio for a K-3 physical education program might focus on the following abilities:

- Engage students in sequenced, integrated motor skill instruction across grade levels
- Promote student understanding of developmentally appropriate cognitive concepts and principles of movement
- Involve students in classroom-level, formative assessment to promote achievement of all students
- Use the results of assessment to inform instructional decision making and to make judgments about program effects
- Engage students in purposeful instruction that supports equitable access to learning and promotes student interaction and reflection
- Promote physical activity across the life span and raise students' awareness of the value of physical activity and healthful living
- Show the impact of student achievement through collaboration with families and the community

Showcase Portfolio

The showcase portfolio can be customized to provide a professional overview of the personality and abilities of the practicing physical education teacher. A limited number of artifacts is selected to serve a particular purpose. For example, although showcase portfolios used for supervisor evaluation, certification or license renewal, goal monitoring, or job enhancement would be different in terms of content, they would all, nonetheless, "showcase" particular aspects of the teacher's competence. They would also offer a basis for summative assessment.

Organization and Management

Once practicing teachers decide on the purposes of their professional portfolio, they need to choose an organizational scheme that is clear and meaningful to other professionals. A plan should also be developed for handling the logistics of the portfolio process. The following section describes a set of teacher standards that can be used as the basis for organizing the professional portfolio. Some management techniques are provided that might help in constructing, managing, and storing the portfolio, as is a discussion of the use of technology. In addition, some processes for involvement are suggested to facilitate the development of a high-quality portfolio.

Focus on Standards

In many instances, the purpose of the professional portfolio will dictate its organizational scheme. For example, if the purpose is to monitor goals, then the actual short- and long-term goals become the organizing center. To satisfy teacher evaluation procedures, the portfolio would be organized around preestablished performance criteria. The portfolio would be organized

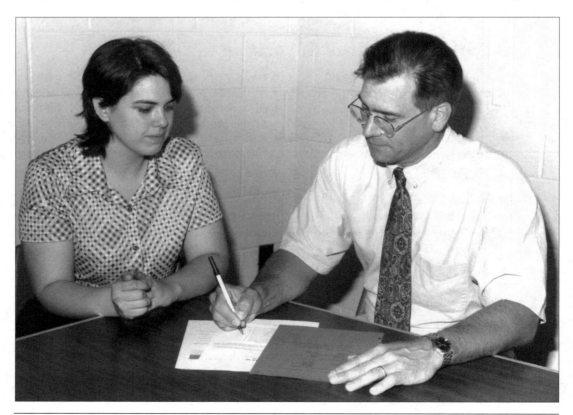

The showcase portfolio is useful for the assessment conference.

around the elements of a mission statement if teachers were showing their contributions to that mission. In general, however, a universal set of standards around which to organize professional portfolios—one that could be used across disciplines and grade levels—would be practical. Fortunately, some relatively clear standards for proficient teaching exist that incorporate the essential knowledge, skills, and dispositions that allow teachers to practice at a high level, thus advancing student achievement.

Because they represent a professional consensus on the aspects of practice that distinguish accomplished teachers, the core propositions and supporting standards of the National Board for Professional Teaching Standards (1999) are recommended as the organizing framework for professional portfolios (step 3 of the portfolio-designing process). The origin of the NBPTS was described in chapter 1, and the five core propositions and supporting standards were identified in table 1.3.

The artifacts selected should provide tangible evidence that each proposition has been met. Collectively, the propositions cover a broad set of teacher competencies: (1) knowledge of the subject to be taught, skills to be developed, and curricular materials that organize the content, (2) knowledge of general and content-specific strategies for teaching and evaluating, (3) knowledge of human development, (4) skills in effectively teaching students from diverse backgrounds, and (5) dispositions to use such knowledge and skills in the best interest of students. They will also be used in subsequent sections of this chapter that deal with item selection and assessment.

The five core propositions were translated into a set of advanced standards for physical education teachers of students ages 3 to 18+. In addition, two National Board Certifications for physical education teachers were created covering the following age ranges: early and middle childhood physical education (student ages 3-12) and early adolescence through young adulthood physical education (student ages 11-18+). The physical education standards describe in observable form what accomplished teachers should know and be able to do, and they support the certification review and assessment process (NBPTS, 2001). The 13 physical education standards, as described in table 4.1, are also recommended to facilitate the organization of professional portfolios for practicing teachers.

Another benefit to using the NBPTS physical education standards is that a teacher who applies for National Board Certification must satisfy comprehensive assessment requirements including a school-site portfolio reflecting various facets of teaching. The portfolio must contain written commentaries describing the teaching and learning in the teacher's classroom, videotapes of interactions with students, and samples of student work with the teacher's written comments. The assessments are designed to evaluate the complex knowledge and teaching behaviors described by the standards (NBPTS, 2004). Additional information is accessible through the NBPTS Web site at www.npbts.org.

Management Techniques

The practicing teacher must assume responsibility for assembling, managing, storing, and updating the professional portfolio throughout the process (step 4 of portfolio-designing process). Decisions about the method of construction, when to "manage" portfolios, how and where to store portfolios, and how to get feedback depend on the purpose and type of portfolio. Although there are many ways to assemble portfolios, some suggestions are provided to handle these logistics. Consideration is given to both the working repository and the professional growth and showcase portfolios.

Organizing Tools

Even experienced teachers may not be good at organizing all of what they collect. They may have a good collection of artifacts, but could use some tools to help manage the loose ends.

- *Dividers.* Whatever kind of container is used, divided notebook folders or divider pages can be used to separate artifacts according to the professional standards or any other category that makes sense (e.g., goals, criteria, program mission statements). A filing system should be created so that the standards are easily identified. Each section could be labeled with a shortened version of the standard.

Table 4.1 Standards of Accomplished Practice for Physical Education Teachers

Standard	Description
1. Knowledge of students	Accomplished physical education teachers use their knowledge of students to make every student feel important. They communicate through a humane, sensitive approach that each child, regardless of ability, can succeed and will benefit from a physically active, healthy lifestyle.
2. Knowledge of subject matter	Accomplished physical education teachers have a deep and broad understanding of the content and principles of physical education, which enables them to devise sound and developmentally appropriate instructional activities.
3. Sound teaching practices	Accomplished physical education teachers possess a thorough comprehension of the fundamentals of physical education and a broad grasp of relevant principles and theories that give their teaching purpose and guide them as they carry out a flexible, yet effective, instructional program responsive to students' needs and developmental levels.
4. Student engagement in learning	Through their own passion for teaching and their personal example, accomplished physical education teachers inspire their students to learn and to participate in and appreciate physical education.
5. High expectations for learners	Accomplished physical education teachers tenaciously maintain a stimulating, productive setting that encourages participation, discovery, goal setting, and cooperation and that holds all students to the highest expectations.
6. Learning environment	Accomplished teachers of physical education create and sustain a welcoming, safe, and challenging environment in which students engage in and enjoy physical activity. They establish an orderly atmosphere with established protocols and expectations conducive to providing maximum learning for all students.
7. Curricular choices	Accomplished physical education teachers select, plan, and evaluate curriculum in a continuous process meant to ensure a sensible, properly structured, positive physical education program that meets students' needs and results in student learning.
8. Assessment	Accomplished physical education teachers design assessment strategies appropriate to the curriculum and to the learner. They use assessment results to provide feedback to the learner, to report student progress, and to shape instruction.
9. Equity, fairness, and diversity	Accomplished physical education teachers model and promote behavior appropriate in a diverse society by showing respect for and valuing all members of their communities and by having high expectations that their students will treat one another fairly and with dignity.
10. Reflective practice and professional growth	Accomplished physical education teachers participate in a wide range of reflective practices that foster their creativity, stimulate personal growth, contribute to content knowledge and classroom skill, and enhance professionalism.
11. Promoting an active lifestyle	Accomplished physical education teachers recognize the multiple benefits of a physically active lifestyle and promote purposeful daily activities for all students that will encourage them to become lifelong adherents of physical activity.
12. Collaboration with colleagues	Accomplished physical education teachers do not work in isolation but function as members of a large learning community. Recognizing that their responsibilities extend beyond their own classrooms, they contribute purposely to enhancing instructional programs and improving the professional culture of their field.
13. Family and community partnerships	Accomplished physical education teachers create advocates for physical education by providing opportunities for family involvement and the involvement of the broader community in the physical education program.

- *Color codes.* To facilitate management, colored dots or colored files could be used to code entries in the portfolio. Artifacts could also be coded using different color markers. A code for the colors needs to be included.

- *Artifact registry.* A sheet could be maintained for each standard on which practicing teachers could record the date, item, and reason for either adding or deleting an item. Because the registry is supposed to chronicle when and why items are removed or replaced, teachers engage in a dynamic form of reflection. An artifact registry form is shown on page 242.

- *Work log.* A biography of work could show the evolution of a long-term project such as a portfolio. This would help in making necessary changes or shifting directions. The log could be as simple as a dated entry that traces all activities and decisions associated with the portfolio.

- *Index.* An alphabetical index of items could be compiled as the portfolio evolves. Such an organizational tool would help in the cross-referencing of artifacts that represent more than one standard, and vice versa. The index could be placed in the front of the portfolio like a table of contents.

- *Self-stick notes.* Artifacts need to be cataloged so ideas are not lost over time. A self-stick note or index card could be attached to each artifact to identify the standard. The card could contain a brief statement explaining why it was collected. Specific descriptors from the standard statement may help later in connecting the artifact to the standard. Using a self-stick note or index card also protects original works.

Storage Options

The actual container for collecting artifacts is a matter of personal preference. Some options include notebooks, expanding and accordion files, hanging files, large file box, folders, satchels, pockets for electronic documents, a large notebook divided into sections, and file drawers in a cabinet. The working repository may require considerable space because it stores all materials connected to teaching and learning. Items for the professional growth and showcase portfolios would be drawn from this collection. Because the showcase portfolio is a more concise representation of accomplishments (e.g., goals achieved, criteria met, professional standards), the number of items is limited. Thus, an accordion file or satchel is all that may be needed depending on who is going to review the portfolio (e.g., supervisor, certification or licensing renewal committee, prospective employer). Ultimately, materials can be scanned for storage on computer disks or stored on computer internal hard drives. Refer to chapter 1 for additional information about the use of technology for storage.

Use of Technology

The section in chapter 1 titled Technology Use in Portfolio Development should be referenced (pages 31-47). The information about hardware, storage, and software has general applicability to developing electronic-based professional portfolios for practicing teachers. Because electronic-based portfolios are an extension of paper-based portfolios, the information in this chapter on organization and management is also applicable (pages 241-243). However, some additional information is important to the development of portfolios for practicing physical education teachers.

Technology Standards

The national educational technology standards for teachers (NETS-T) developed by the International Society for Technology in Education (ISTE) consist of competencies standards and corresponding performance indicators that practicing teachers should know and be able to do (ISTE, 2002). The standards and corresponding performance indicators are identified in table 4.2 (see page 245). In addition, the National Board for Professional Teaching Standards includes technology competence and understanding in its standards (NBPTS, 1999, 2001). Practicing teachers who create an electronic-based or Web-based professional portfolio instead of a paper-based portfolio can demonstrate competency related to these sets of standards simultaneously.

Artifact Registry

Standard/goal/purpose: _____

Add	Delete	Date	Item	Reasons

From *Professional and Student Portfolios for Physical Education, Second Edition,* by Vincent J. Melograno, 2006, Champaign, IL: Human Kinetics.

Table 4.2   Educational Technology Standards and Performance Indicators for Teachers

Standards	Performance indicators
Standard I: Technology operations and concepts Teachers demonstrate a sound understanding of technology operations and concepts.	Teachers: • demonstrate introductory knowledge, skills, and understanding of concepts related to technology. • demonstrate continual growth in technology knowledge and skills to stay abreast of current and emerging technologies.
Standard II: Planning and designing learning environments and experiences Teachers plan and design effective learning environments and experiences supported by technology.	Teachers: • design developmentally appropriate learning opportunities that apply technology-enhanced instructional strategies to support the diverse needs of learners. • apply current research on teaching and learning with technology when planning learning environments and experiences. • identify and locate technology resources and evaluate them for accuracy and suitability. • plan for the management of technology resources within the context of learning activities. • plan strategies to manage student learning in a technology-enhanced environment.
Standard III: Teaching, learning, and the curriculum Teachers implement curriculum plans that include methods and strategies for applying technology to maximize student learning.	Teachers: • facilitate technology-enhanced experiences that address content standards and student technology standards. • use technology to support learner-centered strategies that address the diverse needs of students. • apply technology to develop students' higher order skills and creativity. • manage student learning activities in a technology-enhanced environment.
Standard IV: Assessment and evaluation Teachers apply technology to facilitate a variety of effective assessment and evaluation strategies.	Teachers: • apply technology in assessing student learning of subject matter using a variety of assessment techniques. • use technology resources to collect and analyze data, interpret results, and communicate findings to improve instructional practice and maximize student learning. • apply multiple methods of evaluation to determine students' appropriate use of technology resources for learning, communication, and productivity.
Standard V: Productivity and professional practice Teachers use technology to enhance their productivity and professional practice.	Teachers: • use technology resources to engage in ongoing professional development and lifelong learning. • continually evaluate and reflect on professional practice to make informed decisions regarding the use of technology in support of student learning. • apply technology to increase productivity. • use technology to communicate and collaborate with peers, parents, and the larger community in order to nurture student learning.
Standard VI: Social, ethical, legal, and human issues Teachers understand the social, ethical, legal, and human issues surrounding the use of technology in PK-12 schools and apply those principles in practice.	Teachers: • model and teach legal and ethical practice related to technology use. • apply technology resources to enable and empower learners with diverse backgrounds, characteristics, and abilities. • identify and use technology resources that affirm diversity. • promote safe and healthy use of technology resources. • facilitate equitable access to technology resources for all students.

Reprinted with permission from *National Educational Technology Standards for Teachers: Preparing Teachers to Use Technology,* copyright © 2002, ISTE (International Society for Technology in Education), iste@iste.org, www.iste.org. All rights reserved.

Portfolio Management

Practicing teachers develop their professional portfolios whenever possible at work or at home. Teachers either store their electronic-based portfolios on a CD, USB drive, or the internal hard drive on their own computer. Teachers are responsible for backing up their electronic-based portfolio so that if the original is damaged, another copy is available. Some K-12 schools are networked and teachers are assigned storage space on the network. In this case, teachers can store their electronic-based portfolio on the school network. Sometimes this network is accessible from outside the school, making it very convenient for teachers to work on their electronic-based portfolios at anytime from anywhere. If the teacher cannot access the network from home, then working off a USB drive is suggested with backup onto the school network for safety. Practicing teachers can also develop Web-based portfolios much like the ones described for teacher candidates (page 68). The availability of the resources needed in terms of hardware and software will obviously vary from school to school and from person to person.

Processes for Involvement

Whether the portfolio is used to demonstrate professional growth or to showcase specific accomplishments, there are other considerations in developing a high-quality portfolio. Certain processes for involvement should be built into the system including reflection, self-assessment, and conferences (step 5 of the portfolio-designing process).

Reflection

Artifacts collected for the working repository should be thoughtfully examined and labeled to reveal their meaning and value to the entire portfolio. At the very least, practicing teachers will

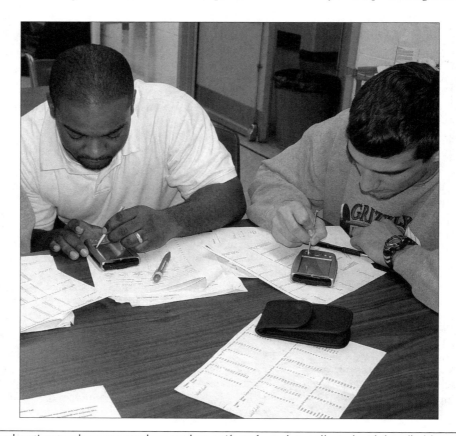

Physical education teachers can produce student artifacts from data collected with handheld computers.

avoid having to determine later why they collected particular items. Through the process of reflection, teachers can determine why they collected artifacts for particular standards, goals, or purposes. The reflection, which can be brief, should not summarize the artifact. It should state what the artifact is; why it fits the standard, goal, or purpose; and what it says about the teacher's competence. A sample reflection cover sheet appears on page 248. These reflection sheets can remain with those items selected for the showcase portfolio.

Self-Assessment

In addition to reflecting on individual items, practicing teachers should review the entire collection of artifacts with reference to short- and long-term goals or how the portfolio covers the professional standards. The process of self-assessment is usually an informal self-check to determine what is not well documented by artifacts. The teacher should become a "collector" in looking for ways to document a goal or standard that is incompletely documented. Teachers should keep these missing areas in mind as they complete professional activities (e.g., school or community projects, student exhibits, teacher-made materials, seminars, personal growth conferences, unit plans). The artifacts self-assessment checklist shown on pages 249-250 can be used to identify professional standards that are well documented (Good), standards that are satisfactorily evidenced (OK), and standards for which goals and artifacts are needed along with a target completion date (Artifacts needed). Review of the professional growth and showcase portfolios will be covered in the subsequent section of this chapter that deals with assessment.

Conferences With Colleagues

An independent, neutral review of one's portfolio is almost always worthwhile. Receiving feedback while organizing and managing the portfolio can be invaluable. It is reasonable to assume that more and more experienced physical educators and other school personnel will be involved in professional portfolios. As a result, opportunities for meaningful dialogue are expanded. Conferencing with colleagues offers an excellent chance for feedback about the portfolio. In addition, these professional connections should foster relationships with colleagues and a collaborative environment. When planning a conference, the following questions should be answered: What are the goals of the conference? What reflections are needed? What questions should be prepared for the conference? When will it be held? At the conference, the following basic questions could be asked: What have you learned about yourself? What aspects of the portfolio are you particularly proud of? If you could publish one thing in your portfolio, what would it be and why? What aspects of your teaching need some attention? How do you plan to deal with these needs?

Item Selection

Ultimately, decisions must be made about what to include in the professional portfolio and what to exclude from it (step 6 of the portfolio-designing process). The selection process is related closely to the type of portfolio. Even for the working repository, criteria should be predetermined or formalized to avoid an overabundance of artifacts. The purposes of the professional growth and showcase portfolios dictate the selection of specific items. The process of selection answers several important questions: *What* items should be included? *How* will the items be selected? *Who* will select these items? *When* will these items be selected?

Most artifacts will be derived from school and community activities, professional development experiences, teacher-made materials, curriculum plans including units and lesson plans, and student work products. The practicing teacher must decide what is essential to the types of professional portfolios in accordance with their purposes. Consideration should always be given to the professional teacher standards when making selection decisions.

Reflection Cover Sheet

Name: _____ Date: _____

Standard/goal/purpose: _____

Name of artifact: _____

Source: _____

Rationale statement: _____

_____

_____

_____

_____

_____

_____

_____

_____

_____

_____

_____

_____

_____

_____

_____

_____

Artifacts Self-Assessment Checklist

Name: _____ Date: _____

Core proposition	Standard	Good	OK	Artifacts needed
1. Teachers are committed to students and their learning.	(a) Recognize individual differences in students and adjust practice accordingly			Goal: Target date:
	(b) Understand how students develop and learn			Goal: Target date:
	(c) Treat students equitably			Goal: Target date
	(d) Extend mission beyond developing the [psychomotor] capacity of students			Goal: Target date:
2. Teachers know the subjects they teach and how to teach those subjects to students.	(a) Appreciate how knowledge in subjects is created, organized, and linked to other disciplines			Goal: Target date:
	(b) Command specialized knowledge of how to convey subject to students			Goal: Target date:
	(c) Generate multiple paths to [learning]			Goal: Target date:
3. Teachers are responsible for managing and monitoring student learning.	(a) Call on multiple methods to meet goals			Goal: Target date:
	(b) Orchestrate learning in group settings			Goal: Target date:

(continued)

Core proposition	Standard	Good	OK	Artifacts needed
3. Teachers are responsible for managing and monitoring student learning. *(continued)*	(c) Place a premium on student engagement			Goal: Target date:
	(d) Regularly assess student progress			Goal: Target date:
	(e) Are mindful of principal objectives			Goal: Target date:
4. Teachers think systematically about their practice and learn from experience.	(a) Are continually making difficult choices that test judgment			Goal: Target date:
	(b) Seek advice of others and draw on education research and scholarship to improve practice			Goal: Target date:
5. Teachers are members of learning communities.	(a) Contribute to school effectiveness by collaborating with other professionals			Goal: Target date:
	(b) Work collaboratively with parents			Goal: Target date:
	(c) Take advantage of community resources			Goal: Target date:

From *Professional and Student Portfolios for Physical Education, Second Edition*, by Vincent J. Melograno, 2006, Champaign, IL: Human Kinetics.

Artifact Possibilities

A wide range of artifacts can be selected for the working repository. Many artifacts may be selected for one or more of the different kinds of showcase portfolios. The artifact possibilities briefly explained here show the range of options that exists, but this list does not include all the possibilities. In fact, experienced physical educators will probably have numerous alternative artifacts from which to select.

- *Philosophy statement:* A position paper or statement of philosophy about teaching or physical education; includes underlying beliefs about practices in physical education that enhance student learning.

- *Goals statement:* The perception of one's role as a physical education teacher; provides information about the direction one wants to take professionally and the means for getting there; includes list of accomplishments in relation to goals.

- *Videotapes or video clips of teaching:* Recordings of actual teaching episodes; document management and motivation techniques, communication modes, accommodation of diverse students, alternative teaching strategies, and student assessment procedures.

- *Teacher-made instructional materials:* Custom-made teaching aids; include multimedia projects, transparencies, charts, posters, videotapes, games, and equipment; show creativity in planning and teaching; photographs of materials may be necessary.

- *Lesson plans:* Document instructional planning and use of multiple methods; components include goals, objectives, student activities, teaching strategies, resources, time schedules, and evaluation standards and procedures.

- *Unit plans:* Comprehensive plans for instruction on specific content areas covering several days or weeks; include organizing centers, content goals, learning objectives, content outlines, learning activities, evaluation methods, and resources.

- *Integrated units:* Units in which physical education is integrated with other subjects; might include health, art, music, science, math, social studies, and language arts; include lesson plans or resource materials that fit a central theme (e.g., science of movement, Greek mythology, measuring human performance); show how physical education contributes to the overall theme.

- *Technology resources:* Samples of materials representing how state-of-the-art technology is incorporated into physical education (e.g., e-mail, electronic bulletin boards, information databases, interactive video); include computer software used or incorporated into teaching (e.g., computer-assisted instruction, HyperStudio, digitized video).

- *Student works:* Samples of student products or exhibits generated in physical education, including individual and class portfolios, learning contracts, projects, and performance evaluations; show a range of learning experiences based on diagnostic review.

- *Case studies:* In-depth analyses of anonymous students' development in physical education over certain time periods; show an understanding of growth and development and an ability to maintain student learning.

- *Community and extracurricular involvement:* Interactions with students, parents or guardians, school personnel, and community members that maintain positive school–community collaboration; includes volunteer experiences and services and responsibilities with clubs, intramurals, and interscholastic athletics.

- *Professional growth activities:* Lists and descriptions of seminars, in-service training, or personal conferences attended; participation in professional organizations and committees; and coursework completed.

- *Professional readings:* Written reactions to issues and concepts covered in a list of professional readings; includes article summaries and critiques and subscriptions to professional publications.

- *Awards, honors, and commendations:* Documents (e.g., letters, certificates) that verify outstanding contributions to the field of education or physical education; include community, professional, and volunteer recognition.

- *Letters:* Written statements from students, parents or guardians, school personnel, and community members in support of teaching practices; reference should be made to professional commitment and responsibility along with comments about professional practice.

- *Photographs:* Document teacher competence and accomplishments that cannot be physically included in a portfolio; show active learning, special events and projects, bulletin boards, learning centers, and movement exhibitions.

- *Logs and journals:* Highlight professional activities and identify professional problems, how the problem was dealt with, the strategy chosen to solve the problem, and the results of implementing the problem-solving strategy; document instructional strategies, management and motivation skills, and collaboration with family and community.

- *Reflections and self-assessments:* Thoughtful examinations of artifacts contained in the professional portfolio (reflection) and a review of the entire collection of artifacts in reference to short- and long-term goals (self-assessment).

Although the working repository is an all-inclusive documentation of teaching competence, it is assembled primarily for personal use as the sum of artifacts. The showcase portfolio, however, should be streamlined and targeted. Depending on its purpose, other kinds of items may be essential, such as the following:

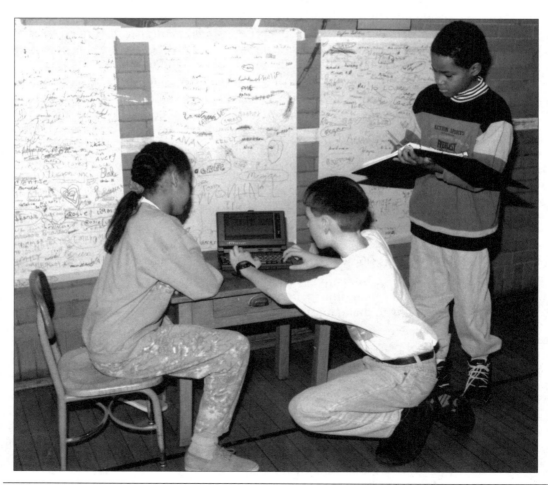

Computer-assisted instruction can be documented in the professional portfolio.

- Cover letter (i.e., introduce self; describe some pertinent experiences; point out areas of portfolio that are exemplary; justify job candidacy, if appropriate)
- Creative cover
- Table of contents or index
- Biographical sketch
- Resume
- Certification or licensing documents (e.g., copy of certificate, transcripts)
- Letters of recommendation
- List of relevant courses (i.e., title, credits, grade, professional standard to which course relates)

Link to Professional Standards

The applicability of the general teacher standards for experienced and accomplished teachers to physical educators can be established through the professional portfolio. Therefore, strong consideration should be given to the link between the standards and the artifacts selected to represent these standards. A broad array of artifacts should be selected for the working repository to facilitate the task of selecting a more limited number of items for the professional growth and showcase portfolios. The greater the variety of representative artifacts, the easier it should be to serve the purposes of these portfolios (e.g., show professional growth, satisfy goals, meet evaluation criteria, qualify for a new job). Table 4.3 links artifacts in physical education with professional standards (NBPTS, 1999). Possible artifacts are indicated for each standard. Many of these possibilities can also be connected to the specific physical education standards identified previously in table 4.1 (page 242).

Assessment

To be thorough in assessing their competence, practicing teachers will need to communicate their accomplishments to others and receive assessment feedback (step 7 of the portfolio-designing process). The contents of the showcase portfolio should undergo continual review. This does not include the built-in review by a supervisor for evaluation purposes or by a prospective employer when seeking a new job. Rather, review in this context refers to feedback during the progressive stages of portfolio development and refinement. Periodic reviews are not only essential, but also natural to a professional portfolio system and a career development plan.

The professional portfolio is an assessment tool itself. The individual artifacts and the entire portfolio should be reviewed according to established purposes. Criteria should focus on the portfolio's content and quality. The two primary sources of assessment feedback are colleagues and self.

Colleague Feedback

A common practice among professional educators is to share ideas or materials and to solicit informal opinions about them. This approach would likely be the most practical way to handle individual artifacts for the working repository. For the professional growth and showcase portfolios, however, a more structured approach is recommended.

Several feedback and assessment constructs can be used, including reflection, conferences, and performance assessment. Each is described here with techniques for providing feedback and assessment data to practicing teachers. Colleagues who provide such reviews should be experienced, trustworthy, and willing to offer objective, constructive feedback. In addition, for illustrative purposes, the teacher standards outlined in the previous chapter section should serve as the basis for these reviews.

Table 4.3 Teacher Standards and Physical Education Artifacts

Supporting standards	Possible artifacts
CORE PROPOSITION 1: TEACHERS ARE COMMITTED TO STUDENTS AND THEIR LEARNING.	
(a) Teachers recognize individual differences in their students and adjust their practice accordingly.	Reflective journal describing accommodations and response to self-control strategies for five students with mild behavior disabilities in a sport education teaching unit
(b) Teachers have an understanding of how students develop and learn.	Project for a graduate course titled How Children Learn Motor Skills showing how principles and concepts are applied to an elementary physical education program
(c) Teachers treat students equitably.	Case studies showing development in physical education for a student of cultural origin different from most members of a class, a student at risk, and a student who is gifted and talented
(d) Teachers' mission extends beyond developing the [psychomotor] capacity of their students.	Observational checklists for determining students' tendencies toward self-responsibility, respect for others, sense of fair play, and higher-order thinking in movement awareness activities
CORE PROPOSITION 2: TEACHERS KNOW THE SUBJECTS THEY TEACH AND HOW TO TEACH THOSE SUBJECTS TO STUDENTS.	
(a) Teachers appreciate how knowledge in their subjects is created, organized, and linked to other disciplines.	Integrated unit plan with language arts and speech titled Communicating Through Movement
(b) Teachers command specialized knowledge of how to convey a subject to students.	Self-appraisal worksheets and inventories for health-related components of fitness (i.e., cardiorespiratory endurance, muscular strength and endurance, flexibility, body composition)
(c) Teachers generate multiple paths to [learning].	Videotape of series of teaching episodes in which a variety of instructional strategies is used (e.g., problem solving, simulations, self-check, reciprocal)
CORE PROPOSITION 3: TEACHERS ARE RESPONSIBLE FOR MANAGING AND MONITORING STUDENT LEARNING.	
(a) Teachers call on multiple methods to meet their goals.	Student portfolio work samples representing different intelligences (e.g., linguistic, mathematical, kinesthetic, spatial, personal, musical) for a six-week unit on Creative Use of Leisure Time
(b) Teachers orchestrate learning in group settings.	Guidelines for group work at fitness stations, participation in team drills, and role playing a sensitive problem (e.g., mocking others' ability, respecting officiating calls of opponent)
(c) Teachers place a premium on student engagement.	Floor plans and setups for gymnasium and outdoor space showing arrangement of equipment and materials and locations of students that maximize active learning
(d) Teachers regularly assess student progress.	Scoring rubrics for a set of sequential lessons on manipulative skills (e.g., dribbling, kicking, throwing, catching, volleying, striking)
(e) Teachers are mindful of their principal objectives.	Lesson plans that link explicit learning objectives with specific student activities and performance standards

Supporting standards	Possible artifacts
CORE PROPOSITION 4: TEACHERS THINK SYSTEMATICALLY ABOUT THEIR PRACTICE AND LEARN FROM EXPERIENCE.	
(a) Teachers are continually making difficult choices that test their judgment.	Descriptions of how the rules and strategies of traditional games (e.g., soccer, volleyball, basketball) are modified to encourage greater participation and teamwork
(b) Teachers seek the advice of others and draw on education research and scholarship to improve their practice.	Annotated bibliography of the principles and applications of "cooperative learning" specific to physical education instruction at the middle school level
CORE PROPOSITION 5: TEACHERS ARE MEMBERS OF LEARNING COMMUNITIES.	
(a) Teachers contribute to school effectiveness by collaborating with other professionals.	Individualized education plans (IEPs) showing the motor development component for a group of students with learning disabilities
(b) Teachers work collaboratively with parents.	Reflection sheet for use by parents and guardians to review and comment on a videotape of a choreographed dance routine
(c) Teachers take advantage of community resources.	Photographs from an elective course conducted at a local state park titled Outdoor Pursuits (e.g., camping, backpacking, hiking, orienteering, cross-country skiing)

Reflection

Because other practicing teachers may be involved in their own professional growth plans or portfolio development, they are qualified to review the work of physical education teachers and provide feedback. Self-reflection was described previously on page 246 as a technique to help manage the portfolio. In a similar manner, reflection by colleagues serves as a cross-check. Colleagues should be asked to (1) offer constructive or encouraging words, (2) disagree with an idea rather than the teacher, and (3) assess the quality of work based on the established standards. The sample colleague reflection sheet that appears on page 256 could be used for this purpose.

Conferences

As mentioned previously , another way to connect with professional colleagues is at a conference using the portfolio as the basis for discussion. The conference could be planned as a general process that answers questions such as, What have you learned about yourself by putting together a professional portfolio? What artifacts are particularly meaningful and why? What areas of your teaching performance need further improvement?

Conferences at this level are meant to be somewhat judgmental. The focus should be on the teacher standards and how artifacts in the portfolio document accomplishments and professional competence related to the standards. Direct personal communication is a legitimate form of assessment if structured properly. Conferences could compare the practicing teacher's perceptions and the colleague's opinion regarding (1) the person's overall strength as a physical education teacher, (2) artifacts that represent "holistic" abilities and dispositions toward teaching, (3) how the portfolio verifies that the professional teacher standards have been met, and (4) what standards need further justification as revealed by the portfolio. Colleagues could focus their feedback around answers to the following reflective stems:

- The part of the portfolio I like best is _____ because . . .
- The part I'm not really clear about is _____ because . . .
- The part you need to tell me more about is . . .
- You could improve your portfolio by . . .
- My overall impression is . . .

Colleague Reflection Sheet

Date: _____

To: _____

From: _____

Please review the items contained in my professional portfolio and provide feedback. Thanks!

1. Which teaching standard is documented the most effectively? Why?

2. What teaching standard is documented the least effectively? Why?

3. What artifacts really made an impression on you? Why?

4. What artifacts do you feel need the most work? Why?

5. What is your overall impression of the organization and presentation of artifacts?

Signed: _____ Date: _____

From *Professional and Student Portfolios for Physical Education, Second Edition,* by Vincent J. Melograno, 2006, Champaign, IL: Human Kinetics.

Performance Assessment

Some physical educators may not feel comfortable asking colleagues to render a more formal rating of their portfolio. Likewise, some colleagues may feel uncomfortable giving one. However, a truly professional relationship should allow such an activity without any repercussions. The showcase portfolio represents the most concise view of the practicing teacher's professional competence. Its assessment should consider the generic teacher standards and general criteria such as organization, form and quality, and evidence of understanding. Colleagues can use the portfolio rating form on pages 258-259.

Self-Analysis

The sample checklist on pages 249-250 for reviewing the teacher standards represents an informal self-check of the entire collection of items. The checklist offers a good way to determine the status of the working repository and to establish goals for standards that are missing documentation. In addition, teachers should analyze the working repository to determine whether there is a need to diversify the different kinds of artifacts. For example, the teacher may have relied too heavily on curriculum units to represent many standards. The artifacts analysis chart on page 260 can be used for this purpose. Check marks, dates, or both could be entered to record the range of artifacts in support of the five core propositions and 17 supporting standards.

For the showcase portfolio, any self-assessment scheme should incorporate explicit content and quality criteria. Because the showcase portfolio is a professional profile, it should receive careful scrutiny. Practicing physical education teachers can use the showcase portfolio rating form on page 261 to assess their own showcase portfolios. The list of portfolio contents would vary depending on the purpose of the portfolio.

Summary

Have you achieved the expected outcomes (see page 236) for this chapter? You should have acquired the knowledge and skills needed for developing professional portfolios for practicing teachers in physical education. The professional portfolio is an authentic way for practicing physical education teachers to document their competence and accomplishments. Developing and implementing a portfolio system includes the following steps:

1. Determine the primary and secondary purposes of the professional portfolio for practicing teachers.
2. Distinguish between the professional growth and showcase types of portfolios.
3. Use the advanced standards for accomplished teachers as the basis for organizing the professional portfolio.
4. Identify options for organizing, managing, and storing the professional portfolio for practicing teachers.
5. Select the processes of involvement that will be used in developing the professional portfolio.
6. Decide *what, how, who,* and *when* relative to the selection of artifacts for the professional portfolio.
7. Develop feedback procedures that will provide a formative and summative review of the professional portfolio for practicing teachers.

The professional portfolio provides a way for practicing physical education teachers to recognize their achieved competence. Through the professional growth and showcase portfolios, accomplished teachers can document their knowledge, skills, dispositions, beliefs, and practices. The showcase portfolio can be used to satisfy assessment procedures, monitor goals, guide career paths,

Portfolio Rating Form

Name: _____ Date: _____

Instructions: Use the following scale to rate each portfolio item according to the following criteria.

4 = Outstanding   3 = Good   2 = Satisfactory   1 = Fair   0 = Poor

Organization: Follows guidelines; completeness of items; clear layout; overall creativity

Form and quality: Writing mechanics; expressiveness; visual appeal; spelling, punctuation, and grammar

Evidence of understanding: Explicit demonstration of knowledge, skills, and dispositions required by the standard; application of ideas

Core propositions, supporting standards, and artifacts	Organization	Form and quality	Evidence of understanding

1. Commitment to students and their learning

    (a) Recognize individual differences in students; adjust practice accordingly

    Artifact:

      Name: _____ _____ _____ _____

    (b) Understand how students develop and learn

    Artifact:

      Name: _____ _____ _____ _____

    (c) Treat students equitably

    Artifact:

      Name: _____ _____ _____ _____

    (d) Extend mission beyond developing the [psychomotor] capacity of students

    Artifact:

      Name: _____ _____ _____ _____

2. Knowledge of subjects taught and how to teach those subjects to students

    (a) Appreciate how knowledge in subjects is created, organized, and linked to other disciplines

    Artifact:

      Name: _____ _____ _____ _____

    (b) Command specialized knowledge of how to convey subject to students

    Artifact:

      Name: _____ _____ _____ _____

    (c) Generate multiple paths to [learning]

    Artifact:

      Name: _____ _____ _____ _____

Core propositions, supporting standards, and artifacts	Organization	Form and quality	Evidence of understanding

3. Responsibility for managing and monitoring student learning

   (a) Call on multiple methods to meet goals

   Artifact:

   Name: _____ _____ _____ _____

   (b) Orchestrate learning in group settings

   Artifact:

   Name: _____ _____ _____ _____

   (c) Place premium on student engagement

   Artifact:

   Name: _____ _____ _____ _____

   (d) Regularly assess student progress

   Artifact:

   Name: _____ _____ _____ _____

   (e) Are mindful of principal objectives

   Artifact:

   Name: _____ _____ _____ _____

4. Think systematically about practice and learn from experience

   (a) Are continually making difficult choices that test judgment

   Artifact:

   Name: _____ _____ _____ _____

   (b) Seek advice of others and draw on education research and scholarship to improve practice

   Artifact:

   Name: _____ _____ _____ _____

5. Are members of learning communities

   (a) Contribute to school effectiveness by collaborating with other professionals

   Artifact:

   Name: _____ _____ _____ _____

   (b) Work collaboratively with parents

   Artifact:

   Name: _____ _____ _____ _____

   (c) Take advantage of community resources

   Artifact:

   Name: _____ _____ _____ _____

Artifacts Analysis Chart

Kind of artifact (e.g., lesson plans)	Name of artifact (e.g., series on movement exploration)	Core propositions/supporting standards															
		1				2			3					4		5		
		a	b	c	d	a	b	c	a	b	c	d	e	a	b	a	b	c

Showcase Portfolio Rating Form

Name: _____ Date: _____

Portfolio Contents

Components of the professional portfolio should be verified according to the following indicators:

+ = Fully developed ✓ = Included, but incomplete 0 = Not included

_____ Cover letter   _____ Certification/licensing documents

_____ Table of contents/index   _____ Letters of recommendation

_____ Biographical sketch   _____ List of relevant courses

_____ Resume   _____ Artifacts representing the teaching standards

Comments: _____

_____

_____

_____

_____

Portfolio Quality

The professional portfolio should evidence an acceptable level of quality. Use the following scale to rate each characteristic and artifact:

2 = High quality;   1 = Satisfactory quality;   0 = Low quality;
above expectations   meets expectations   below expectations

_____ Organization   _____ Artifact 7: _____

_____ Layout/visual appeal   _____ Artifact 8: _____

_____ Creativity/expressiveness   _____ Artifact 9: _____

_____ Spelling, punctuation, grammar   _____ Artifact 10: _____

_____ Artifact 1: _____   _____ Artifact 11: _____

_____ Artifact 2: _____   _____ Artifact 12: _____

_____ Artifact 3: _____   _____ Artifact 13: _____

_____ Artifact 4: _____   _____ Artifact 14: _____

_____ Artifact 5: _____   _____ Artifact 15: _____

_____ Artifact 6: _____   _____ Artifact 16: _____

From *Professional and Student Portfolios for Physical Education, Second Edition,* by Vincent J. Melograno, 2006, Champaign, IL: Human Kinetics.

261

and enhance new job opportunities. Advanced professional standards for experienced teachers are recommended as the basis for organizing the professional portfolio. Also, techniques for managing the portfolio include organizing tools, storage options, and the use of technology. Processes for involvement are suggested such as reflection, self-assessment, and conferences. In addition, the selection of artifacts from a wide range of possibilities should consider the type of portfolio and the professional teacher standards. Finally, assessment feedback about the professional portfolio can be derived from colleagues through reflection, conferences, and performance assessment and from self-analysis through artifacts review and the application of established criteria.

Sample Professional Portfolio System

To synthesize the information presented in this chapter, a sample portfolio system is provided for use by practicing physical education teachers. Although the system is hypothetical in nature, the portfolio elements are applicable to teachers in actual physical education settings. The system incorporates the concepts and principles advanced in this chapter. It is structured in the form of a manual for professional development. The manual (describing a showcase portfolio) could be used independently by physical educators or by any school committed to improving and recognizing the successful practices of physical educators.

In addition, the CD-ROM accompanying the book provides a template (portfolio builder) to create an electronic-based professional portfolio for practicing teachers using Microsoft Power-Point®. Instructions are provided for navigating through the slides that include hyperlinks for access to the necessary files. When the portfolio is completed, it can be copied to a CD for distribution and review. It can also be uploaded to the Internet for access as a Web-based portfolio. The following components are used to organize the portfolio:

- Table of contents
- Introduction
- Resume
- Professional development
- Standards for accomplished teachers
- Lesson plan sample
- Student work samples
- Gallery (pictures, video clips)
- Letters of recommendation
- Teaching evaluations

Professional Development Manual

How to Design and Manage the Showcase Portfolio

CONTENTS

I. RATIONALE AND PURPOSES

As a practicing professional physical educator, your desires to achieve certain teaching goals and to pursue your own professional growth are commendable. Accomplished teachers continually look for ways to improve and bring distinction to their successful practices. Because your effectiveness often goes unrecognized and unrewarded, a process is needed to document growth and achieved competence in the complex act of teaching. That process is the professional portfolio.

For experienced teachers, the incentives for maintaining effectiveness are professional success and personal satisfaction. Although the skills, dispositions, beliefs, and practices that characterize effective physical education teachers are substantial, they need to be documented. The process of gathering information about your work through portfolios can be a rewarding experience. However, given the real-world demands on physical education teachers, some solid reasons are needed for spending time and energy on portfolios. The primary purpose of the professional portfolio is to verify the wide range of knowledge, skills, and dispositions acquired through teaching experience, professional development, advanced training, and reflection. Secondary purposes are to help you (1) grow professionally, (2) monitor your goals, and (3) satisfy evaluation procedures.

II. ORGANIZATION

The ongoing, systematic collection of teaching-related artifacts, including student work samples, is referred to as a working repository. It serves as the complete collection of artifacts from which items are selected for the showcase portfolio, which is a customized overview of your professional abilities as a physical educator. Ideally, the showcase portfolio could be organized around some universal set of teaching competencies. Fortunately, performance categories that describe teaching proficiency do exist. These categories, known as core propositions, are supported by teacher standards that have widespread acceptance and general applicability. The showcase portfolio should be organized around the following core propositions and standards (National Board for Professional Teaching Standards, 1999):

Core Proposition 1: Teachers are committed to students and their learning.

    a. Teachers recognize individual differences in their students and adjust their practice accordingly.

    b. Teachers have an understanding of how students develop and learn.

    c. Teachers treat students equitably.

    d. Teachers' mission extends beyond developing the [psychomotor] capacity of their students.

Core Proposition 2: Teachers know the subjects they teach and how to teach those subjects to students.

    a. Teachers appreciate how knowledge in their subjects is created, organized, and linked to other disciplines.

    b. Teachers command specialized knowledge of how to convey a subject to students.

    c. Teachers generate multiple paths to [learning].

Core Proposition 3: Teachers are responsible for managing and monitoring student learning.

    a. Teachers call on multiple methods to meet their goals.

    b. Teachers orchestrate learning in group settings.

    c. Teachers place a premium on student engagement.

d. Teachers regularly assess student progress.

e. Teachers are mindful of their principal objectives.

Core Proposition 4: Teachers think systematically about their practice and learn from experience.

a. Teachers are continually making difficult choices that test their judgment.

b. Teachers seek the advice of others and draw on education research and scholarship to improve their practice.

Core Proposition 5: Teachers are members of learning communities.

a. Teachers contribute to school effectiveness by collaborating with other professionals.

b. Teachers work collaboratively with parents.

c. Teachers take advantage of community resources.

There is also professional consensus on the aspects of practice that distinguish accomplished physical education teachers. Thus, consideration should be given to these advanced standards specific to what physical education teachers should know and be able to do. The showcase portfolio should integrate the following standards (National Board for Professional Teaching Standards, 2001):

1. Knowledge of students
2. Knowledge of subject matter
3. Sound teaching practices
4. Student engagement in learning
5. High expectations for learners
6. Learning environment
7. Curricular choices
8. Assessment
9. Equity, fairness, and diversity
10. Reflective practices and professional growth
11. Promoting an active lifestyle
12. Collaboration with colleagues
13. Family and community partnerships

III. MANAGEMENT

You must assume responsibility for storing, maintaining, and updating your professional portfolio. Therefore, you will need to decide how to handle the logistics of portfolios (i.e., the method of construction, how and where to store the portfolio, when to manage it, and how to analyze it). These aspects are covered in the following sections.

A. Storage

The actual container for collecting artifacts is a matter of personal preference. Some options include notebooks, expanding and accordion files, hanging files, large file box, folders, satchels, pockets for electronic documents, a large notebook divided into sections, and file drawers in a cabinet. The working repository may require considerable space because it includes the total collection of artifacts. Items for the showcase portfolio would be drawn from this collection. Because the showcase portfolio is a more concise representation of accomplishments, the number of items is limited. Thus, an accordion file or satchel is all that may be needed for paper-based storage. It may be more practical, however, to scan materials for storage on computer disks or on computer internal hard drives.

B. Tools

You may be good at collecting work samples and exhibits but need help managing the portfolio. These organizational tools may be helpful: (1) dividers (to separate artifacts according to teacher standards or incomplete works), (2) color codes (to code entries with colored dots, colored files, or markers), (3) artifact registry (to record the date, item, and reason for either adding or removing an item), (4) work log (to list activities and decisions about the portfolio with dates), (5) table of contents (to list categories and subcategories of items), and (6) self-stick notes (to attach to each artifact to identify standard and explain why it was collected).

C. Reflection

Each collected artifact should be thoughtfully examined and labeled to reveal its meaning and value to the working portfolio. By reflecting on your work samples and exhibits, you arrive at a better understanding of why you collected certain items for particular standards. The reflection cover sheet on page 267 can be used and should remain with those items selected for the showcase portfolio.

D. Self-Analysis

You should review your collection of artifacts to make sure you have appropriately documented the teacher standards. As you complete professional activities, you should keep areas that may be missing documentation in mind. The form on page 268 can be used. The specific teacher standards that support each core proposition should be considered. Where artifacts are needed, indicate your goal for filling the void and a target completion date.

IV. ITEM SELECTION

Ultimately, you must decide what to include and exclude from your professional portfolio. Most artifacts are derived from school and community activities, professional development experiences, teacher-made materials, and curriculum plans that include units and lesson plans. A broad array of artifacts is available for the working repository. As an experienced physical educator, you will have numerous alternatives from which to select, including the following:

1. Statement of philosophy
2. Goals statement
3. Videotape or video clips of teaching
4. Teacher-made instructional materials
5. Lesson plans
6. Unit plans
7. Integrated units
8. Technology resources
9. Student works
10. Case studies
11. Community and extracurricular involvement descriptions
12. Professional growth activities list
13. Professional readings list
14. Awards, honors, and commendations
15. Letters
16. Photographs
17. Logs and journals
18. Reflections and self-assessments

Reflection Cover Sheet for Showcase Portfolio Artifacts

Name: _____ Date: _____

Standard: _____

Name of item: _____

Source: _____

Rationale statement: _____

_____

_____

_____

_____

_____

_____

_____

_____

_____

_____

_____

_____

_____

_____

_____

_____

_____

_____

_____

_____

_____

_____

_____

_____

_____

_____

_____

From *Professional and Student Portfolios for Physical Education, Second Edition*, by Vincent J. Melograno, 2006, Champaign, IL: Human Kinetics.

Artifacts Self-Check for the Showcase Portfolio

Name: _____ Date: _____

Core propositions	Good	OK	Artifacts needed
1. Is committed to students and their learning			Goal: Target date:
2. Knows subject and how to teach it			Goal: Target date:
3. Is responsible for managing and monitoring student learning			Goal: Target date:
4. Thinks systematically about practices and learns from experiences			Goal: Target date:
5. Is a member of learning communities			Goal: Target date:

The task of selecting items for the showcase portfolio should focus on the established teacher standards. A strong link should exist between the standards and the artifacts selected to represent them. The following is a list of the *minimum* expectations for the showcase portfolio relative to the core propositions and standards:

1. Commitment to students and their learning
   - Performance checklist for students who exhibit difficulty in a movement or sport skill
   - Case study showing a student's development in a physical education unit
   - Frequency index scale for an affective behavior (e.g., cooperation, tolerance, interpersonal relationships)
2. Knowledge of subject and how to teach it
   - Integrated unit plan with at least two other subject areas
   - Teacher-made rating scales
   - Videotape or video clips showing at least three kinds of instructional strategies (e.g., guided discovery, practice, role play, cooperative learning)
3. Responsibility for managing and monitoring student learning
   - Student work samples showing multiple methods
   - Assessment procedures for cognitive, affective, and psychomotor learning
   - Lesson plans that link objectives with learning activities and performance standards
4. Thinking systematically about practices and learning from experiences
   - Organization schemes for learning areas (e.g., gymnasium, outdoor field)
   - Results of an action research project
   - Annotated list of professional readings over the past year
5. Being a member of learning communities
   - Motor development component from three IEPs
   - Handouts used for Parents Night
   - Materials written as a member of a curriculum development team

V. FEEDBACK AND SELF-ASSESSMENT

During the progressive stages of portfolio development and refinement, periodic reviews are not only essential, but natural to any system directed toward professional growth. Evaluative criteria should focus on the portfolio's *content* and *quality*. Feedback from colleagues and self-analysis are the best sources for evaluation.

A. Feedback From Colleagues

Because practicing teachers may be involved in their own professional growth plans, they are qualified to review the work of others. Several feedback constructs can be used with the showcase portfolio—reflection, conferences, and performance rating. Colleagues who provide feedback should be experienced, trustworthy, and willing to offer objective, constructive information.

Like self-reflection, *reflection* by colleagues serves as a valuable cross-check. With the established teacher standards as the basis, the reflection sheet on page 270 can be used.

Conferences with colleagues offer another way to acquire feedback and, at the same time, foster relationships in a collaborative environment. The focus should be on the teacher standards and how artifacts document accomplishments and professional competence related to the standards. Conferences should compare your perceptions and your colleague's opinion regarding (1) your overall strength as a physical education teacher, (2) artifacts that represent "holistic" abilities and dispositions toward teaching, (3) how the portfolio verifies that the teacher standards have been met, and (4) what standards need further justification as revealed by the portfolio. Colleagues could focus their feedback around answers to the following statements:

Colleague Reflection Sheet of the Showcase Portfolio

To: _____

From: _____

1. What teaching standard is documented most effectively? Why?

2. What teaching standard is documented least effectively? Why?

3. What artifacts made an impression on you? Why?

4. What artifacts need the most work? Why?

5. What is your overall impression of the organization and presentation of artifacts?

Signed: _____ Date: _____

The part of the portfolio I like best is _____ because . . .

The part I'm not really clear about is _____ because . . .

The part you need to tell me more about is . . .

You could improve your portfolio by . . .

My overall impression is . . .

Assuming that a truly professional relationship exists, a colleague can also provide a more formal *performance rating* of the showcase portfolio. Its review should consider the established teacher standards and general criteria such as organization and form and quality of documentation. The rating form on page 272 can be used for this purpose.

B. Self-Analysis

The previous discussion of self-assessment described an informal self-check of the working repository to establish goals for standards lacking documentation. For the showcase portfolio, you should also try to diversify the kinds of artifacts selected. There may be a tendency to rely too heavily on one kind over another, such as curriculum units. The chart on page 273 can be used to record, with check marks or dates, the range of artifacts in support of the five core propositions and 17 supporting standards. A similar chart could be created for the 13 physical education standards.

From *Professional and Student Portfolios for Physical Education, Second Edition,* by Vincent J. Melograno, 2006, Champaign, IL: Human Kinetics.

271

Rating Form for Showcase Portfolio

Name: _____

Reviewer: _____

Rating scale: + = Impressive; ✓ = Acceptable; 0 = Needs work

	Organization and form Clear layout; writing mechanics; visual appeal	Quality of documentation Expressiveness; explicit link to standard
Is committed to students and their learning		
Artifact 1: _____	_____	_____
Artifact 2: _____	_____	_____
Artifact 3: _____	_____	_____
Knows subject and how to teach it		
Artifact 1: _____	_____	_____
Artifact 2: _____	_____	_____
Artifact 3: _____	_____	_____
Is responsible for managing and monitoring student learning		
Artifact 1: _____	_____	_____
Artifact 2: _____	_____	_____
Artifact 3: _____	_____	_____
Thinks systematically about practices and learns from experiences		
Artifact 1: _____	_____	_____
Artifact 2: _____	_____	_____
Artifact 3: _____	_____	_____
Is a member of learning communities		
Artifact 1: _____	_____	_____
Artifact 2: _____	_____	_____
Artifact 3: _____	_____	_____

From *Professional and Student Portfolios for Physical Education, Second Edition*, by Vincent J. Melograno, 2006, Champaign, IL: Human Kinetics.

Analysis Chart for Showcase Portfolio Artifacts

Kind of artifact	Name of artifact	CORE PROPOSITIONS OR SUPPORTING STANDARDS														
		1				2			3					4		5		
		a	b	c	d	a	b	c	a	b	c	d	e	a	b	a	b	c

From *Professional and Student Portfolios for Physical Education, Second Edition,* by Vincent J. Melograno, 2006, Champaign, IL: Human Kinetics.

REFERENCES

Arter, J., & McTighe, J. (2001). *Scoring rubrics in the classroom.* Thousand Oaks, CA: Corwin.

Black, P., Harrison, C., Lee, C., Marshall, B., & Wiliam, D. (2004). Working inside the black box: Assessment for learning in the classroom. *Phi Delta Kappan, 86* (1), 9-21.

Black, P., & Wiliam, D. (1998). Inside the black box: Raising standards through classroom assessment. *Phi Delta Kappan, 80* (2), 139-144, 146-148.

Bruininks, R.H. (1978). *Bruininks-Oseretsky test of motor proficiency.* Circle Pines, MN: American Guidance Service.

Burke, K. (2000). *How to assess authentic learning* (3rd ed.). Palatine, IL: IRI/Skylight.

Burke, K., Fogarty, R., & Belgrad, S. (2001). *The portfolio connection* (2nd ed.). Palatine, IL: IRI/Skylight.

Campbell, D.M., Cignetti, P.B., Melenyzer, B.J., Nettles, D.H., & Wyman, R.M. (2003). *How to develop a professional portfolio: A manual for teachers* (3rd ed.). Boston: Allyn & Bacon.

Carnegie Task Force on Teaching as a Profession. (1986). *A nation prepared: Teachers for the 21st century.* New York: Author.

Cleveland State University, College of Education and Human Services. (2005). *The teacher education conceptual framework.* Retrieved November 1, 2005, from the World Wide Web: www.csuohio.edu/coehs/college/model/TeacherEducationFramework.pdf.

Cooper Institute for Aerobics Research. (2004). *Fitnessgram* (3rd ed.). Champaign, IL: Human Kinetics.

Darling-Hammond, L. (Ed.). (1992). *Model standards for beginning teacher licensing and development: A resource for state dialogue.* Washington, DC: Council of Chief State School Officers, Interstate New Teacher Assessment and Support Consortium.

Educational Testing Service. (1992). *The Praxis Series: Professional assessments for beginning teachers.* Princeton, NJ: Author.

Educational Testing Service. (2001). *Praxis III: Classroom performance assessments—orientation guide.* Princeton, NJ: Author.

Evans, R. (2001). *The human side of school change: Reform, resistance, and the real-life problems of innovation.* San Francisco: Jossey-Bass.

Gardner, H. (1999). *Intelligence reframed: Multiple intelligences for the 21st century.* New York: Basic Books.

Glatthorn, A.A. (1993). *Learning twice: An introduction to the methods of teaching.* New York: HarperCollins.

Hopple, C.J. (1995). *Teaching for outcomes in elementary physical education: A guide for curriculum and assessment.* Champaign, IL: Human Kinetics.

Hopple, C.J. (2005). *Elementary physical education teaching & assessment: A practical guide.* Champaign, IL: Human Kinetics.

International Society for Technology in Education. (2000). *National educational technology standards for students: Connecting curriculum and technology.* Eugene, OR: Author.

International Society for Technology in Education. (2002). *National educational technology standards for teachers: Preparing teachers to use technology.* Eugene, OR: Author.

Jacobs, H.H. (1997). *Alternative assessment.* Upper Saddle River, NJ: Prentice Hall.

Kelly, L.E., & Melograno, V.J. (2004). *Developing the physical education curriculum: An achievement-based approach.* Champaign, IL: Human Kinetics.

Linn, R. (2000). Assessment and accountability. *Educational Researcher, 29* (2), 4-16.

Loovis, E.M., & Ersing, W.F. (1979). *Assessing and programming gross motor development for children.* Bloomington, IN: Tichenor.

Lund, J.L. (2000). *Creating rubrics for physical education* (NASPE Assessment Series). Reston, VA: National Association for Sport and Physical Education.

Lund, J.L., & Kirk, M.F. (2002). *Performance-based assessment for middle and high school physical education.* Champaign, IL: Human Kinetics.

Marmo, D. (1994, April). *'Sport'folios—On the road to outcome-based education.* Paper presented at the AAHPERD National Convention, Denver, CO.

McTighe, J., & Ferrara, S. (1994). *Assessing learning in the classroom.* Washington, DC: National Education Association.

Melograno, V.J. (1994). Portfolio assessment: Documenting authentic student learning. *Journal of Physical Education, Recreation & Dance, 65* (8), 50-55, 58-61.

Melograno, V.J. (1996). *Developing the physical education curriculum* (3rd ed.). Champaign, IL: Human Kinetics.

Melograno, V.J. (1997). Integrating assessment into physical education teaching. *Journal of Physical Education, Recreation & Dance, 68* (7), 34-37.

Melograno, V.J. (1999). *Preservice professional portfolio system* (NASPE Assessment Series). Reston, VA: National Association for Sport and Physical Education.

Melograno, V.J. (2000a). Designing a portfolio system for K-12 physical education: A step-by-step process. *Measurement in Physical Education and Exercise Science, 4* (2), 97-115.

Melograno, V.J. (2000b). *Portfolio assessment for K-12 physical education* (NASPE Assessment Series). Reston, VA: National Association for Sport and Physical Education.

Metzler, M.W. (2000). *Instructional models for physical education.* Boston: Allyn & Bacon.

Mohnsen, B.S. (2004). *Using technology in physical education* (4th ed.). Cerritos, CA: Bonnie's Fitware.

Murphy, S., & Smith, M. (1992). *Writing portfolios: A bridge from teaching to assessment.* Markham, ON: Pippin.

National Association for Sport and Physical Education. (1992). *Outcomes of quality physical education programs.* Reston, VA: Author.

National Association for Sport and Physical Education. (1995a). *Moving into the future: National standards for physical education: A guide to content and assessment.* Reston, VA: Author.

National Association for Sport and Physical Education. (1995b). *National standards for beginning physical education teachers.* Reston, VA: Author.

National Association for Sport and Physical Education. (2003). *National standards for beginning physical education teachers* (2nd ed.). Reston, VA: Author.

National Association for Sport and Physical Education. (2004). *Moving into the future: National standards for physical education* (2nd ed.). Reston, VA: Author.

National Board for Professional Teaching Standards. (1996). *An invitation to national board certification.* Southfield, MI: Author.

National Board for Professional Teaching Standards. (1999). *What teachers should know and be able to do.* Southfield, MI: Author.

National Board for Professional Teaching Standards. (2001). *NBPTS physical education standards.* Southfield, MI: Author.

National Board for Professional Teaching Standards. (2004). *Early and middle childhood physical education scoring guide.* Southfield, MI: Author.

National Commission on Excellence in Education. (1983). *A nation at risk: The imperative of educational reform.* Washington, DC: U.S. Government Printing Office.

National Commission on Teaching & America's Future. (1996). *What matters most: Teaching for America's future* (summary report). Woodbridge, VA: Author.

O'Connor, K. (2002). *How to grade for learning: Linking grades to standards* (2nd ed.). Glenview, IL: Pearson/Skylight.

Rudner, L.M., & Boston, C. (1994). Performance assessment. *The ERIC Review, 3* (1), 2-12.

SBE Design Team. (1997). *Facilitator's guide and workbook: Common ground in the standards-based education classroom.* Longmont, CO: Northern Colorado Boards of Cooperative Educational Services (BOCES).

Schiemer, S. (2000). *Assessment strategies for elementary physical education.* Champaign, IL: Human Kinetics.

Senge, P., Kleiner, A., Roberts, C., Ross, R., Roth, G., & Smith, B. (1999). *The dance of change: The challenges of sustaining momentum in learning organizations.* New York: Doubleday.

Siedentop, D. (2004). *Introduction to physical education, fitness, and sport* (5th ed.). Mountain View, CA: Mayfield.

Siedentop, D., Hastie, P.A., & van der Mars, H. (2004). *Complete guide to sport education.* Champaign, IL: Human Kinetics.

Stiggins, R.J. (2002). Assessment crisis: The absence of assessment FOR learning. *Phi Delta Kappan, 83* (10), 758-765.

Stiggins, R.J., Arter, J.A., Chappuis, J., & Chappuis, S. (2004). *Classroom assessment for student learning: Doing it right—using it well.* Portland, OR: Assessment Training Institute.

Strand, B.N., & Wilson, R. (1993). *Assessing sport skills.* Champaign, IL: Human Kinetics.

Tierney, R.J., Carter, M.A., & Desai, L.E. (1991). *Portfolio assessment in the reading–writing classroom.* Norwood, MA: Christopher-Gordon.

Ulrich, D. (2000). *Test of gross motor development* (2nd ed.). Austin, TX: Pro-Ed.

U.S. Department of Education. (1991). *America 2000: An education strategy.* Washington, DC: Author.

Winnick, J.P., & Short, F.X. (1999). *Brockport physical fitness test.* Champaign, IL: Human Kinetics.

ABOUT THE AUTHOR

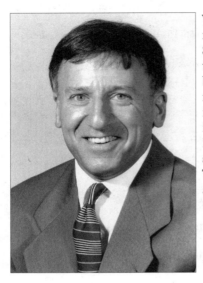

Vincent J. Melograno, EdD, is chairperson and professor in the department of health, physical education, recreation, and dance at Cleveland State University. Besides the first edition of this book, Melograno has written four other texts in the area of curriculum design, coauthored another book, and written chapters for other books and monographs on topics related to teaching and assessment. He has also written numerous articles in professional journals and has presented nationally at AAHPERD and internationally at respected conferences in Australia, Brazil, Germany, Hong Kong, Israel, Japan, Singapore, and South Korea. A department chairperson for 22 years, he is in the International Who's Who in Sport Pedagogy Theory and Research. In his leisure time, he enjoys tennis, fitness training, and softball.